Cognitive Science

Integrative Synchronization Mechanisms in Cognitive Neuroarchitectures of Modern Connectionism

Harald Maurer

University of Tübingen
Balingen-Frommern, Germany

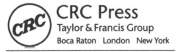

CRC Press
Taylor & Francis Group
Boca Raton London New York

CRC Press is an imprint of the
Taylor & Francis Group, an **informa** business

A SCIENCE PUBLISHERS BOOK

First edition published 2021
by CRC Press
6000 Broken Sound Parkway NW, Suite 300, Boca Raton, FL 33487-2742

and by CRC Press
2 Park Square, Milton Park, Abingdon, Oxon, OX14 4RN

Library of Congress Cataloging-in-Publication Data applied for

ISBN: 9781138487086 (hbk)
ISBN: 9780367638917 (pbk)

Typeset in Times New Roman
by Radiant Productions

Dedication

If you seriously want to work scientifically, you should avoid a "somehow" at all costs.
Prof. em. Dr. rer. nat. Dr. phil. Walter Hoering (1933–2019)

Foreword

This book is a completely revised version of my Ph.D. thesis, which I wrote in the Department of Philosophy of Science at the University of Tübingen.

This book offers a comprehensive and fundamental introduction to connectionist cognitive science from the perspectives of theoretical neuroinformatics, computational and cognitive neuroscience, theoretical neurophilosophy and neurolinguistics. The focus is on the presentation of a variety of extremely influential cognitive neuroarchitectures of modern connectionism. In both (visual) perception and language processing, these neuroarchitectures try to solve convincingly, the binding problem in neurophysiology, in the context of mathematical models or computer simulation models with integrative, temporal synchronization mechanisms.

The new "fluent" theory of neurocognition used in this context of a modern, system-theoretical connectionism is grounded in two methods. On the one hand, analyses within the theory of nonlinear dynamic and complex systems are used. A neurocognitive system can be described using (a system of) (non-)linear differential equations based on convergent, transient vector fields and vector flows in n-dimensional state spaces. These include a distributed representational format in the form of vector constructions (so-called "vectorial form"). On the other hand, information-theoretical analyses with reference to the concept of information entropy are used.

The book is aimed primarily at students from the disciplines of cognitive science, computational and cognitive neuroscience, neuroinformatics, neurophilosophy and neurolinguistics, as well as those interested in the field of artificial intelligence.

It also offers students a basic introduction to connectionism and the theory of artificial neural networks as well as information theory, the (mathematical) theory of nonlinear dynamic systems and the binding problem in neural coding theory in the cognitive neurosciences.

While I would especially like to thank Prof. (em.) Dr. Peter Schroeder-Heister (Department of Logic and Theory of Language at the University of Tübingen), I would also thank the other lecturers to whose lectures and/or courses I was invited, and/or who gave me valuable suggestions for my understanding of the topics concerned, so that this book could be written:

Prof. Dr. Martin Bogdan
(Department of Computer Engineering at the University of Leipzig)

Priv. Doz. (em.) Dr. habil. Kurt Bräuer
(Department of Theoretical Physics at the University of Tübingen)

Prof. (em.) Dr. Michael Heidelberger
(Department of Philosophy of Science and Logic at the University of Tübingen)

Prof. (em.) Dr. Walter Hoering
(Department of Philosophy of Science at the University of Tübingen and the LMU Munich)

Prof. (em.) Dr. Kemmerling
(Department of Philosophy of Mind at the University of Heidelberg)

Prof. Dr. Holger Lyre
(Department of Theoretical Philosophy at the University of Magdeburg)

Prof. (em.) Dr. Klaus Mainzer
(Department of Philosophy and Philosophy of Science at the Technical University of Munich)

Prof. Dr. Hanspeter Mallot
(Department of Cognitive Neuroscience at the University of Tübingen)

Prof. Dr. Thomas Metzinger
(Department of Theoretical Philosophy at the Johannes Gutenberg University Mainz)

Prof. Dr. Catrin Misselhorn
(Department of Philosophy of Science and Technology at the University of Stuttgart)

Prof. Dr. Andreas Nieder
(Department of Animal Physiology at the University of Tübingen)

Prof. Dr. Michael Pauen
(Department of Philosophy of Mind/Berlin School of Mind and Brain at the Humboldt-University of Berlin)

Prof. (em.) Dr. h.c. mult. Wolf Singer
(Max Planck Institute for Brain Research Frankfurt/Main and Frankfurt Institute for Advanced Studies (FIAS))

Prof. Dr. Markus Werning
(Department of Philosophy of Language and Cognition at the University of Bochum)

My special thanks go to Prof. Dr. Andreas Zell (Department of Cognitive Systems at the University of Tübingen) and Prof. Dr. Martin Bogdan (Department of Computer Engineering at the University of Leipzig), who aroused my interest in neuroinformatics and artificial intelligence with their lectures "Theory of Artificial Neural Networks," "Genetic Algorithms and Evolutionary Strategies," "Neural Computing," "Robotics," "Signal Processing" and "Machine Learning".

My special thanks also go to Prof. Dr. Brian McLaughlin (Department of Philosophy and Cognitive Science at Rutgers University), who encouraged me during the Vienna International Summer University (VISU) on "Mind and Computation" to write my M.A. thesis on Smolensky's ICS architecture.

Finally, my special thanks go to Prof. Dr. Dr. Walter Hoering (Department of Philosophy of Science at the University of Tübingen and the LMU Munich), who gave me optimal support during my studies, my M.A. thesis and my Ph.D. thesis, and who will always be a role model for me as a person and a scientist.

I would also like to thank the students for the exciting and interesting discussions in my courses at the universities of Tübingen, Magdeburg and Heidelberg.

Furthermore, I would like to thank my fellows and Ph.D. students for stimulating conversations and tips, especially Dr. Thomas Piecha, Dr. Antje Rumberg, Asst. Prof. Dr. John Michael, PD Dr. Matthias Neuber, Prof. Dr. Jochen Sautermeister, Andreas Jahnke M.Sc., Ph.D. student David Klindt, StD Tobias Herrmann, Regina Sommer M.A., Jürgen Sommer M.A., Christian Dinger and Ass. jur. Heinrich Dietz.

I would also like to thank warmly Ph.D. student Alexander Green and computer science student Maximilian Maurer B.Sc. for proofreading the English manuscript.

I would also like to thank Dr. Antje Rumberg and Dr. Thomas Piecha for their valuable advice on the LateX programming of the manuscript.

Finally, I would like to thank most warmly my wife StB Renate Maurer, Degree in Business Economics (BA), and tax consultant, who made the development of this work possible with a maximum of support, patience and forbearance, and finally, my mother, for proofreading the German manuscript.

Tübingen, Autumn 2020   Harald Maurer

Preface

At this point I would like to give some hints to the reader to get the most out of the book.

In the first part, certain basics which are necessary for the understanding of the second part, are explained. Those who have not yet acquired basic knowledge on the subjects of cognitive science, theory of dynamic systems, connectionism and theory of artificial neural networks, cognitive and computational neuroscience and information theory should first read the respective chapters before studying the various cognitive neuroarchitectures.

I have, in most cases, made the following classification in the footnotes:

1. In the case of original literature that is fundamental to a subject area, the phrase "For fundamental information, see e.g. (...)" or "For basic information, see e.g. (...)" is used.
2. If it is original literature that deals with a subject area in depth, assuming that the reader has some prior knowledge, the phrase "For detailed information, see e.g. (...)" or "For a detailed discussion, see e.g. (...)" is used.
3. In the case of literature that introduces a subject area in which it is assumed the reader has little prior knowledge, the phrase "For an introduction, see e.g. (...)" is used.
4. If the literature provides an overview of a subject area, the phrase "For an overview, see e.g. (...)" or "For a review, see e.g. (...)" is used.
5. In the case of literature that describes a subject area without any previous background i.e. literature which can be called popular science, the phrase "For a beginner's guide, see e.g. (...)" is used.

Any remaining errors and inadequacies are, of course, exclusively attributable to me. In this regard I am always very grateful for hints, suggestions, improvement proposals and constructive criticism, which you can send me via email. The e-mail address, harald.maurer@uni-tuebingen.de, is available for letters.

Tübingen, Autumn 2020 Harald Maurer

Contents

Part II: Cognitive Neuroarchitectures in Neuroinformatics, in Cognitive Science and in Computational Neuroscience

Introduction
Theory of an Integrative Neurocognition

Since the 1970s and 1980s, with the emergence of the theory of nonlinear dynamic systems and the associated development of system-theoretical connectionism in the cognitive neurosciences and cognitive science, a tendency to carry out the analysis and modeling of neural information processing in the human brain using methods that correspond to this system-theoretical paradigm has been observed. This book attempts to consider the model construction of the neural system and the associated neurocognitive functions from this perspective of a nonlinear system dynamic. In the years which followed a multitude of cognitive neuroarchitectures have been developed in connectionism, based on empirical-experimental data mainly from neurophysiology, which try neurobiologically, neurophysiologically and neuropsychologically, to model plausible, perceptual, linguistic and (neuro-)cognitive performances of humans in the context of the binding problem, especially with their integrative (synchronization) mechanisms. Thus, the dynamic binding character of human neurocognition can be adequately considered. This means that perception, thinking, speaking, reasoning and decision-making can be represented by fluent patterns as a flowing occurrence in time.

In the present book, the aim is to build on the main theme of the solution of the binding problem by means of temporal and integrative synchronization mechanisms (with reference to perception and language cognition, especially with reference to the problems of compositionality and systematicity). I will sketch the construction of an integrative theory of neurocognition that is still to be fully developed, on the basis of the representative format of a so-called "vectorial form." Thus, the attempt is made to make plausible the idea of the human brain as a self-organized, dynamic, flexible and adaptive organismic system, by means of the computational performances of the most neurobiologically plausible neuroarchitectures based on internal mental representations in the form of nonlinear dynamic vector fields. In my opinion, these theoretical models will be able to adequately capture the liveliness of a biological organism in the near future by means of these "fluent, liquid or fluid" neurocognitive operations, algorithms and (synchronization) mechanisms.

The first part of this book introduces cognitive science (chap. 1), and its influencing (general) theory of (nonlinear) dynamic systems from mathematics and the natural sciences (chap. 2). Thus, the required prior knowledge, based on the corresponding basic concepts and statements, is available to discuss the two basic cognitive paradigms in cognitive science, classical symbol theory and the theory of (system-theoretical) connectionism (chap. 3). Subsequently, the general binding problem in cognitive neuroscience, especially in neurophysiology, is described (chap. 4.1–4.3), as is the empirical-experimental evidence for the temporal integrative (synchronization) mechanisms for the solution of the binding problem (chap. 4.4). Furthermore, the basics of information theory are presented (chap. 5), as far as they are necessary for the understanding of information-theoretical neuroarchitectures (chap. 10). Finally, in the second part of this book, the mathematical core structure of the cognitive neuroarchitectures and their methods are analyzed, and the models are described in an simple and accessible manner (chap. 6–10), and there will be some final considerations, evaluations and discussions (chap. 11).

Abbreviations

AI	Artificial Intelligence
AIP	Anterior intraparietal (area)
AIT	Algorithmic Information Theory
AM	Amplitude modulation
ANN	artificial neural network
ART	Adaptive Resonance Theory
ASSC	Association for the Scientific Study of Consciousness
BA	Brodmann area
BBE	Brain-Body-Environment
BBS	Binding-By-Synchrony (Hypothesis)
BMU	Best-Matching Unit
BP	Backpropagation (algorithm)
CBMM	Convolution-Based Memory Models
chap.	chapter
CI	Cluster Index
CNN	Convolutional Neuronal Networks
corr.	corrected
CRUM	Computational-Representational Understanding of Mind
CSP	Constraint Satisfaction Problem
CTC	Communication Through Coherence (Hypothesis)
CTR	Communication Through Resonance (Hypothesis)
DAI	Distributed Artificial Intelligence
DCH	Dynamic Core Hypothesis
DL	Deep Learning
DLA	Dynamic Link Architecture
DLM	Dynamic Link Matching
DNF	Dynamic Neural Fields
DST	Dynamic Systems Theory
DFT	Dynamic Field Theory
ed.	editor
eds.	editors
Ed.	Edition
EEG	Electro-encephalography
e.g.	exempli gratia (= "for example")
EMG	Electromyography
EPSP	Excitatory postsynaptic potential
ESN	Echo State Network
esp.	especially

et al.	et alii/et aliae (= "and others")
Ext.	Extended
FEP	Free-Energy Principle
FFNs	feedforward networks
fig.	figure
FIT	Feature Integration Theory (of [Visual] Attention)
fMRI	functional Magnetic Resonance Imaging
fn.	footnote
FPH	Field Potential Histogram
FSE	Free Synaptic Energy
G(D)ST	General (Dynamic) Systems Theory
HRRs	Holographic Reduced Representations
Hz	Hertz
ICS	Integrated Connectionist/Symbolic ([Cognitive] Architecture)
IDE	Integro-differential equation
IP	Intrinsic Plasticity
IT	Inferior-temporal (area)
ITT	Information Integration Theory (of Consciousness)
(j)PSTH	(Joint) Peri-Stimulus-Time Histogram
LFP	Local Field Potentials
LGN	Lateral geniculate nucleus
LI(A)F	Leaky Integrate-And-Fire (Model)
LIP	Lateral intraparietal (area)
LMS	Least-Mean-Square (error)
LOT	Language of Thought
LSM	Liquid State Machine
LTM	Long-term memory
MCA	Multivariate Cluster Analysis
MEG	Magnetoencephalography
MI	Mutual Information
MIP	Medial intraparietal (area)
MML	Micro-Macro Link problem
MNN	Modular Neural Networks
MRI	Magnetic Resonance Imaging
MSSM	Modified Synaptic Stochastic Model
MST	Medial superior temporal (area)
NCC	Neural Correlates of (visual) Consciousness
NFT	Neural Field Theory
NEF	Neural Engineering Framework
NENGO	Neural Engineering Objects
OT	Optimality Theory
PDP	Parallel Distributed Processing
PM	Phase modulation (patterns)
PMLS	Posteromedial lateral suprasylvian (area)
Pr.	Print
PSA	Purely Symbolic Architecture
PSSH	Physical Symbol System Hypothesis
pSTG	posterior superior temporal gyrus

PSTH	Peri-Stimulus-Time Histogram
PTC	Proper Treatment of Connectionism
Rev.	Revised
RGB	red, green, blue (color)
RM-SORN	Reward-Modulated Self-Organizing Recurrent Neural Network
RM-STDP	Reward-modulated Spike-Timing-Dependent Plasticity
RNNPB	Recurrent Neural Networks with Parametric Biases
RRP	Rapid Reversible Synaptic Plasticity
RT(h)M	Representational Theory of Mind
SFC	Synfire Chain (Model)
SN	Synaptic Normalization
SNN	Spiking Neural Networks
SOC	Self-Organized Criticality
SO(F)M	Self-Organizing (Feature) Map
SORN	Self-Organizing Recurrent Network
SPA	Semantic Pointer Architecture
SPAUN	Semantic Pointer Achitecture Unified Network
SRN	Simple Recurrent-Network
SSN	Synaptic Stochastic Model
STDP	Spike-Timing-Dependent Plasticity
STM	Short-term memory
Suppl.	Supplement
TEO	Temporal-occipital (area)
TM	Turing Machine
TPR	Tensor Product Representation
VARS	Vector Approach to Representing Symbols
VIP	Ventral intraparietal (area)
vol.	volume
vs.	versus
VSA	Vector Symbol Architectures
WTA	Winner-Takes-All (function)
XOR	eXclusive-OR

Part I

Foundations of Cognitive Science

1 Cognitive Science: Integrative Theory of Cognition, Cognitivism and Computationalism

This chapter introduces the basic concepts, statements, subject area and methods of cognitive science (chap. 1.1, 1.3 and 1.5), including a list of cognitive science's subdisciplines (chap. 1.2). This will provide the background needed to adequately address the two main alternative approaches to a theory of cognition in cognitive science: the classical symbol theory (chap. 3.1) and the connectionist theory (chap. 3.2). The basic assumption is that a theory of neurocognition – in its structural core – can best be described by mathematical and logical computation operations. Finally, the goal of this introductory book in connectionist cognitive science is to present a comprehensive and appropriate theory of neurocognition in modern (system-theoretical) connectionism (chap. 1.4). This means that this book primarily takes account of empirical evidence from the cognitive neurosciences (chap. 4) and the theoretical concepts of neuroinformatics and computational neuroscience (chaps. 6–10), and is oriented towards them.

1.1 BASIC CONCEPTS, STATEMENTS AND SUBJECT AREA OF COGNITIVE SCIENCE

1.1.1 NEUROCOGNITION AND NEUROCOGNITIVE SYSTEM

Cognitive science[1], which has emerged since the so-called "cognitive turn" in the human sciences (chap. 1.5), is as an integrative transdisciplinary research program

---

[1]For a basic introduction, see e.g. Bermúdez 2014, Thagard 2005, 1998, von Eckardt 1993, Friedenberg and Silverman 2012, Dawson 2001, Sobel and Li 2013, Stainton 2006, Harré 2002, Polk and Seifert 2002, Sobel 2001, Lepore and Pylyshyn 1999, Pfeifer and Scheier 1999, Green and Others 1996, Osherson 1995-1998, Stillings et al. 1995, Varela 1988/1993.
For a brief introduction, see e.g. Thagard 2014, Bechtel and Herschbach 2010, von Eckardt 2003, Rapaport 2000, Simon and Kaplan 1989.
For an introduction to the history of cognitive science, see e.g. Dupuy 2009, Brook 2007, Boden 2006, Harnish 2002, Bechtel et al. 1998, Leahey 1991, Scheerer 1988.
For a brief introduction to the history of cognitive science, see e.g. Bechtel and Herschbach 2010, Thagard 2005.
For an introduction to the methodology and methods of cognitive science, see e.g. Bechtel 1990.

(Mittelstrass 2003), concerned with the study of mental, brain-based intelligent performances, abilities and skills of humans. In other words, it is concerned with the study of (neuro-)cognition.[2] The terms "neurocognition" or "neurocognitive" mean that (connectionist) cognitive neuroarchitectures are treated taking into account to a large extent, the recent neuroscientific empirical evidence. In other words, these neuroarchitectures are more neurobiologically plausible than the classical symbolic models. This includes the fact that the computational transformation processes in the cognitive neuroarchitectures consist of (1) vectorial structures, e.g. semantic, syntactic or sensory concepts in the form of vectors or tensors, and (2) functions like vector additions, vector multiplications, tensor products or oscillation functions.

The first use of the term "neurocognition" was made by the German neuroinformatician Werner Dilger:

"The first question to be answered is what is *cognition*. According to the usual understanding of cognitive science, it is the sum of all cognitive activities, that is, the sum of all mental activities that have something to do with cognition. In a broader sense, the subject area of cognitive science is the investigation of the phenomenon of intelligence. In this sense, cognition could also be understood as the sum of all intelligent activities. Intelligent activities include speaking, thinking, understanding, reasoning, planning, learning, memory and more.

Neurocognition is about explaining how these activities are realized in the brain, or rather, in the nervous system. Since the processes occurring there are very complex, they can not be described in detail. But one can form models of these processes that provide very plausible explanations for many phenomena. They are all based on artificial neural networks (ANN). The subject area of neurocognition should therefore be the investigation of the realization of cognitive processes of the brain with the help of suitable forms of ANN" (Dilger 2003/2004).

For an introduction to cognitive science and (non-linear) dynamic systems theory, see e.g. Haykin 2012, Beer 2000.

For an introduction to cognitive science and computer science, see e.g. Fresco 2014, Marcus 2001.

For an introduction to cognitive science and psychology, see e.g. Elman et al. 1998.

For an introduction to cognitive science and philosophy, see e.g. Samuels et al. 2012, Bechtel and Herschbach 2010, Bechtel 2009, von Eckardt 2003.

For an introduction to cognitive science and embodied cognition, see e.g. Shapiro 2011, Varela et al. 1993, Clark 2001, 1999, Chrisley and Ziemke 2003.

For encyclopedias, dictionaries and manuals on cognitive science, see e.g. Nadel 2003, Wilson and Keil 1999, Frankish and Ramsey 2012, Dawson and Medler 2010, Calvo and Gomila 2008, Houdé 2004, Bechtel and Graham 1998, Posner 1989.

[2]For the definition of the task of cognitive science, see e.g. Urchs 2002, Harré 2002, Rapaport 2000, Strohner 1995, Pfeifer and Scheier 1999, Gold and Engel 1998, Gold 1998, Helm 1998, Metzinger 1998, Green et al. 1996, Duch 1994, Simon and Kaplan 1989.

In addition, the concept of the "neurocognitive model" is increasingly being used in the neurosciences and the cognitive sciences. For an introduction, see e.g. Jacobs and Hofmann 2015 with reference to Price and Friston 2005 and Jacobs et al. 2006.

For the concepts of "cognition" and "cognitive", see e.g. Stephan and Walter 2013, Strube et al. 2000, Strube 1996a, Strohner 1995, Prinz 1976.

The terms "cognition" and "cognitive" derive from the Latin word "cognoscere" or from the Greek word "γιγνώσκειν (*gignóskein*)," English "to recognize, to perceive, to experience, to become acquainted, to know."

In other words, the term neurocognition refers to the analysis of the internal self-organizing principles of the cognition of an information-processing system[3] from the perspective of the more recent scientific empirical and theoretical results of (1) neuroinformatics and computational neuroscience, (2) cognitive neuroscience, (3) neurophilosophy, (4) cognitive neuropsychology and neurolinguistics, based on the mathematical theory of (nonlinear) dynamical complex systems.[4] Accordingly, those theoretical models of the cognitive neuroarchitectures[5] are taken into consideration which try to consider and replicate the newer neuroscientific, empirical evidence to a high degree. In other words, those neuroarchitectures have a high degree of neurobiological plausibility in the context of the cognitive neurosciences.

These neurocognitive functions or capacities can be assigned to a very broad spectrum, ranging from the ability to concretely, associatively process perceptual stimuli (lower, mostly unconscious cognition, so-called "low-level cognition") to abstract, symbolic learning, knowledge and reasoning, including memory and language processing as well as the control of behavior and action (higher, mostly conscious cognition, so-called "high-level cognition").

On the basis of the signal, data and information processing paradigm, however, cognitive science is concerned not only with the cognitive functions or capacities in natural neurocognitive systems, such as in humans, but also in artificial or technical neurocognitive systems, such as robots and in computer simulations (Strohner 1995). The general assumption is that the neurocognitive models and the cognitive neuroarchitectures, with their structures, processes, and mechanisms, can be described or explained by computational operations, the so-called "computations", on the basis of formal transformations of certain representational structures, the so-called (internal) "representations" ("computationalism"[6] and "cognitivism") (Pacherie 2004,

---

[3]For an introduction, see e.g. Haykin 2012, Camazine 2003, Urchs 2002, Strube 1996a.
For the definition of an information-processing neurocognitive system, see e.g. Strohner 1995: "Cognitive systems are those natural adaptive systems that process information using a central nervous system, or such artificial systems that simulate such information processing."
For the exact definition of a (dynamic) system, see chap. 2.

[4]For an introduction to neuroinformatics, see e.g. Hammer 2013, Mallot et al. 1992.
For a beginner's guide to computational neuroscience, see e.g. Gómez Ramírez 2014, Eliasmith 2007, Sejnowski 1999, Sejnowski et al. 1988, Trappenberg 2010.
For an introduction to cognitive neuroscience, see e.g. Rothkopf 2013, Pipa 2013, Smith Churchland and Sejnowski 1989.
For an introduction to neurophilosophy, see e.g. Northoff 2014, Walter 2013a, Brandl 2013.
For an introduction to cognitive neuropsychology, see e.g. Bublak and Finke 2013, Beller 2013, Schultheis 2013.
For an introduction to neurolinguistics, see e.g. Bosch 2013, Alexiadou 2013, Krause 2013, Schröder 2013.
For an introduction to the mathematical theory of (nonlinear) dynamical complex systems, see e.g. Schöner 2013.
On the influence of the metaphor of self-organization for cognitive science, see e.g. Strohner 1995.

[5]For an introduction to the concept of a "(cognitive) architecture", see e.g. Thagard 2012, Vernon et al. 2007, Anderson 2007, Sloman 1999, McCauley 1998, Newell et al. 1989, Rumelhart 1989.

[6]For a detailed discussion on the concept of "computation" in computationalism, in connectionism, in dynamism and in computational neuroscience, see Fresco 2014.
For an introduction, see e.g. Piccinini 2009, Stufflebeam 1998.

Strube 1996b, Sun 2008, Stephan and Walter 2013). The general form of a neu-rocognitive computation scheme can be defined with reference to the construction of the algebraic structure in mathematics, and is thus closely related to the formal mathematical-scientific minimal definition of a dynamical system[7]: An algebraic structure Σ is defined as the tuple $\Sigma = \langle A, f_i \rangle$ or $\Sigma = \langle A, R(a) \rangle$, consisting of a set of fundamental i-ary operations f_i or a set of fundamental relations $R(a)$ imprinted on a nonempty carrier set A with $a = \{a_1, a_2, ..., a_n\}$, so that A is closed under each of these operations or relations, and this structure is invariant to various transformations (so-called "homomorphism" or "isomorphism").[8]

Consequently, in a first step towards an analysis of an information-processing, adaptive and dynamic system, one can distinguish between

(1) the (system) operands of a (system) operation, where these themselves can be computational results of an operation or of a neurocognitive process, i.e., the neurocognitive objects, for example the modeled semantic, syntactic and visual-sensory activation patterns in the form of vectors or tensors or in the form of vector coordinates in the system state space, and

(2) the (system) operations in the form of neurocognitive relations or in the form of neurocognitive transformation or transfer functions. For example, the vec-tor additions and the vector multiplications in the activation, propagation and learning functions (see chap. 3.2.1), or the tensor products in the tensor product representation (see chap. 6.1.3), and so on.[9]

It should be noted that, as far as the ontological or epistemic status of an algebraic structure is concerned, the meaning of the neurocognitive objects is only of a derived

---

[7]For a (minimal) definition of a (nonlinear) dynamic system, see chap. 2.2.2 and chap. 1.4.

Strohner emphasizes that, in the end, the optimal methodological strategy would be to seek a synthesis of theoretical structuralism with empirical functionalism in order to adequately consider – by means of a complete system analysis – both the internal structures of a system and the functional, situative interactions with its constantly changing system environment (so-called "systemism"; Strohner 1995 with reference to Bunge 1979): "In particular, a systemic analysis indicates that information processing does not simply activate an existing knowledge structure based on input, but reorganizes cognitive models from existing components with new structures that are optimally suited to input and knowledge. The formation of a cognitive representation is accordingly always a system formation with emergent cognitive properties.

An important prerequisite for system formation is the interrelationship of the components involved, their coherence, which determines to what extent the system appears to be an integrated unit. The tectonic coherence aspect can therefore be called the integrity of the system. Integrity also implies whether a certain knowledge is given meaning on the basis of its intentionality.

The systemic analysis of cognitive representation is based on the integrity of a cognitive system consisting of an external system function and an internal system structure."

For the concept of a (general) system theory and the concept of system analysis, see also chap. 2.1.

[8]For fundamental information, see e.g. Birkhoff 1936a/1976a, 1936b/1976b.

For an introduction, see e.g. Burris and Sankappanavar 1981/2012, Ihringer 1993, Werner 1978, Grillet 2007, Erk and Priese 2000.

See also Gómez Ramírez 2014, Lyre 2006, Klir 1991.

See also chap. 1.1.6, 2.2.2.

[9]For a detailed discussion, see chap. 1.1.2 and 1.1.3.

See the formal mathematical-scientific minimal definition of a "dynamic system" in chap. 2.2.2.

nature, since these can only be individuated via relations or functions ("structural realism").[10]

Furthermore, in the context of developing an integrative theory of neurocognition, the following question arises: How can natural intelligence and artificial intelligence be explained as uniformly and convincingly as possible by means of mental or neurocognitive structures, processes and mechanisms? According to the prevailing opinion[11] (for example, the more recent theoretic developments in embodied cognition, emotional cognition, situated cognition, social cognition and extended cognition) affective, motivational, volitional, actional, social, and ethical phenomena are to be summarized – as a supplement to the original subject area – under the concept of a system-theoretical neurocognition.[12]

1.1.2 NEUROCOGNITIVE STRUCTURE

Following the basic idea that one defines a general neurocognitive computation scheme with reference to the construction of the algebraic structure, one can therefore formulate the definition of a "neurocognitive structure" such that it means the static structure of system objects. For example, the structure of semantic, syntactic and visual sensory activation patterns in the form of vectors, tensors or vector coordinates in the system state space. However, since the cognitive neuroarchitectures analyzed here are designed as dynamic systems, and their central system function, (the fast and flexible synchronization binding mechanism), is a dynamic system capacity, a neurodynamic analysis is preferred. Therefore, a neurocognitive structure is more likely to be understood as the dynamic informational flow of computation by means of dynamic (transformation and transfer) functions that govern changes in state variables over time, by means of the tensor product and the vector addition in the tensor product representation, for example (see chap. 6.1.3).

---

[10]In contemporary philosophy of science under the subheading of "structural realism", one understands that, in scientific theories (true) knowledge about theoretical entities is decisively obtained on the basis of theoretical terms which, in the context of the construction of (abstract) models or model classes, refer to particular facts of reality in such a way that the interpretation of these model constructions is ensured by means of relational structures or relational functions of the model objects.
For an introduction, see e.g. Lyre 2006, Landry 2007.
See also Strohner's "Systemic Realism" (1995) with reference to Bunge 1979.

[11]See e.g. Stephan and Walter 2013, Clark 1998, 1999, Strohner 1995 with reference to a methodological "systemism".
For an introduction, see e.g. Lyre 2013, Lyre and Walter 2013, Walter 2013b, Kyselo 2013, Scholz 2013, Slaby 2013.

[12]For a more extensive discussion of the approach of "embodiment" or "embodied cognition", see e.g. Shapiro 2011, Pfeifer et al. 2008, Gibbs 2007, Ziemke 2003, Anderson 2003, Wilson 2002, Pfeifer and Scheier 1999, Clark 1999.
For an introduction, see e.g. Wilson and Foglia 2011, Chrisley and Ziemke 2003, Varela et al. 1993.
For an introduction to the approach of "social cognition", see e.g. Lambert and Chasteen 1998.
For an introduction to the approach of "extended cognition", see e.g. Clark and Chalmers 1998, Shapiro 2011.
See also Strohner 1995.
For a beginner's guide, see e.g. Bermúdez 2014, Lenzen 2002.
For an overview of the topic, see e.g. also Stephan and Walter 2013, Maurer 2014a.

1.1.3 NEUROCOGNITIVE PROCESS AND NEUROCOGNITIVE FUNCTION

Thus, in the definition of a neurocognitive computational scheme, the definition of the "neurocognitive (learning, control and regulatory) process"[13] acquires a more fundamental meaning from the dynamic system operations, for example, from circular convolution (see chap. 6.2) or nonlinear oscillation functions (see chap. 8.14). These operations are ultimately responsible for providing the central (mental) system function of the information-processing system to be considered, whereby adaptive learning processes with both top-down and bottom-up directed feedback mechanisms are of fundamental importance (von Eckardt 2003, Strohner 1995). In the present case, the respective desired synchronization capacities of the cognitive neuroarchitectures under investigation constitute the computational basis—as the fundamental causal mechanism—for adequately and convincingly solving the general binding problem in the cognitive neurosciences and in cognitive science (see chap. 1.1.4, 4.3).

Furthermore, within the framework of a dynamic-systemic analysis method, the system dynamics of the cognitive neuroarchitectures are acquired increasing importance in processual simulation models. This is evident, for example in the presentation of system state changes in the form of the attractor dynamics of converging trajectories in n-dimensional system phase spaces (see chap. 2.2.3, 7) (McClelland 2009, Strohner 1995).

1.1.4 NEUROCOGNITIVE SYNCHRONIZATION MECHANISM

In an effort to be guided by scientific explanatory methods and models in cognitive science, and in theoretical neurophilosophy, one endeavors to use the term "mental mechanism"[14] or "neurocognitive mechanism" to scientifically explain the mental behavior of an information processing system. In addition, among other things in the cognitive neurosciences, especially in medical neurophysiology, it is being investigated how integrative synchronization mechanisms attempt to solve the (general) binding problem (see chap. 4.3, 4.4). Building on this, a variety of approaches in neuroinformatics, neurolinguistics, cognitive science, and computational neuroscience have been developed since the 1980s to construct integrative synchronization mechanisms in cognitive neuroarchitectures that theoretically and technically model this neural mechanism in the field of visual perception and language cognition (see chap. 6–chap. 10).

---

[13] Accordingly, a neurocognitive process can be understood as an actual and real-time proceeding realization mechanism of (process) algorithms or of computational procedures stored in the neurocognitive system.
See chap. 1.1.5.

[14] For an introduction, see e.g. Glennan 2008, Craver and Bechtel 2006, Machamer et al. 2000.
For a more in-depth discussion, see e.g. Bechtel 2008, Craver 2007, Piccinini 2007, Bechtel 2006, Abrahamsen and Bechtel 2006, Bechtel and Abrahamsen 2005.

According to the American philosopher of science Carl F. Craver, this newer explanatory term[15] of a (causal, reproductive) mechanism leads one to understand, especially in the cognitive neurosciences, an analytic description of a fact, according to which a mechanism consists of (Craver 2007, Craver and Darden 2013):

(1) constitutive entities (that is, of components) and
(2) activities (that is, processes or interactions between these components).

These activities have such an active organizational structure that they can explain the target phenomenon over several levels or fields of description with necessary causal relevance, so that the individual components can be the subject of a targeted, operational manipulation control.

According to the American philosopher of science William Bechtel, in a new philosophy of the life sciences, a neurobiological or mental mechanism, identified by a phenomenon to be explained, is defined as a reductionist, active and causal structure[16] that has a specific function with respect to

(1) its structural components,
(2) its cyclic, recursive and autocatalytic (process) operations (in the sense of state changes in time), and
(3) its proper organization which is subject to a structural or a functional mechanistic decomposition:

"A mechanism is a structure performing a function in virtue of its component parts, component operations, and their organization. The orchestrated functioning of the mechanism is responsible for one or more phenomena." (Bechtel 2008)

1.1.5 COMPUTATION AND COMPUTATIONAL (PROCESS-)ALGORITHM

Unless one abstracts from the physical implementation of these mental and neurocognitive structures, processes, and mechanisms, the central theme of cognitive science lies in finding formally mathematical and/or logical "(process) algorithms"[17] or "computational procedures" (in the sense of computational (procedural) rules[18] or

---

[15]For general information on the notion of scientific explanation in cognitive science, see e.g. von Eckardt 2003.

[16]Note the – probably intended – reference to the general concept of an algebraic structure. See chap. 1.1.1.

[17]See e.g. Lenzen 2002 with reference to Neisser 1974.
For an introduction, see e.g. Strube 1996d.
On the term "algorithm" in cognitive science, see e.g. Ranhel et al. 2017, Lappi and Rusanen 2011, Fetzer 2002, Dietrich 1999, Steedman 1996, Pylyshyn 1989.
On the term "algorithm" in theoretical computer science and mathematics, see e.g. Erk and Priese 2000, Kleene 1967.
For an introduction, see e.g. Harel 2004.

[18]On the concept of the (computational) rule in classical symbol theory and in connectionism, see e.g. Horgan and Tienson 2006, 1999, 1998, 1996, 1994b with reference to Garson 1994, Horgan and Tienson 1994a, 1992b, 1991a, b, 1990, 1989, Hatfield 1991, Dorffner 1991.
For a general overview, see Maurer 2014a.

in the sense of operating (procedural) instructions[19]).[20] These mental algorithms or purely mechanical procedures, located between the sensory and motor skills of a neurocognitive system, operate on data structures or on information structures in the form of internal "mental representations" in the context of computational processes or processual operations ("Computational-Representational Understanding of Mind (CRUM)" (see Box 1.1.5) (Thagard 2005).

This corresponds to the general form of a neurocognitive computation scheme, as already defined (see chap. 1.1.1). Here, for example, in the context of the general Hebb algorithm (see chap. 3.2.1), or more specific learning algorithms such as the Kohonen algorithm (see chap. 3.2.4.4) or the Grossberg algorithm (see chap 3.2.4.5)), several operations or mathematical functions are linked together with a plurality of operands in the form of variables (as in the form of synapses or input vectors), and with a plurality of constants (as in the form of learning constants).

The classical computational method and concept of computation[21] (in the sense of computability and decidability theory in the framework of theoretical computer science[22]) is described in the so-called "Turing Machine (TM)"[23] (see Fig. 1.1), named after the British logician, mathematician and cryptanalyst, Alan M. Turing. The simplified, mathematical function and working procedure of a computer, modeled by this machine has been transferred to the functioning of human cognition by a variety of cognitive scientists[24]: The Turing machine thus represents an algorithm or a mechanical computer program that manipulates (alphabetical) symbols by way of a computational procedure or by way of an operating instruction. That is, according to a finite, well-defined set of computational rules, certain characters of a well-defined set of a working alphabet are read in from a storage tape and written back to that

---

[19]See Thagard 2005, Lenzen 2002.

[20]For an introduction to the problem of "functionalism" in cognitive science on the basis of philosophy of science, see e.g. Bermúdez 2014, Urchs 2002, Lenzen 2002.

[21]For an introduction, see e.g. Piccinini 2012, von Eckardt 2003, Rapaport 2000, Stufflebeam 1998. See also Miłkowski 2018, Favela and Martin 2017.
For a more extensive discussion, see Fresco 2014, Pylyshyn 1989.
In contrast, the term "neural computation" has recently been used in the sense of a nonlinear encoding of sensory information as well as a linear decoding of neural information in the form of spike trains in computational neuroscience, for example in Eliasmith 2007.
For a detailed discussion, see chap. 4.2.1, 6.3.

[22]According to prevailing opinion, the standard definition of computation or computability is defined on the basis of the typical operationality of a Turing machine (see Fig. 1.1).
For a brief discussion, see e.g. Sipser 2013, Erk and Priese 2008, Schöning 2008, Hopcroft et al. 2006.

[23]For a fundamental discussion, see e.g. Turing 1936, 1938, Copeland 2004.
For a more in-depth discussion, see Fresco 2014, Wells 2004, Eliasmith 2002, Lappi and Rusanen 2011, Cutland 1980.
For an introduction, see e.g. Erk and Priese 2008, Schöning 2008, Hopcroft et al. 2006, Kleene 1967.
For the formal definition of a (determined) Turing machine, see e.g. Erk and Priese 2008.
For a beginner's guide, see e.g. Walter 2014, Sobel and Li 2013, Friedenberg and Silverman 2012, Bermúdez 2014, Mainzer 2003, Urchs 2002, Lenzen 2002, Harnish 2002, Pfeifer and Scheier 1999, Dawson 2001.

[24]For an introduction, see e.g. von Eckardt 2003.
For a detailed discussion, see Zylberberg et al. 2011, Lappi and Rusanen 2011, Wells 1998.

tape. Thus, a specific character string is mapped by means of a systematic transformation into a resulting character string. In other words, the Turing machine thereby describes a mathematical function and, if such a function can actually be computed using a Turing machine, it is called Turing-computable.

Box 1.1.5   Hard Rules vs. Soft Laws:

The commitment of classical symbol theory to the use of "hard rules" to manipulate and transform symbol representations (in the sense of the "logical form") has now been widely criticized, above all by the American philosophers and philosophers of science, Terence Horgan and John Tienson. According to them, it is neither necessary nor desirable for connectionism to adapt to the use of such rules. On the other hand, it is plausible that the connectionist models, with their "soft laws" in the framework of a psychological theory, create an alternative type of causal interaction in which the causal connections work together as in a "collective," and in which the causal consequences of individual neuronal connections can often be overruled by the opposing influence of other connections (so-called "soft-weight satisfaction"). An example of the soft laws are the local and subrepresentational activation and propagation functions performed between the individual neurons in an artificial neural network. This would provide the basis for a more appropriate non-classical cognitive theory, one in which the mathematical constructs of dynamic systems theory applied at the algorithmic level ("algorithmic-level rules") refine the hard rules of classical symbol theory applied at the representational level ("Programmable Representation Level [PRL] Rules").

In contrast to classical symbol theory, which represents a "Rules and Representations (RR)" conception, the new paradigm of connectionism, according to Horgan and Tienson, represents a "Representation without Rules (RWR)" conception.

For an introduction, see e.g. Horgan and Tienson 1991b.

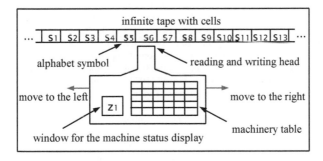

Figure 1.1: Schematic diagram of a Turing machine: The Turing machine consists of a (potentially) infinite band divided into cells that may be empty or contain a single alphabet symbol. At a given time, only the character on which the writing head and the reading head are currently located can be edited. Namely, a character can be read, deleted or replaced by a new character. Then, in another computing step, the machine writing head and reading head can then be moved one place to the left or to the right, wherein the machine state changes after each working step. A machine board with instructions determines how the Turing machine behaves (according to Schöning 2008, Cutland 1980, Dawson 2001).

1.1.6 INTERNAL MENTAL REPRESENTATION

Finally, a fundamental concept in cognitive science is the concept of "(internal) mental representation"[25], which is usually defined in analogy to the computer with its data structures and associated algorithms. By understanding and supplementing the definitions of the neurocognitive structure, the neurocognitive process and the computational algorithm, one understands in general

(1) a mental (informational) structure which, in the optimal case, is a homomorphic[26] or isomorphic[27] transformation relation, adequately representing an informational structure of the system environment, and

[25]For an introduction to cognitive science, see e.g. Thagard 2014, 2005, Sobel and Li 2013, von Eckardt 2012, 2003, 1999, 1993, Egan 2012, Denis 2004, Lloyd 2003, Lenzen 2002, Billman 1998.
For a more extensive discussion, see e.g. Strohner (1995), who complementarily combines both structural and functional methodologies in the context of an (eco-)systemic cognitive analysis, and thus strives for an empirically founded theory of cognitive representation against the background of a systems theory of cognition, consisting of the subareas of sensomotorics, syntax, semantics and pragmatics.
For an introduction to cognitive psychology, see e.g. Anderson 2015, Engelkamp and Zimmer 2006, Mielke 2001, Engelkamp and Pechmann 1993, Glaser 1993, Herrmann 1993; see also Eysenck and Keane 2010.
For an introduction to linguistics, see e.g. Sucharovski 1996.
For an introduction to cognitive neuroscience, see e.g. Walsh and Laughlin 2006.
For an introduction to philosophy, see e.g. Strasser 2010.
For the discussion on a general definition of the representation against the background of theoretical linguistics according to Peirce, see e.g. von Eckardt 1993.
See also in neurophilosophy the so-called "Emulation Theory of Representation" according to Grush 2001, 2004.
For a reference to various definitions of mental representation in neuroinformatics, neurophilosophy, neurolinguistics and cognitive psychology, see, in detail, e.g. von Eckardt 1993.
The history of the concept of representation can be summarized as follows: Within the framework of neo-behaviorism, C.E. Osgood (1957) formulated a theory of representation (also J. Bruner [1957], who was a representative of the "new-look" movement in perceptual psychology). Thanks to these approaches, early cognitive psychology already had a terminology of mental representation at its disposal. Nevertheless, it continued to be completely determined by the word field around the term "code" until the end of the 1960s. The term "representation" spread in psychology at the beginning of the 1970s, but without displacing the code terminology. Cognitive psychology has not developed an independent concept of representation, but its advancement is due to the reception of impulses from some other disciplines. For example, from linguistics by J. Katz and J.A. Fodor (1963) and N. Chomsky (1980), from Artificial Intelligence (AI) research in computer science by A. Newell (1973), and from the analytic philosophy of mind by J.A. Fodor (1976). Fodor's book "The Language of Thought" started the integration of philosophy into cognitive science.
In this tradition, the expression "representation," has, essentially, the four following meanings (Scheerer 1992): 1. an "idea" in the broader sense, that is, a state of consciousness with a cognitive character, 2. an "idea" in the narrower sense, that is, a state of consciousness which refers to or is derived from an earlier state, 3. a "representation," that is, a structure-identical representation through images and signs of all kinds, and 4. a "substitute."

[26]For an introduction to the concept of "homomorphism" in the sense of a linear mapping in mathematics, see e.g. Dummit and Foote 2004, Huppert and Willems 2010, Bosch 2006, Wolff et al. 2004, Pareigis 2000, Ihringer 1993.
See also, Dekkers 2017, Gómez Ramírez 2014.

[27]For an introduction to the concept of "isomorphism" in the sense of a bijective linear mapping in mathematics, see e.g. Dummit and Foote 2004, Storch and Wiebe 1990, Bosch 2006, Kowalsky and Michler 1995, Wolff et al. 2004, Pareigis 2000, Ihringer 1993.
See also, Dekkers 2015, Gómez Ramírez 2014.

(2) an associated computational, algorithmic and mental (informational) procedure that operates on those mental structures.[28]

In the paradigm of classical symbol processing theory (see chap. 3.1) one starts from the assumption that these mental structures can be modeled as discrete, logical or linguistic propositions, concepts, individual variables or individual constants, and the mental procedures can be modeled as logical or linguistic operations (such as junctors or quantor-logical, n-ary predications or relations). Conversely, in the paradigm of the system-theoretical connectionism (see chap. 3.2), one assumes that it is best to dynamically model these mental structures as computer-simulated, continuously vector-described and distributed activation patterns[29] in a self-organized, recurrent artificial neural network. The mental procedures are dynamically modeled here as their vectorial activation functions, propagation functions and adaptive learning functions (so-called "vectorial representations" [Dilger 2003/2004, Goschke and Koppelberg 1990, Hatfield 1991]).[30]

This trend away from a static, discrete format to a new continuous, dynamic, distributed and transient representation format[31] based on vector and attractor constructions (which can be used to describe a cognitive agent through permanent interactions embedded in its environment, thereby constituting cognitive structures[32]), can thus be characterized by the following aspects:

(1) dynamism with flow equilibrium character (see especially chap. 1.4, 2, 3.2.6, 7.4,
(2) systemism with a vectorial form (see especially chap. 1.4, 2, 3.2.6, 6.1, 7.4, 7.5, 8.1),
(3) the principle of self-organization (see especially chap. 2.3, 3.2.4.4, 3.2.4.5, 4.4, 8.1, 8.2, 10.3),
(4) temporalism or synchronism (see especially chap. 4.2.3, 4.4, 8, 9),
(5) holism (see especially chap. 2, 3.2, 4.4, 6.2, 7.1), and
(6) pragmatism (see especially chap. 1.4, 3.2.6, 10.3).

1.2 SUBDISCIPLINES OF COGNITIVE SCIENCE

Since, in view of the scope of research, a distribution of tasks among various subdisciplines of cognitive science was undertaken, it is possible to name six classical subdisciplines, as recommended by H. Strohner (1995), B. von Eckardt (2003), J.L.

---

[28] For a thorough discussion, see e.g. Gómez Ramírez 2014, Haselager et al. 2003. See also, Thagard 2014, Lenzen 2002, Thagard 2005, Markman 2003, von Eckardt 1999.

[29] It is also referred to as distributed activation states.

[30] For an introduction, see e.g. Vernon et al. 2007, von Eckardt 2003, Markman 2003, Lloyd 2003, Bringsjord and Yang 2003, von Eckardt 1993, van Gelder 1999b, d, 1992a, 1991a, b, 1990b.

[31] See Friedenberg and Silverman 2012 with reference to Peschl 1997. For a more extensive discussion, see also, Peschl 1996b, Spivey 2007, Eliasmith 2007.
For an introduction to the notion of representation format in cognitive science, see e.g. Billman 1998.

[32] On the pragmatic turn in cognitive science, see e.g. Engel et al. 2016, Engel et al. 2013a.

Bermúdez (2014) with reference to H. Gardner (1986), A. Stephan and S. Walter (2013):[33]

1. (cognitive) psychology,
2. (cognitive) neurosciences, consisting of medical neuropsychology and (cognitive) neurology, neurophysiology, (cognitive) neurobiology, cognitive psychology and (cognitive) neuropsychology,
3. (cognitive) linguistics or psycholinguistics,
4. (cognitive) anthropology,
5. (neuro-) philosophy, and
6. neuroinformatics and Artificial Intelligence (AI) - Research.

1.3   METHODOLOGY AND METHODS OF COGNITIVE SCIENCE

In order to integrate these sub-disciplines into a homogeneous discipline of cognitive science, one will have to strive for a scientific-theoretical reflection in order to be able to standardize the cognitive-scientific terminology and method.[34]

As for the methodological analysis of a cognitive phenomenon, the literature[35] generally refers to the British mathematician, physiologist and neuroscientist, David Marr (1982), who proposed to distinguish three general levels of cognitive science analysis ("The Tri-Level Hypothesis"[36]):

(1) the "computational level," which is concerned with a semantic, theoretical and abstract analysis of a specific problem to be solved by a particular competence of the neurocognitive information processing system (for example, the [general] binding problem in cognitive science and the neurosciences),

(2) the "algorithmic level," which deals with the question of which mathematical-formal structure of an algorithm can be used in the context of a (mechanistic) "functional analysis"[37], so that the relevant information processing problem can be solved in the best possible way. For example, the binding problem being

---

[33]Based on the report of the SLOAN Foundation in 1978.
For an review of the various subdisciplines, see e.g. Sobel 2001, Stillings et al. 1995, Simon and Kaplan 1989.

[34]On a detailed description of the cognitive science method or methodology, see e.g. Bechtel 1990, 1988/1991, McCauley 1998.
For an introduction to the cognitive science method or methodology, see e.g. Stillings et al. 1995, Thagard 2005, Strohner 1995, Strube et al. 2000, von Eckardt 1993.
On the methods in the subdisciplines of cognitive science, see Thagard 2005.
On a unified cognitive scientific terminology in the sense of the (dynamic) system theory, see e.g. Strohner 1995.

[35]See e.g. Dawson 2003, 2001, Houng 2003 also refer to the similar classification of the analysis levels in Pylyshyn 1985.
See also the similar classification of the analysis levels in Simon 2003 and in Stillings et al. 1995.
See also Horgan and Tienson 1996.

[36]For a detailed discussion, see Dawson 2001.
For an introduction, see Bermúdez 2014, von Eckardt 2003, Clark 2001.

[37]On the concept of "functional analysis" in cognitive science, see e.g. Dawson 2001 with reference to Cummins 1975, 1983.
See also Krieger 1996.

solved by means of integrative synchronization mechanisms in the form of vector and tensor constructions or attractor constructions, the associated differential equation systems or in the form of oscillation functions, and

(3) the "implementational level" which finally deals with the physical, that is, the anatomical-physiological or physical-technical factors that must be present in order to implement the functional mathematical procedures and mechanisms. In the case of the connectionist cognitive neuroarchitectures these factors are, for example, the corresponding neuronal activation, propagation and learning functions implemented in (humanoid) robots.

One of the most important methods of realization of cognitive neuroarchitectural models in cognitive science, especially in the field of "Artificial Intelligence (AI)",[38] is "computer simulation."[39] In this one tries to emulate, describe and explain human cognitive processes with the help of mathematical models, computer programs, and (based on the latter), computer-generated simulations (Thagard 2005). The concept of internal mental representation (as already stated [see chap. 1.1.6.]), is thereby of fundamental importance for "cognitive modeling" [40] in a cognitive theory. Whereas in the "symbol-oriented classical artificial intelligence" (the "symbolism" [see chap. 3.1]) mental representations are regarded as syntactically structured symbols, in the "subsymbol-oriented new artificial intelligence" (the "connectionism" [see chap. 3.2]) the notion of mental representation is applied to self-organized, recurrent and dynamical artificial neural networks.[41]

An important distinguishing feature between symbolism and connectionism is the model-technical construction[42] of neuronal information processing (Romba 2001), in other words, the answer to the question: How does the intelligent processing of information by humans work?

---

[38]For a comprehensive discussion, see e.g. Haugeland 1985, Bickhard and Terveen 1995, Iida et al. 2004.
For an introduction, see e.g. Sun 1998, 2001.

[39]For a detailed discussion, see Maurer 2014b, Weber 1999.
For an introduction, see e.g. Strube et al. 2000.

[40]For a comprehensive discussion, see e.g. Rathgeber 2011, who outlines a "general constructive model theory" of cognition.
See also Plaut 2000, McClelland 1999, Lewis 1999, Dawson 2001, Pylyshyn 1989.
For this topic, see also in general Friedenberg 2009, Harré 2002, Strohner 1995, Schmid and Kindsmüller 1996.
On a historical overview of the different model approaches in cognitive sciences, see e.g. Shiffrin 2010.
For an introduction, see e.g. McClelland 2009, who presents a very balanced summary of the various approaches, Sun 2008, who focuses on "Computational Cognitive Modeling", Friedenberg 2009, who gives an overview of "Dynamical Modeling", and Walter 2014, who, in addition to the traditional cognitive modeling of symbolism, connectionism and dynamism, sets out the newer modeling approaches, such as "Situated Cognition", "Embodied Cognition", "Extended Cognition", "Distributed Cognition", and "Enacted Cognition".

[41]For an introduction, see Shapiro 2011, Harré 2002, Mielke 2001, Pfeifer and Scheier 1999, Dawson 2001, Clark 2001, Rapaport 2000, Varela et al. 1993, Strube et al. 2000, Strube 1996a, Green et al. 1996, Simon and Kaplan 1989.

[42]For a detailed discussion, see chap. 3.1 and 3.2.
On the discussion, in philosophy of science, about the methodological principles in the analysis and construction of theoretical system models in the neuro- and cognitive sciences, see e.g. Gómez Ramírez 2014, Bermúdez 2014.

1.4   COGNITIVE SCIENCE AND (NONLINEAR) DYNAMICAL SYSTEMS THEORY

Since the middle of the 1990s[43], cognitive science (oriented towards [system-theoretical] connectionism[44]) has become increasingly used to the methods and conceptions from the (mathematical) "Dynamic Systems Theory (DST)" in the analysis of adaptive, self-organized (neuro-)cognitive systems and the corresponding development of cognitive neuroarchitectures: (1) "The Dynamic(-al) (System) Challenge"[45], (2) "The Dynamical Approach"[46], (3) "(Noncomputable) Dynamical Cognition (NDC) Approach"[47], (4) "Dynamical (Systems) Hypothesis (D(S)H)"[48], (5) "The Brain-Body-Environment (BBE) Systems Approach"[49], and (6) "The Complex Systems Approach"[50] (see chap. 2.2).[51] These neurocognitive systems with their cognitive neuroarchitectures, as well as the neurocognitive agents concerned in computer simulation experiments, are based on (non-linear) differential equation systems[52], which can more adequately model the continuous self-organization dynamics[53] of complex neuronal information processing in the context of human (neuro-)cognition. Above all, it is stressed that the time aspect for the in-depth understanding of (human) cognition is of utmost importance. Since cognition takes place *in* the continuous real-time of processual events, it is reflected in quantitative time variables in dynamic models, as well as in a transient, dynamic representation format (Van Gelder 1999d). This is also compatible with a dynamic-mechanistic

---

[43]For a groundbreaking book, see Van Gelder and Port 1995.

[44]For a detailed discussion, see e.g. Van Gelder 1998b with his "Dynamical (Systems) Hypothesis (DH)", Abrahamsen and Bechtel 2006, Van Gelder and Port 1995, Bechtel 1998, Horgan and Tienson 1992b.
For an introduction, see e.g. Van Gelder 1999d, Thagard 2005, Strube 1996a, Strohner 1995, Clark 2001. For a beginner's guide, Lenzen 2002, Bermúdez 2014.
A detailed overview can be found in e.g. Beer 2000, Van Leeuwen 2005.

[45]See Thagard 2005, Clark 1997, 1999.

[46]See e.g. Pfeifer et al. 2008, Haselager et al. 2003, Malmgren 2006.

[47]See Horgan and Tienson 1996, 1992b.

[48]For a fundamental discussion, see e.g. Van Gelder and Port 1995, Van Gelder 1998b, a, 1999c, a.
For an introduction, see e.g. Van Gelder 1999d, 1997, Port 2003.
For critical information, see e.g. Eliasmith 1996/1998a, 1998b.

[49]See e.g. Beer 1992a, b, 1995, 1997, 2008, 2014.

[50]See e.g. Scott Jordan et al. 2015, Gray 2012, Silberstein and Chemero 2012, Dixon et al. 2012, Riley et al. 2012, Gibbs and Van Orden 2012.
For an introduction, see e.g. Eliasmith 2012.

[51]For an introduction, see e.g. Gómez Ramírez 2014, Friedenberg and Silverman 2012, Fusella 2013 with reference to Van Gelder 1998a, b and Gray 2012, Shapiro 2011, Schneegans and Schöner 2008, Thagard 2005, Pfeifer and Scheier 1999, Elman 1998.
For a detailed discussion, see e.g. Favela and Martin 2017, Spivey 2007, Hotton and Yoshimi 2011, Pfeifer et al. 2008, Chemero and Silberstein 2008.
For an introduction to psychology, see e.g. Friedenberg 2009.
On the influence of (eco) system theory for cognitive science see e.g. Strohner 1995.

[52]According to Thagard 2005, the nonlinear differential equations are characterized by the fact that the various system variables of a differential equation, fed back together reciprocally in certain circumstances, can interact with each other.

[53]On the influence of the metaphor of self-organization for cognitive science, see e.g. Strohner 1995.

explanatory approach in the philosophy of (neuro-)cognitive science (Abrahamsen and Bechtel 2006; see also chap. 1.1).

1.5 EXCURSION: COGNITIVE TURN IN PSYCHOLOGY

In the first half of the 20th century, a distinction was made in the history of psychology between J.B. Watson's "orthodox behaviorism" (Watson 1913, Thorndike 1911) and the "neo-behaviorism" propounded by C.L. Hull, E.C. Tolman and B.F. Skinner (Hull 1943, Tolman 1948, Skinner 1953). Since the beginning of the 1960s, the dominance of neo-behaviorism in psychology has declined, and psychology is becoming "cognitive." This means that on the one hand, research development is shifting towards cognitive processes such as thinking, and on the other hand, psychic phenomena (including behaviour) are preferentially explained through internal cognitive variables. These new approaches and new developments, summarized with the catch phrase the "cognitive turn",[54] are altogether too varied and diverse to be precisely determined by their uniform and common features (Ulich 2000). The efforts ranged from simply improving orthodox behaviorism-oriented model constructs by including additional "intervening (cognitive) variables" (Tolman 1938) to attempting to overcome and replace (neo-)behaviorism by the postulation of the self-responsible "reflexive subject" (Groeben and Scheele 1977). However, most of the cognitively oriented psychologists of (neo-)behaviorism have adhered to the long-standing goal of psychology: that experience and behavior should be explained and predicted by generalizing assumptions, and should be changed and "optimized" by the control and variation of the underlying external situational factors that condition behavior and experience.

In view of these behavior-controlling conditions, however, a clear reversal of the perspective and the question took place: the behavior is controlled by not (only) the external situation factors but also – tendentially – by the person himself. This departure from the behavioristic approach of a passive reacting organism towards a knowledge-processing, self-controlling, self-acting and perceiving individual has been termed the "cognitive turn" or the "cognitive revolution" in psychology.

Thus, while at the time of (neo-)behaviourism one was concerned with the learning of behavior, in the view of modern cognitive psychology all learning, thinking, feeling, and acting are subject to control by knowledge or information processing in the broadest sense. Modern cognitive psychology puts issues of acquisition, mapping, retrieval and application of knowledge or information at the center. It usually maintains the functionalist perspective: the contributions that thoughts, actions, knowledge acquisition and knowledge make to the fulfillment of specific tasks and to the solution of specific problems, i.e. "adaptation" in the broadest sense, continue to be of interest.

---

[54]For detailed information to the cognitive turn, see e.g. Sturm and Gundlach 2013, Bermúdez 2014, Strube 1996b, Strohner 1995.
It is often also referred to as the "cognitive revolution". See e.g. Leahey 1991, Stephan and Walter 2013 with reference to Gardner 1985 and Miller 2003.

It should be noted, however, that from a historical perspective of psychology, the term "turn" applies more to psychology in the USA than to Europe, especially to Germany, in which the perceptual, gestalt, holistic and thinking psychological tendencies always had higher importance than in the USA (Lück 2013, Scheerer 1988).

The labeling of theories as "cognitive" has evolved from the learning theory discussion. For a preliminary characterization of this type of theory, it is best to follow a provisional negative definition by Donald O. Hebb: Someone practices cognitive psychology when he argues that the behavioral approach with its stimulus-response relations is not sufficient to explain more complex behaviors. As a rule, however, this rather generous provision is somewhat limited in that the term "cognitive" is reserved only for those approaches that – as mediating conditions between the stimulations and the reactions – allow links that are not themselves again self-internalized connections of this stimulus-response scheme. This narrower concept of a "cognitive theory" thus excludes those theories with intervening variables of neo-behaviorism, which are based on only the "stimulus-response formula" (Hebb 1960).

In the tradition of North American psychology, the neo-behaviorist Tolman is regarded as the main representative of the cognitive tendency within classical learning theories (Tolman 1932/1949, 1938, 1948). In the succession of his cognitive learning theory in the sixties and seventies, two theoretical traditions can now be distinguished, both of which describe themselves as "cognitive" and set themselves apart from the theories of (neo-)behaviorism, but no longer exclusively in the field of learning. In somewhat simplified terms, these two fields of research can be juxtaposed as cognitive theories with a structuralist or a functionalist accent. What both have in common is that they emerged from fusions between theoretical traditions of (neo-)behaviorism and theoretical systems of European provenance. Cognitive theories with a structuralist accent focus on the determination of cognitive structures. K. Lewin, with his "Topological Psychology," was the first to present a reasonably closed theory for the identification of cognitive structures, but his situation analyses achieve hardly anything beyond a description (Lewin 1936). J. Piaget's structural-genetic system with its complementary mechanisms of assimilation and accommodation is regarded as a model case of a structurally oriented cognitive theory (Piaget 1970, Piaget and Inhelder 1969). Among the American research groups that have been strongly influenced by the reception of Piaget's theory, J.S. Bruner's approach, in which the concept of "representation" plays a key role, is particularly noteworthy (Bruner et al. 1967). Cognitive theories with a functionalist accent are concerned with understanding, as far as possible, the functioning of the processing units to be assumed between stimulation and reaction on the basis of processes. The initial starting point was the discovery of conditions of perception independent of stimuli. The second starting point is seen in the English "Human Performance" research, whose investigations by D.E. Broadbent also gave rise to the postulation of mediating processing stages (Broadbent 1958). At the end of the sixties, the main components of both research approaches were combined under the name "Cognitive Psychology", first by U. Neisser (1967), then by D.E. Broadbent (1971). As an additional constitutive element of his cognitive theory, Neisser emphasizes the special value of concepts and ideas from the field of information sciences (Neisser 1967).

In addition, there are those cognitive theories that give preference to cybernetic constructs. This is mainly done with the aim of being able to include the dimension of action often used by opponents as a missing dimension in cognitive psychology, as in the model of G.A. Miller, E. Galanter and K.H. Pribram. They received a one-year grant from the Ford Foundation in 1958 to test the benefits of cybernetics for psychology. The result of this work was the book "Plans and the Structure of Behavior", published in 1960. Cybernetics interprets a purposeful behaviour as a behaviour aimed at the approximation of the behaving system to another, whereby the movement of approximation can be controlled by two process patterns: positive and negative feedback. For the description of negative feedback, for example, it may be assumed that the following are defined: (1) a given set value that is to be reached (the target value of the system), and (2) a value describing the current state of the system (the actual system value). If the measurement of the actual value deviates from the setpoint adjustment, the output quantity of the reference junction (determined by the measuring element) sends a specific message to the controlling element, which readjusts the actual value to the setpoint value (again) via the controlled system. The authors apply this cybernetic model of a feedback control system to humans: the human being is influenced not only by stimuli, but also by "plans" that he pursues to reach his goals, which are based on his knowledge of himself and his environment. During the action, the human constantly checks whether the desired final state is reached through a feedback loop. Their conception of human action as a multi-faceted network of control loops promised to resolve the long-running controversy as to whether behavior was more a result of external environmental conditions or inner goals of action, by integrating both into the cybernetic model (Miller et al. 1960/1970, Neisser 1967).

Cognitive psychology (with the involvement of computer science, neurophysiology, linguistics and other disciplines including cognitive science and artificial intelligence) dealt in the sixties, and especially in the seventies and eighties, with the questions of the "functioning" of cognitive structures and processes. This meant, for example, reviewing what preconditions must be met for the processing of information and how information processing can be improved under certain circumstances, assuming that perception and attention, memory and thinking are inseparably linked. Within the framework of this research development, "the independent theoretical psychology was replaced by the hasty adoption of models and concepts provided by information and computer technology" (Neumann 1985). But even without computer analogy, the psychological model of information processing, i.e. the modern cognitivist position that all learning, thinking, acting and feeling is controlled by information processing, was a consequence of the adoption of the system-theoretical paradigm in psychology (Ulich 2000). The question therefore arose, of what is meant by an "information-processing system" in psychology, whereby, for example, the approach of P.H. Lindsay and D.A. Norman in their book "Human Information Processing. An Introduction to Psychology" (1972/1977) was applied. To understand the human being as a "system" means, therefore, to see the different performance areas in an ordered context and to relate their interaction to something "whole", namely the person. The totality of the processes of consciousness and the ways of experience and behaviour are therefore to be imagined as an ordered, composite whole which, under certain circumstances, is capable of self-control in so far as it can adapt its actions to the changed inner states and external environmental conditions, and is thus in constant exchange with the environment. Accordingly, "information processing" is a generic term for all processes by means of which knowledge in the broadest sense is processed, i.e. recorded, stored, retrieved, compared, evaluated and applied, whereby the result can be a decision, an expansion of the knowledge base, an action plan or its modification, and much more. The term "information"[55] refers to any communication or message that has a news value for the recipient.

---

[55] It should be noted, however, that in cognitive psychology the term "information" is not used as a terminus technicus, e.g. in the sense of mathematical information theory according to C.E. Shannon, but is understood more broadly. See e.g. Scheerer 1988.

2 (General) Theory of (Non-Linear) Dynamical Systems and the Paradigm of Self-Organization

The following chapter presents a brief outline of the models, methods, concepts and principles of (general) systems theory (chap. 2.1), and the mathematical theory of (nonlinear) dynamic systems (chap. 2.2), since connectionism (chap. 3.2) is considered to belong to the (nonlinear) dynamical systems in the context of the mathematical model typology (within the framework of Marr's algorithmic [analysis] level (chap. 1.3.)).[56] This includes the concept of self-organization (chap. 2.3), the attractor theory (chap. 2.2.3), the concept of (non-)linearity (chap. 2.2.4), the complexity theory (chap. 2.2.5), and the theory of deterministic chaos (chap. 2.3.2) (as research branches within cognitive science). At the end of the chapter is a listing of the most important authors (chap. 2.4).

2.1 (GENERAL) SYSTEM THEORY AND SYSTEM ANALYSIS

2.1.1 (GENERAL) SYSTEM THEORY

The term "(General) System Theory"[57] is usually understood as a transdisciplinary research program; after the initial approaches in the 1920s, it began to further develop

---

[56]See e.g. Nadeau 2014, Munro and Anderson 1988, Wilson 1999, Horgan and Tienson 1996, 1992b, Smolensky 1988a, Kosko 1992, Clark 1997a, 1997b, Leitgeb 2005, Van Gelder 1999d.

[57]For basic information, see e.g. von Bertalanffy 1950a, 1950b/2010, 1968, 1975, Ashby 1952, Hall and Fagen 1968, Klir 1969, Rapaport 1986.
For an introduction, see e.g. Dekkers 2017, Jantsch 1989, Steinbacher 1990, von Bertalanffy 1972b.
For an introduction to the (general) system theory based on mathematics, see e.g. Zadeh 1969, who designed an abstract, set-theoretical version of systems theory.
For a beginner's guide, see e.g. Jantsch 1979/1980.
For an introduction to philosophy of science, see e.g. Lenk 1975, 1978, Ropohl 1978, 1979, Seiffert 1985.
For an introduction to the historical roots of modern system theory, see e.g. von Bertalanffy 1972a, François 1999, Klir 1969.

from the 1940s. It covers mathematical, scientific, engineering and social science research fields, and includes research areas such as Norbert Wiener's "Cybernetics" (Wiener 1948/1961, 1965).

2.1.2 BASIC CONCEPT OF THE (OPEN) SYSTEM

The basic concept of system theory, the notion of the "(open) system"[58] (derived from the Greek word "σύστημα (sýstēma)"[59]) is generally determined by the following minimal definition: A system, as a functionally closed entity that can be distinguished from its environment, consists firstly of a set of "system elements" between which there are (reciprocal) interrelationships, which also applies to the element features with the corresponding characteristic values. Secondly, a system consists of a set of "system relations" or "system operations" which link the system elements together in a specific way. This spatial, temporal or causal arrangement of the elements with reference to each other is referred to as the "system structure."[60] The "system function" is understood to be the characteristic of all the patterns of relationships that occur. That is, the system function is the overall behavior and performance states of the system in its environment. The elements of a system, in turn, can be considered as the "subsystems". However, the system itself may be considered as an element of a more comprehensive system, the "suprasystem" or "cosystem", so that a system interpretation may be made at various stages of such a "system hierarchy". The concept of the suprasystem serves as a term for the class of all systems with which the considered system, the "reference system", maintains interaction processes, i.e. the "system environment".

2.1.3 SYSTEM ANALYSIS AND SYSTEM TECHNIQUES

In the German-speaking world, the system theory (in the narrower sense) is sometimes distinguished from "system analysis" (Imboden and Koch 2008, Häuslein

---

[58]For fundamental information, see e.g. Hall and Fagen 1968: "A system is a set of objects together with relationships between the objects and between their attributes".
For detailed information, see e.g. von Bertalanffy 1950a, 1950b/2010, 1968, 1975, Asby 1952, Klir 1969, Rapaport 1986, von Bertalanffy and Rapaport 1956.
For an introduction, see e.g. Fieguth 2017, Dekkers 2017, Jantsch 1989, 1980, 1979/1980, Strunk 2000, Strunk and Schiepek 2006.

[59]The English translation of the Greek "sýstēma (syn + histanai)" is given as: composition, connexion, relatedness, merger, assembly; pattern, union, totality, education; also (general) structure, principle of order, uniformly ordered whole.
See Stavropoulos 2008, Gemoll and Vretska 2006, Menge 1913/2001, 1986/1993.
See also e.g. Kornwachs 2008, Gloy 1998a.
On the history of the concept of the system, see Dekkers 2017.

[60]The term "mathematical structure" has been of fundamental importance in modern mathematics and physics since the twentieth century; for example, since the 1930s, the author collective with the pseudonym, Nikolas Bourbaki, has attempted to unify mathematics founded on the axiomatic method of the German mathematician David Hilbert, whereby the structural concept is central ("mathematical structuralism").
For a detailed discussion, see e.g. Dieudonné (1970).
For an introduction, see e.g. Mac Lane 1996, Wussing 2009, Ebeling et al. 1998, Puntel 2006.

2003, van de Wouw et al. 2017) and engineering-oriented "system technology" (Frey and Bossert 2008, Unbehauen 1998, 2002).

2.2 (MATHEMATICAL) THEORY OF (NONLINEAR) DYNAMICAL SYSTEMS

2.2.1 DYNAMICAL SYSTEMS THEORY

The "Dynamic Systems Theory (DST)"[61] describes the behavior of complex dynamic systems with their mathematical functions, concepts, and models, using linear and nonlinear differential equations. This description includes the behavior of the neuronal system of neurons and neuron populations in human neural networks (Köhle 1990). These systems, with their intrinsic dynamics, generate the (stabilization) mechanisms that give rise to certain systemic patterns of behavior; these, with a sufficient degree of stability, can withstand the effects of a complex system environment. Mathematically, this corresponds to the fact that the solution of a finite set of differential equations of a (neural) dynamic system converges to an invariant or (relatively) stable system state (Kosko 1992).

The mathematical definition of a finite set of (ordinary or partial) differential equations, also called a system of differential equations, is given by the following formulas:

$$x_1'(t) = f_1(x_1(t), ..., x_d(t))$$

$$\vdots$$

$$x_d'(t) = f_d(x_1(t), ..., x_d(t))$$

(Hall and Fagen 1968, von Bertalanffy 1950b/2010, Ashby 1952).

---

[61]For fundamental information on dynamic systems theory in mathematics, see e.g. Birkhoff 1927/1966.

For an introduction on dynamic systems theory in mathematics, see e.g. Teschl 2011, Hinrichsen and Pritchard 2010, Perko 2009, Guckenheimer and Holmes 1990, Katok and Hasselblatt 1995, Arrowsmith and Place 1990, Casti 1977, Casti 1985, Hinrichsen 1981/1988, Devaney 1994, Robinson 2009.

For an introduction to the theory of dynamic systems in physics, computer science and neuroscience, see e.g. Gerthsen 1999, Metzler 1998, Scheinerman 2000, Der and Herrmann 2002, Brin and Stuck 2002.

For an introduction to dynamic systems theory in psychology and cognitive science, see e.g. Thelen and Smith 2006, Jaeger 1996, Schöner 2009, 2001, Thagard 2005, Horgan and Tienson 1996, 1992b.

For an introduction to the theory of dynamic systems in all scientific disciplines, see e.g. Fieguth 2017, Mainzer 2004, Jaeger 1996.

For an introduction to the historical roots of modern dynamic systems theory, see e.g. Jaeger 1996.

2.2.2 MINIMAL DEFINITION OF A DYNAMICAL SYSTEM

The formal mathematical-scientific minimal definition of a "dynamical system"[62] with a large number n of elements[63], consists of:

(1) an abstract, d-dimensional so-called "phase space" or "state space" X, whose d system variables $x_1(t), ..., x_d(t)$ in the form of vector coordinates completely describe the overall system state, $x(t)$, in its progression with time t [64], and

(2) a dynamic (transformation) function f, which determines the changes of all "state variables" in time and thus the overall system state, indicated as a triple (T, X, f).

It consists of

1. a set T of time parameters with $T = \mathbb{N}_0$, $\mathbb{Z}$, $\mathbb{R}_0^+$ or $\mathbb{R}$, where the time can be interpreted as a generalized iteration index[65],

2. a non-empty set X, the phase space or state space with a d-dimensional state vector $x(t) = x_1(t), ..., x_d(t)$ of the system with $x(t) \in \mathbb{R}^d$,[66] and

3. a (transformation) function $f^t : T \times X \to X$ with $t \in \mathbb{N}_0$, $\mathbb{Z}$, $\mathbb{R}_0^+$ or $\mathbb{R}$.

One now differentiates two model types of dynamic systems, depending on whether the time parameter is discrete or continuous[67]:

In the first case for $t \in \mathbb{N}_0$ or $t \in \mathbb{Z}_0$ one gets a discrete dynamical system, which can be represented as an iteration of a function:

$$x(0) = x_0, \text{ and} \qquad (2.1)$$

$$x(t+1) = f(x(t)). \qquad (2.2)$$

---

[62]For a compact mathematical definition, see e.g. Teschl 2011.
For a general and detailed mathematical definition, see e.g. Hinrichsen and Pritchard 2010, Hinrichsen 1981/1988, Casti 1977.
For a definition based on the specifications of physics, computer science and neuroscience, see e.g. Metzler 1998, Scheinerman 2000, Der and Herrmann 2002, Brin and Stuck 2002, Ott 2002, Arrowsmith and Place 1990.
The system definition is closely related to the definition of the so-called "algebraic structure" Σ according to $\Sigma = \langle A, f_i \rangle$, consisting of a set of fundamental i-ary operations f_i or relations imprinted on a non-empty carrier set A.
See also, the remarks in chap. 1.1.

[63]The number n of (system) elements determines the number of dimensions d of the state vector, i.e. $n = d$, where one dimension geometrically represents a system variable or a system parameter $x_j(t)$.

[64]Concerning the concept of the (system) state in physics and its relation to its use in the context of the Turing machine, see e.g. Zadeh 1962/1991 with reference to Turing 1936.
A (system) variable $x_j(t)$ is used to mathematically and quantitatively record a (system) element with the index $j = 1, ..., d$ or its element attributes.
See e.g. Hall and Fagen 1968.
A vector coordinate within the phase space geometrically designates a system state that can, in principle, be captured.

[65]See Metzler 1998.

[66]This represents a so-called "metric space".
For an introduction, see e.g. O'Searcoid 2007, Kaplansky 1977, Jänich 2005, Heine 2009, Metzler 1998.
According to Jaeger 1996, the state vector $x(t) = x_1(t), ..., x_d(t)$ of the system specifies "which numeric values have the observed system variables at a given time".

[67]See e.g. Der and Herrmann 2002, Scheinerman 2000, Metzler 1998, Arrowsmith and Place 1990, Teschl 2011, Brin and Stuck 2002.

In the second case for $t \in \mathbb{R}_0^+$ or $t \in \mathbb{R}$ one obtains a continuous dynamical system whose dynamics can be described by (a system of)[68] ordinary differential equations:

$$x(0) = x_0, \text{ and} \tag{2.3}$$

$$X(x) = \frac{d}{dt}x(t) = x'(t) = F(x(t), t). \tag{2.4}$$

Such a system can be regarded as a "vector field" F[69] or as a "vector flow"[70], which describes the "curves" of the vector coordinates on the basis of tangential vectors, the typical "trajectories"[71] or the "orbits," and thus, their movements in the state space during a time course ("phase portrait"[72]) (see Fig. 2.1). This means that the system tracks a "coherent system history, a 'trace in time'" (Jaeger 1996).

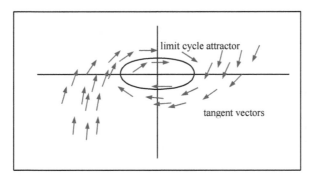

limit cycle attractor

tangent vectors

Figure 2.1: Schematic diagram of a vector field of a limit cycle attractor (shown as an ellipse) with a portion of the corresponding tangent vectors (shown as arrows) in a 2-dimensional phase space (following Jetschke 1989).

---

[68] If a continuous dynamic system has more than one dimension, i.e. $x \in \mathbb{R}^d$ and $f^d : \mathbb{R}^d \to \mathbb{R}^d$ with $d > 1$, the equation (2.4) is to be understood as a system of first-order ordinary differential equations according

$$x_1'(t) = f_1(x_1(t), ..., x_d(t))$$

to: $\vdots$

$$x_d'(t) = f_d(x_1(t), ..., x_d(t)).$$

See, for example, Der and Herrmann 2002.

[69] For a detailed discussion, see e.g. Guckenheimer and Holmes 1990, Khalil 2002, Jetschke 1989, Arrowsmith and Place 1990.
See also, Norton 1995.
For an introduction, see e.g. Königsberger 2002, Scheck 2007.

[70] For the term "phase flow" or "vector stream" see e.g. Jetschke 1989, Arrowsmith and Place 1990, Drin and Stuck 2002.

[71] For an introduction, see Gerthsen 1999, Haken 2004.

[72] See e.g. Perko 2009, Teschl 2011, Khalil 2002, Arrowsmith and Place 1990, Metzler 1998, Jetschke 1989, Robinson 2012, 2009, 2004, Hinrichsen and Pritchard 2010, Der and Herrmann 2002.

A vector field is mathematically defined as follows: A vector field v on a set $\Omega \subset \mathbb{R}^n$ is an mapping that assigns a vector $v(x)$ to each point $x \in \Omega$, $v : \Omega \to \mathbb{R}^n$. If v is a C^k mapping, we speak of a C^k vector field. Geometrically, one interprets a vector field v by thinking that at each point $x \in \Omega$, the vector $v(x)$ is attached; formal: One forms the pairs $(x, v(x))$, $x \in \Omega$. Physically, a vector field is often interpreted as the velocity field of a stationary, i.e. time-independent flow, where $v(x)$ is the velocity vector at point x (Königsberger 2002).

2.2.3 ATTRACTOR THEORY AND STABILITY THEORY IN DYNAMICAL SYSTEMS

A central topic within the framework of the theory of dynamic systems is that of the convergent system processes towards relatively invariant, stable system states, the "attractors"[73] with corresponding "attractor basins". Geometrically interpreted, they correspond to a space area in the phase space to which adjacent trajectories from arbitrary starting points in a certain environment are heading asymptotically, in other words, one which "attracts" these trajectories (see Fig. 2.2).

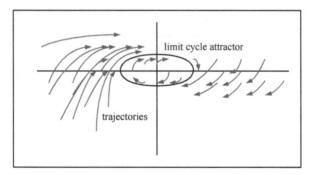

Figure 2.2: Schematic diagram of a phase portrait of a limit cycle attractor (represented as an ellipse), with part of the corresponding trajectories (represented as arrows), in a 2-dimensional phase space. The corresponding orbits are asymptotically stable (inspired by Jetschke 1989, Arrowsmith and Place 1990).

The mathematical-scientific minimal definition of an attractor can be given in relation to a discrete, deterministic dynamic system as follows[74]: Given, an n-fold iteration of a (transformation) function f^n with $f^n(x_1) = x_n + 1$ with $n \in \mathbb{Z}^+$ and

---

[73]For an introduction, see e.g. Jaeger 1996, Mainzer 2010, Schiepek and Strunk 1994, Strunk and Schiepek 2006, Horgan and Tienson 1996, Prigogine and Stengers 1993.
See also, Kolen 2001.
For the mathematical-scientific (minimal) definition of an "attractor", see fn. 74.

[74]For fundamental information, see e.g. Newhouse 1984, Devaney 1994.
For detailed information, see e.g. Metzler 1998, Jetschke 1989, Perko 2009, Guckenheimer and Holmes 1990, Teschl 2011, Der and Herrmann 2002, Brin and Stuck 2002, Robinson 2009.
See also, Ebeling et al. 1990.

$x \subseteq X$, then we call a compact, invariant and attractive set $A \subseteq X$ an attractor, if there is a (fundamental) environment U of A and a distance function d in a metric space such that the following holds:

$$\lim_{n \to \infty} d(f^n(x), A) = 0 \quad \forall x \in U, \, U \text{ neighborhood of } A \subseteq X \tag{2.5}$$

with the two properties

(1) $\equiv_{n \geq 0} f^n(U) = A$ and

(2) $f(\bar{U}) \subseteq U$ with $(\bar{U})$: closure of U.

The mathematical-scientific minimal definition of an attractor can also be given in relation to a stochastic dynamic system with reference to a subset A of system state space X as follows[75]: Given, $A \subseteq X$ with $\forall x_i \in \Lambda, \forall x_j \notin A, \forall n$, then : $f^t(x_i) \in A, M_{ij}^n = 0$ with M as a transition matrix of a Markov chain and $\lim_{n \to \infty} M_{ik}^n = 0$, if $s_k \in A$.

One can now distinguish the following different types of attractors:[76]

(1) "fixed-point attractor"
(2) "limit cycle attractor" (see Fig. 2.1 and Fig. 2.2.)
(3) "torus attractor"
(4) "strange attractor" or "chaotic attractor"

Mathematical "stability theory"[77] deals with an exact analysis of the "structural stability"[78] of a dynamic system in relation to the inner and outer disruptions, the "perturbations," of the system behavior according to A.M. Lyapunov, H. Poincaré and A.A. Andronov (Khalil 2002, Unbehauen 2002, Robinson 2009).

The "stability" of a (non-excited) system, according to A.M. Lyapunov, is mathematically defined as follows: An equilibrium state z_e is called *stable* if and only if there is always a quantity $\delta = \delta(t_0, \varepsilon) > 0$ only dependent on t_0 and ε for arbitrary values t_0 and $\varepsilon > 0$, so that

$$\|\zeta(t ; z(t_0)) - z_e\| < \varepsilon \text{ for all } t \geq t_0 \tag{2.6}$$

if the initial state $z(t_0)$ is selected within the δ-environment of the equilibrium state, so that

$$\|z(t_0)) - z_e\| < \delta. \tag{2.7}$$

Stability thus demands that an environment of initial states $z(t_0)$ always exists around the considered equilibrium state, so that the solutions $\zeta(t ; z(t_0))$ for all $t \geq t_0$ remain within a small environment of the equilibrium state. Of course, there has to be $\delta < \varepsilon$ (Unbehauen 2002).

---

[75] See Heylighen 2003. See also, Berger 2001, Ebeling et al. 1990.
For the concept of the "Markov chains" see the explanations in chap. 10.3.

[76] For an introduction, see e.g. Devaney 1994, Jetschke 1989.
See also, Jaeger 1996, Schiepek and Strunk 1994, Kosko 1992.

[77] For detailed information, see e.g. Perko 2009, Khalil 2002, Arrowsmith and Place 1990, Teschl 2011, Mesarovic and Takahara 1975, Unbehauen 2002.
For an introduction, see e.g. Königsberger 2002.
See also, Ebeling et al. 1990, Jaeger 1996.

[78] See e.g. Devaney 1994, Unbehauen 2002, Jetschke et al. 1989.

2.2.4 (NON-)LINEARITY OF A DYNAMICAL SYSTEM

The "linearity"[79] and the "nonlinearity"[80] of a complex dynamic system is determined from the (transformation) function f used in each case, which corresponds to either the general linear form

$$f(x) = ax + b, \tag{2.8}$$

or the general nonlinear forms, e.g. the polynomial function (formula [2.9]), the exponential function (formula [2.10]) or the logistic function (formula [2.11])

$$f(x) = a_n x^n + a_{n-1} x^{n-1} + \ldots + a_2 x^2 + a_1 x + a_0 \text{ mit } n \notin \mathbb{N}_0 \tag{2.9}$$

and the constant coefficients $a_0, a_1, a_2, \ldots, a_n$, or

$$f(x) = a^x \text{ or } f(x) = e^x \tag{2.10}$$

with $a > 0$ and $a \neq 1$, or

$$f(x) = S \cdot \frac{1}{1 + e^{-kSt}\left(\frac{S}{f(0)} - 1\right)} \tag{2.11}$$

with a threshold S and a constant k.

2.2.5 COMPLEXITY THEORY IN DYNAMICAL SYSTEMS

A further central topic in the framework of the theory of dynamic systems is the (not yet uniformly made) definition of their "complexity"[81], which can be best explained by the notion of complex structure.[82] The theory of complex systems has now, for the first time, been dealt with in statistical physics (according to L. Boltzmann, M. Planck, A. Einstein, and J. von Neumann) (Reichl 2009, Gerthsen 1999). This has

---

[79]For an introduction, see e.g. Fieguth 2017, Unbehauen 2002.

[80]For detailed information, see e.g. Scott 2007, 2005, 1999, Strogatz 2018, Casti 1985, Khalil 2002, Robinson 2004.
For an introduction, see e.g. Fieguth 2017, Argyris et al. 1995, Hooker 2011.
On the history of nonlinear science, see e.g. Scott 1999.
See also Mainzer 1994, 2008, 1999, who explains this topic using numerous examples of complex dynamic systems with nonlinear dynamics from mathematics and the natural sciences.
With respect to nonlinear dynamic systems in connectionism, see Elman et al. 1998.

[81]For detailed information, see e.g. Morin 2008, Mainzer 2007a, Chu et al. 2003, Snooks 2008.
For an introduction, see e.g. Nicolis and Prigogine 1989, Prigogine 1985/1991, Ebeling et al. 1998.
For a beginner's guide, see e.g. Hooker 2011, Mainzer 2010.
For a historical review of the topic of complexity, see e.g. Heudin 2006.

[82]See e.g. Ebeling et al. 1998, with reference to Simon 1962, Grassberger 1989a, 1989b, Lai and Grebogi 1996.

shown that, related to its subsystems, qualitatively new system properties may occur in a system. This is referred to as "emergence"[83] and, according to Mainzer, this condition must be included in the definition (Mainzer 1992, Mainzer and Chua 2013).

In the context of the "complexity theory"[84] a quantitative-mathematical definition has been developed in the form of the so-called "algorithmic complexity" (according to A.N. Kolmogorov 1968a, G.J. Chaitin 1975, and R. Solomonoff, 1964a, 1964b). According to the "Algorithmic Information Theory (AIT)" (A.N. Kolmogorov, G.J. Chaitin and R. Solomonoff), the purpose of a theory is to grasp a (complex) area of reality by means of the most compact and efficient compression of (algorithmic) information within a computer program. This means that if a theory is given in axiomatic form, it is important "to obtain a set of consequences as comprehensive as possible from a small set of sentences by means of logical conclusions."[85]

2.3 PARADIGM OF SELF-ORGANIZATION

2.3.1 PRINCIPLE OF SELF-ORGANIZATION AND EMERGENCE

The Paradigm of Self-Organization[86] (which is closely related to the theory of dynamic systems and describes the spontaneous structure-forming process), can be defined – in a simplified way – by its basic concept of "self-organization" as a (nonlinear) non-equilibrium process. Contrary to the Second Law of Thermodynamics[87], the principle of self-organization is characterized decisively by the fact that

---

[83]For detailed information, see e.g. Stephan 1999, 2003, 2006.
For an introduction, see e.g. Laughlin 2005, Feltz 2006.
For critical information, see e.g. Kornwachs 2008.
The concept of emergence has also been formulated mathematically on the basis of the construction of the "hyperstructure". See, for example, Baas 1997.

[84]For detailed information, see e.g. Klir 1991.
See also Nakamura and Mori 1999.
For an introduction, see e.g. Ebeling et al. 1998, which contains an review on further complexity measures.

[85]For an introduction see e.g. Ebeling et al. 1998, Kanitscheider 2006, Prigogine and Stengers 1993, Lyre 2002.
For critical information, see Prigogine and Stengers 1993.

[86]For detailed information, see e.g. Heylighen 2003, Mainzer and Chua 2013, Kauffman 1993.
For an introduction, see e.g. Dalenoort 1989a, b, Freund et al. 2006, Götschl 2006, Mainzer 1999, 2007b, Neuser 1998, Huett and Marr 2006, von der Malsburg 2003a, Laughlin 2005.
See also, the anthologies of Dalenoort 1989c, Krohn and Küppers 1990, Niegel and Molzberger 1992, Vec et al. 2006, Niegel 1992.
For a historical review, see e.g. Paslack 1991, Krohn et al. 1987, Skirke 1997, Heidelberger 1990.
For a beginner's guide, see e.g. Jantsch 1979/1980, Kratky 1990, Hülsmann et al. 2007, Aizawa 2006.

[87]The Second Principle of Thermodynamics states that the entropy S – in the sense of "disorder" – of a complete system can never decrease. Hence, $\Delta S \geq 0$, so that, according to the German physicist, Rudolf Clausius, the entropy of the universe always strives for a maximum. In contrast, entropy in subsystems can decrease. The tendency towards spontaneous instability of a system thus leads to a development of time, an "arrow of time" (according to the British astrophysicist Arthur S. Eddington), which corresponds to a transition to more and more probable system states.
For an introduction, see e.g. Reichl 2009, Moore 1998, Prigogine 1980, Ebeling et al. 1998, Ebeling 1982.

structures and processes of a class of systems, as a whole, occur spontaneously and are maintained to create global order.[88] With regard to the analysis level of the system components, these qualitatively new "emergent"[89] structures and processes (which are relatively autonomous, spontaneous and stable), cannot be derived or predicted in principle (Heylighen 2003, Ebeling et al. 1998, Schmidt 2008). These spontaneous structure-forming processes result from a dynamic system reaching a higher-order system state via "an export of entropy", so that "entropy production is kept to a minimum" (Reichl 2009, Ebeling et al. 1998, Schrödinger 1944/2012). According to the German philosopher of science Klaus Mainzer (1999, 2007a, 1993, 2005), one has to distinguish between the "conservative self-organization" in thermal equilibrium from the "dissipative self-organization".[90] An open non-equilibrium system (i.e. a system far from thermal equilibrium) is characterized by the fact that its phase transitions and the stability of its structures are determined by a critical balance of non-linear and dissipative mechanisms. This means that new, emergent structures at the macroscopic analysis level are formed by a multitude of complex nonlinear interactions of system elements at the microscopic analysis level. That is so if the exchange of matter, energy and information of the open, dynamic and dissipative system reaches a critical threshold with its environment (Mainzer 1999). The macroscopic dynamics of such a system is defined according to "an equation

$$\dot{z} = f(z, \alpha) + F(t), \qquad (2.12)$$

where future states depend non-linearly on the present state z and a control parameter α for mass and energy exchange. $F(t)$ stands for internal or external fluctuations of the system" (Mainzer 1999).

Based on this, one can now enumerate a necessary, if not sufficient, minimum number of key features of self-organized dynamic systems (Maurer 2017):

(1) Systemic emergence or spontaneous global system organization:

One of the most basic features, that of systemic emergence, is that a spontaneous global system organization of an (open) dynamic system is formed by the local interaction of a sufficiently high number of system elements using a coherence generating process mechanism. This may happen, for example, via a correlative synchronization mechanism (e.g. in the Binding-By-Synchrony (BBS) hypothesis (see chap. 4.4), in the laser or the convection cells in the Bénard experiment (Haken 2004, 1988a,b, Bishop 2008, 2012, Maurer 2014a)). In other words, based on simple physical neighborhood rules, initially random and statistically independent activities of the system components are gradually increased in a causally self-organized manner. Thus, with

---

[88] See e.g. Ashby 1962/2004, Glansdorff and Prigogine 1971, Nicolis and Prigogine 1977, von Foerster 1960, Kauffman 1993.

[89] See e.g. Stephan 1999, 2003, 2006, Hoyningen-Huene 2007, Kornwachs 2008, Gómez Ramírez 2014.

[90] For detailed information, see e.g. Prigogine 1980, Nicolis and Prigogine 1977; see also von Bertalanffy 1950a, Haken 1983, 2004.
For an introduction, see e.g. Jantsch 1981, Mainzer 2007a.

increasing probability, a more complex state of the overall system is established. This is associated with a qualitatively new system behavior on a higher level of analysis which, in turn, is increasingly causally imposed on the individual system components.

(2) Circular-causal, autocatalytic and cross-catalytic system dynamics:

These fluent, processual self-organization mechanisms (also referred to as "process structure") which produce the coherent overall activity of the individual system components, consist of causal, circularly structured, and nested associations of positive or negative feedback loops (Maurer 2006/2009, 2014a, Jantsch 1979/1980, Wolstenholme 1990, Schmidt 2008). Circular-causal autocatalytic or crosscatalytic system dynamics may develop, as in the case of the oscillating chemical reaction systems in the "Belousov-Zhabotinsky reaction" (Prigogine 1980, Nicolis and Prigogine 1977, Maurer 2014a), and in the self-instructive and self-replicative biosynthesis (reaction) cycles (the "hypercycles" in the framework of self-preservation of biological information in biomolecular systems [Eigen 1971, Eigen and Schuster 1977, 1979]).

In general, a self-organization process begins with a self-organizing mechanism with positive, self-reinforcing feedback. This usually leads to a stable system configuration (in terms of a dynamic equilibrium), and proceeds with excessive growth acceleration. Thereafter, such a process with a negative, self-damping feedback returns a disproportionately negatively deviated system behavior to a more stable system configuration as part of an error correction, where, in a circular-causal analysis, a time delay parameter between the circularly arranged causes and effects relationships is observed.

(3) Far-from-equilibrium dynamics or steady state (system) dynamics:

In contrast to the conservative self-organization mechanisms near thermal equilibrium in mostly physical-anorganic (closed) systems (e.g. the dipole orientation of a ferromagnet ("Ising model") or crystallization), the process-circular self-organization mechanisms of (open) dynamic systems produces a system dynamic far-from-equilibrium (also called steady-state (system) dynamic).[91] This dynamic is characterized by the fact that flow patterns are formed within the framework of (positive and negative) feedback loops by continuously replacing system components in exchange with the system environment. Therefore, a continuously maintained flow equilibrium is achieved if the exchange of matter, energy and information of the system with the environment is ensured. In other words, while classical thermodynamics considers a system isolated from the environment whose thermodynamic entropy (according to the Second Principle of Thermodynamics) can only increase until it has been transferred to its equilibrium state due to irreversible processes in time, the Russian-Belgian physicochemist Ilya Prigogine has modeled a non-linear non-equilibrium thermodynamics. An open dynamic system continuously imports

---

[91] See e.g. Prigogine 1980, Nicolis and Prigogine 1977; see also, von Bertalanffy 1950a, Haken 1983, 2004, Schrödinger 1944/2012.
For an introduction, see Mainzer 1999, 1994, 1993, 2005, Jantsch 1981, Huett 2006, Huett and Marr 2006.

free energy with low entropy from the environment in such a way that the internal generation of entropy and the export of entropy to the environment are balanced. In this way, the system is able to maintain its internal system structure under the conditions of "far from equilibrium", i.e. "the system is constantly renewing itself" (Jantsch 1979/1980). This was the first time that spontaneous self-organization processes could be explained in oscillating chemical (reaction) systems, such as the "Belousov-Zhabotinsky reaction". As long as a constant flow of energy through the system takes place, the decrease in entropy is more than compensated for by "dissipative self-organization" as a result of the release of energy with high entropy to the environment. For this reason, the space-time internal structures in these systems are called "dissipative structures".[92]

(4) Relatively autonomous and adaptive system regulation or system control:

On the one hand, constant transport and transformation flow of circulating matter, energy and information through the system enable it to develop a much higher degree of variable and adaptive system behavior. This allows the system to effectively compensate for the perturbations occurring in the system environment. On the other hand, the increasing dependence on external sources of matter, energy and information makes such a system more fragile and sensitive to fundamental changes in the environment (for a similar line of thought, see Heylighen 2003). Therefore, a dynamic system tends to achieve the highest possible degree of operational coherence with its circular process mechanisms so that a global system process can be established. This enables the system to continuously and recursively self-reproduce and self-reconstruct its physical system components ("autopoiesis") (Varela et al. 1974, Varela 1975, 1979, Kampis 1991). In these organizationally closed, autocatalytic or cross-catalytic cycles of bio- and neurochemical processes, the production of each molecule, participating in the respective cycle, is catalyzed by another molecule or molecule compound in the cycle or by an adjacent coupled cycle. These cycles form the basis for a hierarchical system organization with relatively autonomous subsystems in more complex systems, up to a processual global system configuration with a definite system boundary compared to an external system environment (for a complarable line of thought, see Heylighen and Joslyn 2001). The system hierarchy must correspond to an optimal synthesis of the highest possible degree of functional specialization of the individual subsystems and a high degree of functional integration of these subsystems within a system (Tononi et al. 1994, Tononi et al. 1998, Edelman and Tononi 2000).

In addition, a concept of an increased degree of adaptive and basal autonomy in complex dynamic systems as a whole is only guaranteed if a cyclical and recursive metabolic system organization can be maintained. On the one hand, this system organization essentially preserves the global system structure with its operational closure by means of self-constructive process mechanisms. On the other hand, due to the thermodynamic openness of the dynamic system, it generates an efficient system behavior repertoire by the functional implementation of free system energy in an

---

[92]For an introduction, see e.g. Maurer 2014a, Banzhaf 2009.
On the consequences of information processing in neural systems, e.g. von Seelen and Behrend 2016.

optimal, self-referential manner (Kauffman 2000: "Work-Constraint (W-C) Cycle"; Ruiz-Mirazo and Moreno 2004, Ruiz-Mirazo et al. 2004, Barandiaran and Moreno 2006).

(5) Distributed system regulation and robust, stable system functions:

As already indicated, the control and regulation function of the redundant and distributed system organization is distributed decentrally over the dynamic system as a whole. This means that the system elements and the subsystems based on them function relatively autonomously on the basis of the (nested) feedback effects. This is best illustrated in the case of the human brain and its artificial model architectures. Here, the control mechanisms of neuronal organization and dynamics are arranged over a large number of networks with interacting neuronal assemblies; the control mechanisms' neural information is stored in a distributed manner ("Parallel Distributed Processing (PDP)").[93] This means that – in analogy to the functioning of an optical hologram – even in the event of a considerable failure of neurons, it is possible to deal with "noisy," incomplete, inaccurate, contradictory and otherwise disturbed or faulty data ("resistance to noise"), or to compensate for this failure by means of a steady decrease of performance. This implies that through gradual compensation, the model delivers useful, albeit more blurred results ("graceful degradation") (McClelland et al. 1986, Maurer 2014a). In other words, the system has sufficient stability (in the sense of an [only] gradual decrease in global system performance) because it has adequate and appropriate correction mechanisms that can produce and maintain robust and resilient system structures and system functions against (random) perturbations.

(6) Non-linear system functionality and probabilistic system prediction:

As already mentioned, open and dynamic non-equilibrium systems operate with non-linear functions, e.g. with polynomial, exponential or logistical functions. An example of this is the activation functions of technical neurons in cognitive neuroarchitectures (chap. 2.2.4). These non-linear functions mean that relatively small fluctuations can be amplified disproportionately (see above (2)), particularly in the context of (positive) feedback effects (Heylighen 2003). Thus, small differences in the micro-states of the system, i.e. in the initial values of the system variables, can lead to fundamentally different (qualitative) macro-states of the system. In other words, the system is highly sensitive to the initial and boundary conditions (Prigogine and Stengers 1993, Maurer 2014a). A dynamic (chaotic) system is therefore characterized by the unpredictability of the system behavior due to this sensitive dependence on initial conditions, or more precisely, due to the inaccurate knowledge of the initial conditions and the development of the boundary conditions during the ongoing non-linear computation process (Leven et al. 1994). In addition to these limitations, the prediction of a self-organized system is subject to further limitations, for example in neurobiologically plausible cognitive neuroarchitectures. This is given by the use of stochastic synapses, which permit the transition probability only from the previous

---

[93] See Rumelhart and McClelland 1986a, b, Clark 1989, Hinton et al. 1986 ("Distributed Representations"). For an introduction, see Maurer 2014a.

to the next system state (Maass and Zador 1998, 1999, El-Laithy and Bogdan 2009). Thus, although the system development can be traced retrospectively in the context of a deterministic causal analysis, only certain probability predictions can be made at the time of the decision as to which system development path will be taken.

(7) System convergence and internal stable system element configuration:

Using mathematical terminology, this can also be considered under the problem of the stability of a nonlinear self-organized system. Since the nonlinear differential equation systems usually have several solutions, the system can aim for a certain spectrum of different probable stable configurations. The preference for a certain stable internal system structure will also depend, among other things, on stochastic fluctuations. In other words, within the framework of feedback cycles an "avalanche-like" self-reinforcement of already existing system fluctuations occurs, so that a se-lection of a limited number of certain coherent behavior patterns is made, e.g. in the form of a (field) mode (Haken 2004, 1988a). Thus, over a certain range of crit-ical system instability (the so-called "bifurcation"), the entire system dynamics can only be determined on the basis of a small number of dominant system variables, the so-called "order parameters" within the framework of the "enslavement princi-ple" (Haken 2004, 1988a, 1988b). The information about a certain desired system configuration (in the form of a state vector of an n-dimensional system state space) can then be mathematically described as a convergent system process towards rela-tively invariant, stable, system states – the "attractors" with a corresponding "attrac-tor basin". Geometrically interpreted, they correspond to an area in the state space to which neighbouring trajectories are directed asymptotically from any starting point in a certain environment (in other words, a point which "attracts" these trajectories). If interpreted in terms of information theory, this corresponds to a (spontaneous) reduction of statistical information entropy[94], i.e. a reduction of the (medium) un-certainty or indetermination of the prediction of a system's state information in the form of a probability distribution function.

(8) Self-organized or self-generated structural system complexity:

Both, this statistical theory of (potential) information and the algorithmic theory of (current) information[95], attempt to capture a complex system through a minimally compact and efficient compression of (algorithmic) information in the context of a digital computer program. This compressed information can now be used to quanti-tatively define the self-organized or self-generated structural and functional complex-ity of a system (Mainzer 2007a, Morin 2008, Ladyman et al. 2013): In the first case of a statistical entropy-based information theory, this happens within the framework of "Organic Computing" (Schmeck et al. 2011, Branke et al. 2007) and other related approaches (Gershenson and Heylighen 2003, Shalizi and Shalizi 2005, Kreyssig

---

[94] See Shannon 1948, Shannon and Weaver 1949/1963.
For an introduction, see e.g. Lyre 2002, Glaser 2006, Jaynes 2010, Kampis 1991, Maurer 2014a.

[95] See Kolmogorov 1968a, b, Chaitin 1975, Solomonoff 1964a, b.
For an introduction, see Lyre 2002, Maurer 2014a.

and Dittrich 2011), or in the second case within the framework of the "Functional Clustering Model" (Tononi et al. 1994, Tononi et al. 1998, Maurer 2014a) and the "Information Integration Theory (IIT) (of Consciousness)" (Tononi and Sporns 2003, Tononi 2004a, Maurer 2014a).

2.3.2 THEORY OF DETERMINISTIC CHAOS

Self-organization theory is also closely associated with the "Deterministic Chaos Theory"[96] and the associated "Bifurcation Theory"[97], which are characterized by the unpredictability of system behavior due to the sensitive dependence on initial conditions.[98]

This fundamental problem of the predictability of a chaotic process dynamics due to inaccurate knowledge of the initial conditions can be illustrated in the theoretical model using different versions of "strange" or "chaotic attractors"[99]. The best-known models are the "Lorenz attractor", the "Hénon attractor" and the "Rössler attractor". Finally, even biogenetic and social evolution can be regarded as a sequence of cyclical self-organization processes, dominated, for example, by the principle of "Self-Organized Criticality (SOC)" (according to P. Bak[100]) (Ebeling et al. 1998).

---

[96]For detailed information, see e.g. Berger 2001, Leven et al. 1994, Strogatz 2018, Ott 2002, Peitgen et al. 1994, Jetschke 1989, Teschl 2011.
For an introduction, see e.g. Robinson 2004, Argyris et al. 1995, Metzler 1998, Thompson and Stewart 1986.
See also, Kanitscheider 2006, Schiepek and Strunk 1994, Strunk and Schiepek 2006, Kolen 2001, Wildgen and Plath 2005, Prigogine and Stengers 1993.
For a beginner's guide, see e.g. Gleick 1987, Briggs and Peat 1990.
For a historical review, see e.g. Paslack 1991, Morfill and Scheingraber 1991.

[97]For an introduction, see e.g. Perko 2009, Guckenheimer and Holmes 1990, Arrowsmith and Place 1990, Jetschke 1989, Khalil 2002, Teschl 2011, Argyris et al. 1994, Robinson 2009.
See also, Ermentrout and Terman 2010, Kolen 2001, Jaeger 1996, Strunk and Schiepek 2006, Wildgen and Plath 2005.
A "bifurcation" represents a branching in the sense of a "two-way forking" in the system state space during a critical system state, which entails a qualitative change in the system state and thus affects the development of the nonlinear system over time.

[98]For a detailed discussion, see e.g. Peitgen et al. 1994, Ott 2002.
For an introduction, see e.g. Prigogine and Stengers 1993.
For the mathematical definition of the basic features of a chaotic system see e.g. Robinson 2009, 2004.

[99]For detailed information, see e.g. Schuster and Just 2005, Peitgen et al. 1994.
For an introduction, see e.g. Robinson 2004, Metzler 1998, Brin and Stuck 2002, Jetschke 1989, Argyris et al. 1995.
See also Kolen 2001, Strunk and Schiepek 2006, Schiepek and Strunk 1994.

[100]For an essential paper, see e.g. Bak et al. 1987.
For an introduction, see e.g. Bak and Chen 1991, Kauffman 2000, Fieguth 2017.

2.4 MODELS IN THE PARADIGM OF SELF-ORGANIZATION AND IN THE THEORY OF DYNAMICAL SYSTEMS

2.4.1 MODELS IN PHILOSOPHY AND IN PHILOSOPHY OF SCIENCE

In philosophy and philosophy of science, a number of authors have taken up this paradigm of the theory of (non-linear) dynamic systems including self-organization theory.[101] The term "paradigm" is understood in the sense of the American philosopher of science and scientific historian, Thomas S. Kuhn.[102] Below is a brief list of the most important authors (Maurer 2014a). The intention is to stimulate a fundamental research program, in order to embed connectionism (by considering it as a subdiscipline within the theory of nonlinear, complex dynamic systems) into a "General (Dynamic) Systems Theory (G(D)ST)" in the sense of a (to be developed) unified science (Smith Churchland 1986, Padulo and Arbib 1974):

(1) the Austrian theoretical biologist and philosopher, Ludwig von Bertalanffy,
(2) the German philosopher Hans Lenk and the German engineer and (technical) philosopher, Günter Ropohl,
(3) the German philosopher of science, Klaus Mainzer,
(4) the Austrian philosopher of science, Johann Götschl, and
(5) the Australian philosopher and cognitive scientist Timothy van Gelder.

2.4.2 MODELS IN NATURAL, HUMAN, SOCIAL AND CULTURAL SCIENCES

In the natural, human, social and cultural sciences, a large number of authors have established and represented this paradigm of the theory of (non-linear) dynamic systems, including the theory of self-organization in the broadest sense.[103] The most important ones are briefly listed below (Maurer 2014a):

(1) the American mathematician and biophysicist, Alwyn C. Scott,
(2) the American mathematician, Steven Strogatz,
(3) the Russian-Belgian physicochemist, Ilya Prigogine, together with the Belgian engineer, Paul Glansdorff and the Greek-Belgian physicochemist, Grégoire Nicolis,

---

[101] For detailed information, see e.g. Ropohl 1979, Lenk 1975, 1978, Händle and Jensen 1974.
For general information, see e.g. Eilenberger 1990, Kratky 1990.
See also, Huett and Marr 2006, Götschl 2006.
For an review, see e.g. Paslack 1991, Krohn and Küppers 1992, Krohn et al. 1987, Skirke 1997.
For critical information, see e.g. Gloy 1998a, 1998b.
See the remarks in chap. 1.2.4.2.

[102] According to Kuhn (1962/2012), the term "paradigm" refers to the set of key statements (1) on which a theory in empirical science and its historical development are based, (2) which attracts a consistent group of supporters and (3) causes them to form groups in order to devote themselves to the still unsolved problems over a long period of time by being bound by the same rules for scientific research.

[103] For a review, see e.g. Paslack 1991, Jaeger 1996, Jantsch 1979/1980, Skirke 1997, Mainzer 2007a, 1999, 2005, Heylighen 2003.
See also, Krohn and Küppers 1990, Schiepek and Tschacher 1997.

(4) the German theoretical physicist, Hermann Haken,

(5) the English mathematician and neuroinformatician, Michael A. Arbib,

(6) the German neuroinformatician, Gregor Schöner,

(7) the Belgian cyberneticist, Francis Heylighen,

(8) the German biochemist and physicochemist, Manfred Eigen, together with the Austrian theoretical chemist, Peter Schuster,

(9) the American theoretical biologist, Stuart A. Kauffman,

(10) the Chilean neurobiologist and philosopher, Humberto R. Maturana, together with the Chilean neurobiologist, Francisco J. Varela,

(11) the Austrian zoologist, Rupert Riedl, the Austrian zoologist and evolutionary biologist, Günter P. Wagner and the Austrian biologist and philosopher of science, Franz M. Wuketits,

(12) the Swiss developmental psychologist, Jean Piaget,

(13) the German psychologist, Günter Schiepek, the German psychologist and economist, Guido Strunk as well as the German psychologist and psychotherapist, Wolfgang Tschacher,

(14) the German sociologist, Niklas Luhmann.

3 Theoretical Paradigms in Cognitive Science and in Theoretical Neurophilosophy

This chapter provides an introduction to classical symbolic theory (chap. 3.1), including the symbolic information processing method (chap. 3.1.1), the local symbol representation (chap. 3.1.2), the symbolic production systems (chap. 3.1.3), and the standard argument for symbolism (chap. 3.1.4). This is followed by an introduction to the cognitive theory of connectionism (chap. 3.2) as it has developed since the 1980s. The respective basic concepts, statements and subject area will be presented in detail, including the associated connectionistic information processing method (chap. 3.2.1), the representational typology (chap. 3.2.2), the potential landscape-metaphor (chap. 3.2.3), the basic models in connectionism (chap. 3.2.4), the methodical principles (chap. 3.2.5), and the relation between connectionism and dynamical system theory (chap. 3.2.6). Furthermore, the positive motivation and the criticism of symbol theory and connectionism are also discussed (chap. 3.1.4, 3.1.5, 3.2.7 and 3.2.8).

3.1 CLASSICAL SYMBOL THEORY

The main features of the classical Symbol Theory will be presented in this section:

3.1.1 SYMBOLIC METHOD: SYMBOLIC INFORMATION PROCESSING ON THE BASIS OF SYMBOLS AND SYMBOL STRUCTURES

The classic symbol-processing theory[104], "symbolism," considers symbolic information processing (or symbol processing[105]) as the appropriate explanatory approach for cognition and intelligence. It consists of the formal, serial and universal manipulation or transformation of given symbols – characters of a strictly defined alphabet

---

[104]For an introduction, see e.g. Lewis 1999, Anderson and Perlis 2003, Sun 2001, Dyer 1991. See also, Korb 1996.
Classical Symbol Theory in its connection to Classical Artificial Intelligence (AI), by Haugeland (1985), also referred to as "Good Old Fashioned AI (GOFAI)," is described, for example, in Korb 1996, Dorffner 1991, and in Romba 2001.

[105]See e.g. Strube 1996c.

– into other symbols, according to a definite and finite computational method. This method consists of a set of computational rules or axioms ("algorithm" [see chap. 1.1.5.]). In other words, humans are regarded as information processing systems (Newell and Simon 1976, Simon and Newell 1964), just like computers ("Computational Theory of Mind" [see chap. 1.1.5.]). The discrete elementary symbols or the complex symbol structures can designate things in such a way that the system can influence or be influenced by given symbols or symbol structures. These symbols or symbol structures thus serve as internal mental representations of the external environment to which a "symbol system" tries to adapt (for more information on the term "symbol system", see e.g. Newell 1980).

It is now possible to create a symbol-oriented minimum model, either on the basis of "logical form"[106] (proposed by Gottlob Frege, Bertrand Russell and Ludwig Wittgenstein) using "(atomic) predication" and the "(2-ary) relation":

$$F(a) \text{ and } R(a,b) \tag{3.1}$$

or, correspondingly, on the basis of "linguistic form" (proposed by the American linguist Noam Chomsky in his "Generative (Phrase Structure) Grammar"[107]):

$$[S\,[NP]\,[VP]] \text{ and } [S\,[NP]\,[VP\,[V\ NP]]] \tag{3.2}$$

3.1.2   LOCAL SYMBOL REPRESENTATION

At every point in time, such a symbol system contains a collection of these symbol structures, which are composed of a number of instances ("tokens") of individual symbols.[108] These symbols are in a local physical relation to each other, that is, one symbolic token is next to another, so that the definition of a symbol can be defined as follows: A symbol is a uniquely identifiable and localizable unit that acts as a substitute or placeholder for a particular object of reality.[109]

3.1.3   SYMBOLIC PRODUCTION SYSTEMS

In addition to these symbol structures, a symbol system contains a number of "production rules", which is why it is also referred to as a "production (rule) system"[110]

---

[106]For fundamental information, see e.g. Frege 1879/1964, 1891/1994, 1892/1994a, 1892/1994b, Whitehead and Russell 1910-1913/1927, Russell 1918-1919/1986, Wittgenstein 1921/1990, 1929/1993. For an introduction, see e.g. Suppes 1957/1999, Quine 1940/1981, Beckermann 1997, Bucher 1998, Hoyningen-Huene 1998.

[107]For fundamental information, see Chomsky 1957.
For an introduction, see e.g. Bermúdez 2014, Dürscheid 2005, Pelz 2002, Sobel 2001.

[108]Simon and Newell (1964) also speak of "symbol occurrences".

[109]See e.g. Newell and Simon 1976.
For a definition of a symbol, see Romba 2001. Van Gelder (1999b) speaks here of "strictly local".
See chap. 3.2.2.

[110]For an introduction, see e.g. Simon 1999, Schunn and Klahr 1998, Opwis and Lüer 1996.
G. Jones and F.E. Ritter (2003) provides the following (minimal) definition: "Production systems are computer programs that reason using production rules".

(see Fig. 3.1 and Fig. 3.2). In the theory of formal languages a "production rule", also called "production," is a (transforming) rule that determines how to create a combination of new constructs from an already known construct, e.g. a word, by replacing the rule on the left-hand side with the rule on the right-hand side (Fig. 3.1). These productions are, in principle, rules of the form: If the conditions $A_1, ..., A_n$ ("premises") are fulfilled, execute action B ("conclusion") ("material implication").

Accordingly, the interpretation of the symbol structures means that, if a symbol structure is specified, the symbol system is able to execute the relevant syntactic production and transformation processes that can create, convert or remove symbols. The symbol structures can be changed by internal states of the system (that is, by other symbol structures), or by external states, (that is, by the states of real objects) or they can themselves change internal or external states.

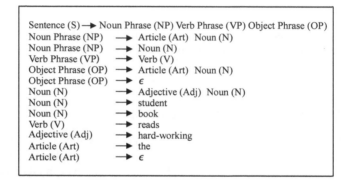

Figure 3.1: Production system with simple production rules for the example sentence 'The hard-working student reads the book.' (following Schöning 2008).

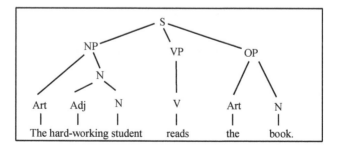

Figure 3.2: Schematic diagram of a syntax tree with a constituent structure for the example sentence 'The hard-working student reads the book.' (following Schöning 2008).

An example of a production system is the "SOAR Production System" by A. Newell (Newell 1990) or the "Adaptive Control of Thought-Rational" (ACT-R 7.0) by J.R. Anderson (Anderson 1983, 1993, 1998, 2002, 2007, Anderson and Lebiere 1998, Anderson et al. 2004, Borst and Anderson 2015; see also Lebiere and Anderson 1993 with a connectionist variant).
For an introduction, see e.g. Solso 2005.

Thus, the definition of a "physical symbol system" is as follows: "A physical symbol system is a machine that produces through time, an evolving collection of symbol structures" (Newell and Simon 1976). The theory of symbol processing, based on the American cognitive psychologists and computer scientists, Allen Newell and Herbert A. Simon, is grounded on the well-founded assumption that every intelligent action and behavior manifests itself in a physical system of symbols. Thus, symbol processing systems are always physical symbol systems. This means that the entire symbol system clearly and exclusively obeys the laws of physics ("Physical Symbol System Hypothesis (PSSH)"[111]): The symbolic information processing system is thus purely physical, and is defined as a system that possesses the necessary and sufficient conditions for intelligent behaviour and action. In other words, "[it (author's note)] specifies a general class of systems within which one will find those capable of intelligent action" (Newell and Simon 1976). Every physical symbol system is therefore an intelligent system; the symbol system hypothesis hence implies "that intelligence will be realized by a universal computer" (Newell and Simon 1976).

3.1.4   POSITIVE MOTIVATION FOR SYMBOLISM: STANDARD ARGUMENT BY J.A. FODOR AND Z.W. PYLYSHYN

According to the American philosopher Jerry A. Fodor and the Canadian philosopher Zenon W. Pylyshyn (1988), the classical symbol oriented model is characterized by (1) a "combinatorial syntax and semantics for mental representations"[112] and (2) mental operations ("structure sensitivity of processes").[113,114] The general structure of the argumentation of these philosophers can be explained as follows.[115] Based on

---

[111] See Newell and Simon 1976: "The Physical Symbol System Hypothesis. A physical symbol system has the necessary and sufficient means for general intelligent action."
See also e.g. Newell 1980. See also Anderson and Perlis 2003.
For an introduction, see e.g. Besold and Kühnberger 2013a, Bermúdez 2014, Urchs 2002.
According to Strube 1996a, Newell and Simon discuss the conditions of the possibility of (artificial) intelligence in the sense of cognition.

[112] According to Fodor and Pylyshyn (1988), one has to postulate a combinatorial syntax and semantics of mental representations and define them as follows, since otherwise certain properties of propositional attitudes would not be explainable:
(1.1) "(...) there is a distinction between structurally atomic and structurally molecular representations";
(1.2) "(...) structurally molecular representations have syntactic constituents that are themselves either structurally molecular or structurally atomic";
The authors describe the first two conditions as the demand for a (syntactic) constituent structure of mental representations.
(1.3) "(...) the semantic content of a (molecular) representation is a function of the semantic contents of its syntactic parts, together with its constituent structure."
The third condition is often referred to as the demand for a compositional semantics.

[113] See Fodor and Pylyshyn 1988.
The classical concept of a structure-sensitive process in cognitive science is the conclusion, the "logical inference."

[114] See Fodor and Pylyshyn (1988) who consider (1) and (2) as the requirements that a classical cognitive model defines, i.e. they constrain the physical realizations of symbol structures in the sense of a physical symbol system according to Newell.

[115] See Goschke and Koppelberg (1990) who provide a very good summary which is essentially followed in this section.

the fundamental principle of the "(syntactic and semantic) constituent structure of mental representations"[116], it is possible to explain the following closely connected basic characteristics of human cognition: productivity, systematicity, compositionality and inferential systematicity. These four central concepts whose formulation has already been produced by the American linguist Noam Chomsky[117] as part of his "Generative (Phrase Structure) Grammar" (see chap. 3.1.1.) are now explained in more detail (Fodor and Pylyshyn 1988).

3.1.4.1 Productivity of Mental Representations

According to Fodor and Pylyshyn (1988), the productivity argument is based on human language competence: mental and linguistic representations are productive, which means that a competent speaker of a natural language can potentially create an unlimited number of different expressions and phrases from a limited number of simple language units. Furthermore, the speaker can also produce and understand an unlimited number of different thoughts, so-called "propositions." [118],[119] However, this is only possible if the speaker has an internal syntactic constituent structure that enables them to competently generate complex mental representations (that is, the symbol structures).

3.1.4.2 Systematicity of Mental Representations

According to Fodor and Pylyshyn (1988), the systematicity argument is also supported by human language production and human understanding of language: The mental and linguistic representations are systematic, i.e. "the ability to produce/understand some of the sentences is intrinsically connected to the ability to produce/understand certain of the others" (Fodor and Pylyshyn 1988). This means that if, for example, a competent speaker understands the sentence 'John loves Mary', he or she will necessarily understand the content-related sentence 'Mary loves John'. Therefore, one has to postulate a generative mechanism that enables the speaker to recognize the same syntactic constituent structure <first individual constant ×

See also, Bechtel and Abrahamsen 1991, Petitot 1994, von Eckardt 1993.

[116]In linguistics, a "constituent" means those parts of a sentence into which a syntactic (de-)construction can be meaningfully decomposed. These are the components which, in their entirety, can be replaced among each other (substitution test), converted (permutation test), omitted (deletion test) and combined (coordination test). Thus, for example, a sentence cannot directly be decomposed into words, but first into groups of words, into the "phrases," which thus represent the constituents.
In symbolic logic, the term "constituent" refers to those syntactical units of a (first-order) predicate logic that are permissible as term or as formula in the context of a calculus based on the alphabet of a language. See e.g. Fromkin 2001, O'Grady 1997, Grewendorf et al. 1993, Meibauer 2002, Vater 2002. See also e.g. Quine 1940/1981, 1970, Sommers 1989, Stegmüller and Varga von Kibéd 1984, Beckermann 2008.

[117]See e.g. Fodor and Pylyshyn 1988, with reference to Chomsky 1965, 1968.

[118]With regard to the terms "proposition" and "propositional attitude", read chap. 3.1.4.5 for further information.

[119]See Fodor and Pylyshyn (1988), who assume that one can only think of a thought that can be expressed through an internal mental representation.

relator × second individual constant> in the two example sentences. That is, the speaker could generate the complex symbol structure *aRb* or *bRa* in terms of formal predicate logic by means of a structure-sensitive substitution operation of the constituents *a* and *b*.[120]

3.1.4.3 Semantic Compositionality of Mental Representations

According to Fodor and Pylyshyn[121], the argument of semantic compositionality concerns semantic systematicity: under the assumption of the syntactic constituent structure of a sentence[122], the meaning of a complex mental representation can be "computed" as a function of the semantic content of its lexical elements and the syntactic structure of its constituents, on the basis of the relevant operations. In this case, the syntax "mirrors" the semantics (Fodor and Pylyshyn 1988). This means that "there is an isomorphism between the causal relations that hold between symbols in virtue of their formal or syntactic properties and the semantic or inferential relations between the contents expressed by the symbols."[123] In other words, correspondence in relation to the constituent structure guarantees an adequate semantic interpretation in terms of "semantic coherence," only if the contribution to the overall meaning of an expression is computed compositionally, i.e., structure-dependently. For this reason (and due to its semantic structure), a complex mental representation stands in a systematic relation to other mental representations.

However, the assumption of a syntactic constituent structure only explains the semantic systematicity if the meanings of the constituents of a complex symbol structure are context-independent ("principle of compositionality").[124] For, "if the meaning of constituents were to vary, depending on the context of the larger expression in which they are embedded, this would make it hard to understand how semantic compositionality is possible" (Goschke and Koppelberg 1990).

---

[120]In the text we follow the notation of Fodor and Pylyshyn (1988). According to usual notational convention in logic, $R(a,B)$ or $R(b,a)$ would have to be written.

[121]See Fodor and Pylyshyn 1988, Fodor 1987.
For an introduction, see e.g. Pagin and Westersthl 2008, 2010.

[122]According to Fodor and Pylyshyn (1988), the principle of (semantic) compositionality presupposes a (syntactic) constituent structure of sentences.

[123]See Goschke and Koppelberg 1990 with reference to Fodor and Pylyshyn 1988.
See also Pylyshyn 1984, 1980.

[124]According to Fodor and Pylyshyn (1988), a lexical element must make approximately the same semantic contribution in every context in which it is embedded, i.e. one needs semantically individuated and stable atomic mental representations.
According to Linke et al. (2001), the principle of compositionality is also called the "Frege's Principle".
On the principle of compositionality see e.g. Frege 1892/1994a, 1923-1926, reprinted in Frege 1923/1976.

3.1.4.4 Systematicity of Inference and Inferential Homogeneity

According to Fodor and Pylyshyn[125], the argument of "systematicity of inference" states that the correspondence of logical and psychological laws can be explained only by the assumption of a logical syntax demanded by classical symbolic theory. For only if the "logically homogeneous class of inferences is carried out by a correspondingly homogeneous class of psychological mechanisms" will it become possible to explain why the cognitive capacity to draw certain logical conclusions does not show gaps so that someone who can draw the conclusion from $P \wedge Q \wedge R$ to P could not draw the conclusion from $P \wedge Q$ to P (Fodor and Pylyshyn 1988). Since the authors assume this inferential homogeneity, however, the logical law that it is possible to infer from a conjunction on the respective conjunction components corresponds to the psychological law that the mental representation $P \wedge Q$ consists of the constituents P, Q and the logical particle $\wedge$. This explains the systematicity of the logical conclusion.

In conclusion, the authors state that if one assumes a theory of structured representation, one is forced to accept representations with a similar or identical structure. In the linguistic case, this structure is the syntactic form and, in the inferential case, it is the logical form. In addition, assuming structure-sensitive mental processes, this theory will predict that similarly structured representations, in general, will play similar roles in thinking (Fodor and Pylyshyn 1988).

3.1.4.5 Representational Theory of Mind and Language of Thought by J.A. Fodor

These theses of the Symbolic Paradigm thus lead to the core thesis of the linguistic structure of mental representations. According to Fodor, the competence to use an "external" language in a productive and systematic way is explained by the fact that humans have an "internal Language of Thought (LOT)"[126] with recursive and combinatorial syntax and semantics on the basis of internal mental representations[127] (so-called "Representational Theory of Mind (RT(h)M)") [128]:

"(...) RTM is the conjunction of the following two claims:
Claim 1 (the nature of propositional attitudes):

---

[125] See Fodor and Pylyshyn 1988.
The term "coherence of inference" is also used. See e.g. Bechtel and Abrahamsen 1991, Petitot 1994.

[126] See Fodor 1976, 2008.
For an introduction to the LOT hypothesis, see e.g. Bermúdez 2014, Rey 2003.
See also e.g. Sterelny 1990, Kurthen 1992.

[127] The minimal definition of the term "mental representation" contains a 3-ary representational relation $R_{mentRep}(Syst, St_{Real}, St_{Syst})$ between (1) an individual information-processing system $(Syst)$, (2) something that is represented by the system in terms of an aspect of the present state of reality (St_{Real}), and (3) something which is represented in terms of a functionally-individuated, internal state of the system (St_{Syst}).

[128] For a detailed discussion, see e.g. Fodor 1976, 1981a, 1981b, 1983, 1987.
See also e.g. Sterelny 1990, Kemmerling 1991.

For any organism O, and any attitude A toward the proposition P, there is a ('computational'/'functional') relation R and a mental representation MP such that MP means that P, and O has A if O bears R to MP.

Claim 2 (the nature of mental processes):

Mental processes are causal sequences of tokenings of mental representations."

Thus, thinking and reasoning are based on the manipulation of syntactically structured symbols in the language of thought. Due to the clear interpretation of the symbols and symbol structures, these symbol transformations (and hence, all tasks to be performed by the symbol system) can be exhaustively described at any time ("symbolic [semantic] transparency" [Clark 1989]). These features are therefore understood as decisive advantages of the symbol-oriented cognitive theory.

According to Fodor (1987), a person has a certain "propositional attitude" (e.g. a belief) if (1) the person has formed an internal mental representation in the form of a "proposition"[129] with certain content, and (2) the person stands in a certain intentional relation to this representation. That is, this representation has a certain functional position in the formal computation or deduction process of the language of thought.

3.1.5 CRITICISM OF SYMBOLISM

Within the context of the "symbolism vs. connectionism debate", the connectionists frequently and strongly criticised symbolism and the models of classical artificial intelligence.[130] For this reason, the most important arguments are only briefly mentioned here:

1. the limitation to explicit, logical or linguistically formalized symbol processing tasks on the basis of propositional representations and the simultaneous neglect of cognitive (classification) problems in the sensor system,
2. the susceptibility of the functionality of rigid symbol processing programs in the case of error-prone program code,
3. the lack of context sensitivity and the resulting so-called "frame problem"[131] in the classification of new available data,
4. the lack of generalization performance in symbol-oriented learning methods and
5. the self-restriction to symbol processing within a single system.

---

[129]Following Frege 1918/1919, reprinted in Frege 1923/1976, a "proposition" in logic and linguistics means the thought or the mental content contained in a statement. In other words, a proposition means what a declarative sentence expresses, i.e. its "sense". In other words, a proposition is the smallest linguistic unit that can form an autonomous statement, i.e. a truth-apt statement, independent of other linguistic units.

[130]For detailed information, see Maurer 2006/2009.
For an overview, see e.g. Eliasmith and Bechtel 2003, Strube 1996a, Horgan and Tienson 1994a, Kurthen 1992.

[131]For an introduction, see e.g. Shanahan 2003.

3.2 THEORY OF CONNECTIONISM

In competition with classical symbolic theory, the main idea behind the connectionist cognition model is that functions, principles and structures are transferred from cognitive neurobiology, medical neurophysiology and cognitive neuropsychology, to the technical information processing systems in neuroinformatics.[132] This means the mathematical, model-theoretical abstraction of the connectionist theory (briefly described in the following subsections), is primarily based on the structure and functioning of the human brain ("brain style modeling" [Strube 1996a]). In comparison to the human brain, however, this is a greatly simplified replication or model construction (Zell 2003).

3.2.1 CONNECTIONISTIC METHOD: CONNECTIONISTIC INFORMATION PROCESSING ON THE BASIS OF VECTORS AND VECTOR STRUCTURES

"Connectionism"[133], the connectionist information processing theory[134], is generally understood as the application of parallel information processing to the topic of (neuro-)cognition, within the theory of artificial neuronal networks. As a result, this approach is also referred to as "Parallel Distributed Processing (PDP)"[135], with ref-

---

[132]The discipline of "neuroinformatics" is an interdisciplinary branch of computer science that is concerned with the internal information processing in neuronal systems, especially in the human brain, in order to convert them into mathematical models, e.g. cognitive neuroarchitectures, and to apply them in technical systems, e.g. in robots.
For an introduction, see e.g. Haykin 1999, Zell 2003, Rojas 1996, Mallot 2013.

[133]For fundamental information, see Rumelhart and McClelland 1986a, b, Smolensky 1988a.
For detailed information, see e.g. Smith Churchland 1986, Churchland 1989, 1995, Bechtel and Abrahamsen 1991, 2002, Clark 1989, 1993, Horgan and Tienson 1996, 1991a, MacDonald and MacDonald 1995, Gärdenfors 2000, Marcus 2001.
For an introduction, see e.g. Kiefer 2019, McLaughlin 1998, Bechtel 1994, Flusberg and McClelland 2017, Feldman and Shastri 2003, McClelland 1999, Ramsey 1999, Sun 2001, Buckner and Garson 2019, Hanson 1999, Kemke 1988, Strube 1990.
For a historical overview, see e.g. Berkeley 2019.
See also, Kralemann 2006, Pospeschill 2004, Dorffner 1991, Helm 1991, Romba 2001, Weldle 2011, Wang and Liu 2005.
See also the remarks in chap. 6.1.5.
The term "connectionism" is derived from the English word "to connect" and, according to Marx (1994), goes back to the American psychologist Edward L. Thorndike.

[134]According to Hatfield (1991), " connectionism is not a theory (...), but a group of theories and approaches that share an interest in computational systems that can be characterized by 'connectionist' primitive operations".

[135]As to the epistemic status of the connectionist theory, which had been discussed mainly in the context of "symbolism vs. connectionism debate", the view of an "eliminative connectionism" is generally held, together with the opinion of P.M. Churchland and P. Smith Churchland. This approach is opposed to J.A. Feldman's and D.H. Ballard's "structured connectionism", D.S. Touretzky's "implementational connectionism", R. Sun's "hybrid connectionism" and P. Smolensky's "integrative connectionism". This also raises the question of which claim for an explanation does the connectionist theory have in comparison with classical symbol-processing theory with regard to the appropriateness of the respective modelling of cognitive processes and structures. Furthermore, it also concerns the question as to which of D. Marr's three different levels of explanation is to be assigned to a particular connectionist view or a cognitive neuroarchitecture.
For fundamental information, see e.g. Smith Churchland 1986, McCloskey 1991, Feldman and Ballard 1982, Feldman 1982, Touretzky 1991, Sun 1995, Smolensky 1995.

erence to the standard work of the connectionist paradigm written by the American psychologists David E. Rumelhart and James L. McClelland, "Parallel Distributed Processing: Explorations in the Microstructure of Cognition" (1986).

An "Artificial Neural Network (ANN)"[136] can be regarded as a directed and weighted mathematical graph[137]. It consists of a large number of single, rather simple processing units, the "nodes", which represent (technical) neurons. These processing units are usually connected in series in several "layers", consisting of the so-called "input units", the "hidden units" and the "output units". An ANN is characterized by parallel and distributed information processing between these processing units which are wired to one another through weighted connections representing (technical) synapses (the "edges") (Zell 2003).

This neuronal information processing is thus based on the functioning of biological neurons and synapses and the neurophysiological processes in the (neo-)cortex (Squire et al. 2008, Bear et al. 2016, Kandel et al. 2013). The model simulates the neurobiological information in the brain that the "membrane potential" of a biological neuron generates along its axon – an "action potential"[138] – from the state of the "resting potential." This means that a neuron generates a neuroelectric impulse (the postsynaptic neuron "fires"). This requires that the temporal and spatial summation of the action potentials of the presynaptic neurons, which are transmitted along their presynaptic axons to the dendrites of the postsynaptic neurons via the neurochemical synapses, exceed a certain "threshold potential". On the basis of the synaptic intensity of neurotransmitter transmissions in the synapse gap, a weighting ("synaptic plasticity" (Bear et al. 2016, Rösler 2011)) of the incoming excitatory or inhibitory impulses ("synaptic integration" [Squire et al. 2008, Kandel et al. 2013]) takes place (see Fig. 3.3).

In the connectionistic model of neuronal information processing, a postsynaptic neuron computes its own actual state of activation $a_j(t+1)$. This consists of a numerical activation value determined by means of a normally nonlinear, sigmoid "activation function" f_{act} (Rey and Wender 2011, Zell 2003, Trappenberg 2010) (see Fig. 3.4):

$$a_j(t+1) = f_{act}[a_j(t), net_j(t), \theta_j].$$ \hfill (3.3)

For detailed information, see e.g. Marcus 1998.

For an introduction, see e.g. Bermúdez 2014, Pospeschill 2004, Hilario 1997, Lange 1992, Wermter and Sun 2000, Sun 1997.

See also Weldle 2011.

See also the remarks in chap. 1.1.3, 2.2.9, 5.1.5, 6.1.5.1.

[136]For an introduction, see e.g. Haykin 1999, 2012, Zell 2003, Rojas 1996, Mallot 2013, Graupe 2008, Müller et al. 1995, Rey and Wender 2011, Anastasio 2010, Davalo and Naït 1991, Grauel 1992, Mallot et al. 2000, Knieling 2007, Köhle 1990, Haun 1998.

See also Bothe 1998, Kasabov 1998, Smith Churchland and Sejnowski 1992.

For the mathematical aspects of artificial neural networks, see e.g. Hammer and Villmann 2003.

For the different types of neurons and network architectures in artificial neural networks, see e.g. Zell 2003, Haykin 1999, Graupe 2008, Rojas 1996.

For the different mathematical models of biological neurons, see e.g. Köhle 1990, Bothe 1998.

[137]For the term "(directed) mathematical graph", see e.g. Balakrishnan and Ranganathan 2012, Krumke 2009.

[138]For the term "action potential", see e.g. Squire et al. 2008, Bear et al. 2016, Kandel et al. 2013.

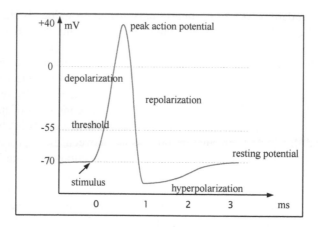

Figure 3.3: Schematic diagram of an action potential (similar to Rösler 2011).

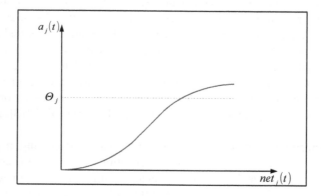

Figure 3.4: Schematic representation of a logistic activation function (similar to Rösler 2011). See formula 3.3.

As a rule, an S-shaped and non-linear sigmoid activation function (or transfer function) which best simulates the activation mode of biological neurons, is used. Some examples are the "logistic activation function"

$$f_{\log}(x) = \frac{1}{1+e^{-x}} \tag{3.4}$$

or the activation function of the "hyperbolic tangent"

$$f_{\tanh}(x) = \tanh(x) = \frac{e^x - e^{-x}}{e^x + e^{-x}}. \tag{3.5}$$

The activation function consists of the previous state of activation $a_j(t)$, the "network input" $net_j(t)$ and the "threshold" ("bias") θ_j (see formula 3.3).

The network input is computed using the "propagation function". This is the sum of the products of the respective connection weights w_{ij}[139] toward the presynaptic neurons N_{i_1} and N_{i_2}, with their outputs $o_i(t)$ or $a_i(t)$[140] (see formula 3.3):

$$net_j(t) = \sum_i o_i(t)w_{ij} \text{ or } net_j(t) = \sum_i a_i(t)w_{ij}.\text{[141]} \qquad (3.7)$$

If the previous state of activation of the postsynaptic neuron, together with its network input, exceeds the threshold, the postsynaptic neuron N_j becomes active (this is the "sigma neuron model") (Rey and Wender 2011, Zell 2003, Hanson 1999) (see Figs. 3.5 and 3.6).

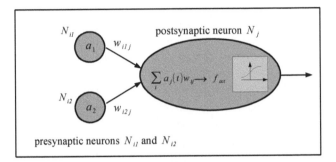

Figure 3.5: Schematic diagram of the mathematical model of information transfer between technical neurons with an activation function, f_{act}, which represents the basis for constructing artificial neural networks (modified accordingly to Haykin 1999, Houghton 2005, and Bothe 1998).

In the "weight matrix" or "connectivity matrix"[143] W, all connection weights of a network are combined. The high connectivity of the neurons is achieved by a large number of weighted connections or links. Like neuroanatomic synapses, these connections have a weighting (or coupling) strength. These weights (modeled by a numerical value) represent either an excitatory or inhibitory influence of a presynaptic neuron on its postsynaptic neuron. Within the context of certain learning rules, it

---

[139] The weight of the connection from unit i to unit j is denoted by w_{ij}.

[140] An alternative network input based on the neurobiological concept of "presynaptic inhibition" within the "Sigma-Pi neuron model" is defined as follows:

$$net_j(t) = \sum_i w_{ij} \prod_k o_k(t). \qquad (3.6)$$

See e.g. Zell 2003, Trappenberg 2010, Köhle 1990, Bothe 1998.

[141] For the simplified case that the outputs of the presynaptic neurons $o_i(t)$ are equal to their activations $a_i(t)$.

[142] See McCulloch and Pitts 1943, 1948.
For an introduction, see e.g. Rojas 1996, Ermentrout and Terman 2010.

[143] For an introduction to the concept of the "weight matrix" or "connection matrix", see e.g. Rey and Wender 2011, Palm 1982.

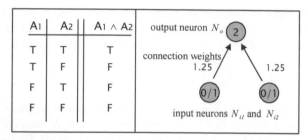

Figure 3.6: Schematic diagram showing the basic functioning of information transfer in an artificial neural network, illustrated by the following example. The logical semantics of a conjunction (represented in the left graphic segment) is transferred to a suitable vector-based connectionistic network structure (represented in the right graphic segment). The technical neurons, as defined by W.S. McCulloch and W. Pitts[142], function as a "logical gate". The output neuron fires when the weighted sum of inputs exceeds the threshold, using operations of vector addition and vector multiplication resulting in the following computations (according to Zell 2003):

$$1 \cdot 1.25 + 1 \cdot 1.25 = 1.25 + 1.25 = 2.50 > 2.00$$
$$1 \cdot 1.25 + 0 \cdot 1.25 = 1.25 + 0.00 = 1.25 < 2.00$$
$$0 \cdot 1.25 + 1 \cdot 1.25 = 0.00 + 1.25 = 1.25 < 2.00$$
$$0 \cdot 1.25 + 0 \cdot 1.25 = 0.00 + 0.00 = 0.00 < 2.00$$

The truth value 'T' corresponds to the activation value '1' of the input neurons N_{i1} and N_{i2}, and the truth value 'F' corresponds to the activation value '0'.

is now possible to learn in an artificial neural network by means of incremental[144] synapse modifications by increasing or decreasing particular connection weights.

The learning rule (also referred to as the "learning method") is an algorithm according to which an artificial neural network learns to yield the desired output for a given input (Rey and Wender 2011, Zell 2003). The "Hebb rule"[145] (named after the Canadian psychologist, Donald O. Hebb) is the basis for most more complex learning rules,[146] and is thus the fundament of the principle of neural plasticity (Smith

---

[144]The term "incremental" generally refers to a gradual increase in the number of a variable. In the case of (imperative) programming languages in computer science, the elementary increment or decrement operator is used to enable loop constructions in the program sequence.

[145]It was formulated as follows in his book "The Organization of Behavior. A Neuropsychological Theory" (1949): "When an axon of cell A is near enough to excite a cell B and repeatedly or persistently takes part in firing it, some growth process or metabolic change takes place in one or both cells such that A's efficiency, as one of the cells firing B, is increased".
For detailed discussion, see e.g. Gerstner and Kistler 2002.
For an introduction, see e.g. Rey and Wender 2011, Zell 2003.

[146]The "delta rule", also called "Widrow-Hoff rule", and the learning method of "backpropagation" are derived from the general mathematical form of Hebb's learning rule, according to Rumelhart et al. 1986b, defined by

$$\Delta w_{ij} = \eta \, h(o_i, w_{ij}) \, g(a_j t_j), \tag{3.8}$$

in which the expected activation t_j, the "teaching input," is added as a parameter.
See e.g. Rey and Wender 2011, Zell 2003, Gerstner and Kistler 2002, Kasabov 1998.

Churchland and Sejnowski 1992, Rösler 2011). The rule says: The synaptic weight is increased if the pre- and postsynaptic neurons are active in subsequent time steps, i.e. if the presynaptic neuron fires and the synapse is "successful" insofar as the postsynaptic neuron also fires:

$$\Delta w_{ij} = \eta o_i a_j, \tag{3.9}$$

where w_{ij} is the change of connection weight Δw_{ij}, η is a constant learning rate, o_i is the output of the presynaptic neuron i and a_j is the activation of the postsynaptic neuron j.

As far as the underlying information is concerned, it is now possible (in principle[147]) to divide the learning processes into two classes. On the one hand, there is the class of "supervised learning" (Haykin 1999, Zell 2003), according to which class an external instance in the learning process specifies the best output template, as well as each input template, as additional information. On the other hand, there is the class of the neurobiologically more plausible "unsupervised learning" (Rojas 1996, Müller et al. 1995, Haykin 1999, Zell 2003). In this case the learning algorithm (e.g. the Kohonen algorithm [see chap. 3.2.4.4] or the Grossberg algorithm [see chap. 3.2.4.5]) tries to determine its statistical distribution independently from the training set of randomly distributed input patterns, by means of probability density functions. For example, in the context of the problem of correct classification of data vectors, it is possible to create a category using a statistical vector-based prototype (McClelland et al. 2010).

A neural network is therefore not programmed in the traditional sense, but rather "trained". Using application examples in a special learning phase (in which prototypical pairs of input and output patterns are presented to the network), the connection weights of the network, which are initially set mostly at random, are adapted[148] to a given problem in the form of data vectors.

In summary, the basic computation in connectionism is carried out by the activation propagation in the neurons, depending on the permanently changing connection weights in the synapses of the artificial neural network (Hatfield 1991).

On the basis of these fundamental algorithms, connectionism is therefore also referred to as a "subsymbolic theory"[149]. This is because it tries to explain the cognitive competence "below" the level of the symbol structures (using a "bottom-up method") (Rumelhart et al. 1986b). As a result, neurocognition is usually based on self-organization processes *without* an external control function that uses program instructions (Dorffner 1991). Rather, neurocognition is modeled by means of subsymbolic microelements. These microelements take the form of mathematical vectors up to more complex, numerical vector, tensor, attractor and oscillator constructions, to be interpreted as symbol structures (the "[dynamic] pattern of activations") (Peschl 1996a, Dorffner 1991).

---

[147]See e.g. Rojas 1996, Köhle 1990.
Sometimes a threefold division is made, so that the "reinforcement learning" is added as a third class. See e.g. Haykin 1999, Zell 2003, Bothe 1998.

[148]For dynamic adaptation in neural networks, see e.g. Arbib 2003.

[149]For the basic concept of the "subsymbol" in Paul Smolensky's subsymbol paradigm, which is explained in "The Coffee Story", please refer to the remarks in Maurer (2006/2009).

3.2.2 CONNECTIONISTIC REPRESENTATION AND REPRESENTATIONAL TYPOLOGY

The information of a connectionist system is encoded by means of the weighted linking patterns between the individual processing units (i.e. in the network architecture, or the network topology). More specifically, it is determined by the type, number, formation and output of the processing units, especially the "hidden (processing) units", the threshold values, the learning rule, and (above all else) the distribution of the connection weights (i.e. the vectorial connection matrix of the network).[150]

Contrary to classical Artificial Intelligence (AI) systems, the representatives of connectionism emphasize that information is usually not stored in localized places in a program. Instead it is decentralized, and located simultaneously in the distributed totality of overlapping connections between several processing units ("informational holism"[151]). It is therefore also referred to as "Parallel Distributed Processing (PDP)"[152], "Distributed Artificial Intelligence (DAI)"[153] or "Multi-Agent Systems"[154]. A distributed representation[155] of a piece of information means that no single processing unit of a network performs a syntactically or semantically determinable subtask alone within the network's mode of operation. Rather, an individual unit processes a portion of the overall task that cannot be determined in advance.[156] Only an assembly of processing units generating a "distributed pattern of activation" can do this (Hinton et al. 1986). The term "parallel" (Hinton et al. 1986) indicates that the process of information processing in an artificial neural network no longer follows a classical von Neumann architecture.[157] This means that each processing step cannot be processed until the previous step has been completed.

---

[150] According to Hatfield (1991), there are two ways of using the concept of representation in connectionism, in relation to the connection weights or the network's evolving activation pattern.

[151] See e.g. Clark 1989, Dreyfus and Dreyfus 1986, who speak of "Holistic Similarity Recognition" with reference to the model of the optical hologram.

[152] Fundamental to the connectionist paradigm was the book by D.E. Rumelhart and J.L. McClelland: "Parallel Distributed Processing: Explorations in the Microstructure of Cognition" (1986).

[153] For an introduction, see e.g. O'Hare 1996.

[154] For an introduction, see e.g. Ferber 1999.

[155] For detailed information, see e.g. Hinton et al. 1986, Van Gelder 1989, 1990b, 1991a, 1992a. For an introduction, see e.g. Plate 2003a, Peschl 1996a.
For the advantages of a distributed representation, see for example, Plate 2003a.
See also, Dorffner 1991, Helm 1991.
One tries not to assign a semantic concept or proposition to a single processing unit, but to distribute it over a group of units. Therefore, one and the same group of units is involved in the representation of several concepts, so that different concepts can be superimposed, allowing conceptual similarities to be expressed directly.

[156] However, this would be the case for the representation type of a "(ultra-)local representation". See below.

[157] See e.g. Korb 1996.
The term "classical von Neumann architecture", named after the Hungarian-American mathematician John von Neumann, is understood, in computer science, as a basic reference model for the functioning of computers used today, according to which, both program instructions and the program data can be stored in a common memory.
For an introduction, see e.g. Rojas and Hashagen 2000.

Following P. Smolensky and G. Legendre (2006a), T. van Gelder (1999b, 1991a, 1992a, 1990b), N.E. Sharkey (1991) and S.J. Thorpe (2003), four basic representation types[158] can now be distinguished in connectionism: (1) "strictly local" or "ultra local", (2) "(fully) local", (3) "semi-local" or "distributed", and (4) "fully distributed" or "strongly distributed". These types cover a spectrum that allows the combination of mental object components, from the discrete local concatenation[159] of symbols (in classical symbol theory) up to the overlapping (the superposition) of fully distributed subsymbolic representations (in the connectionist paradigm).

In the "strictly local" or "ultra local" representational type, a mental object or item, e.g. the word 'coffee', is only represented by a single cell or neuron. The activation state of the other cells is irrelevant, which means that this type can be transformed directly into a symbol concatenation (see Fig. 3.7).

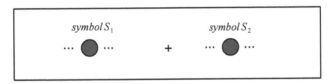

Figure 3.7: Schematic diagram of the representation type "strictly local" or "ultra local" (inspired by van Gelder 1999b).

In the "local" or "fully local" representation type, a mental item is represented by a cell or a neuron, but as a border case of a "sparse distributed representation". This means that the item is now represented in an assembly or "pool" of cells in which only *one* single cell is active, but the activation state of the other cells is now relevant (see Fig. 3.8).

In contrast, in the "distributed-basic notion" or "semi-local" type of representation a mental object is represented by a cell assembly. Here, *all* cells of the assembly participate in the representation, though the cell activation states of other assemblies are irrelevant. This means that two mental objects, e.g. the words 'coffee' in the sense of 'cup with coffee' and 'coffee' in the sense of 'pot with coffee', are represented by two completely separate cell assemblies. This is why there is no overlapping or superposition of the patterns to be learned (see Fig. 3.9).

An overlapping, the "super(-im-)position"[160], occurs only with the fourth representation type: "fully distributed" or "strongly distributed". A mental object is rep-

---

[158]The representation typology is mainly oriented towards T. van Gelder, P. Smolensky and G. Legendre, while S.J. Thorpe partly uses terms that are different from them. A simplified version, based on that of P. Smolensky and G. Legendre, can be found in M. Tye (1988).
See also Trappenberg 2002 in the framework of computational neuroscience.

[159]See Smolensky and Legendre 2006a.
On the concept of concatenation in the sense of theoretical computer science as a 2-ary operation of the algebraic structure of the "monoid" for the generation of character strings, see e.g. Schöning 2008.
On the use of a more general concept of spatial and temporal concatenation, see van Gelder 1990a.

[160]For an introduction, see e.g. Clark 1993 with regard to van Gelder 1991a.
See also, van Gelder 1992a.

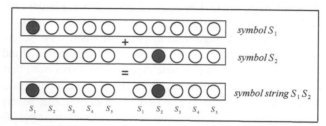

Figure 3.8: Schematic diagram of the representation type "local" or "fully local" (inspired by Smolensky and Legendre 2006a and van Gelder 1999b).

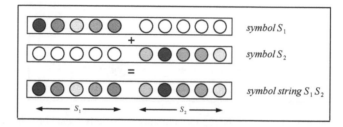

Figure 3.9: Schematic representation of the representation type "distributed-basic notion" or "semi-local" as vector addition of two vectors with, respectively, five active and disjunctive vector components. Gray levels indicate the different degrees of neuronal activity (inspired by Smolensky and Legendre 2006a and van Gelder 1999b).

resented by a cell assembly, in such a way that a pattern to be learned is not solely represented by the cells of a *single* cell assembly. In addition, the same cell assembly (and thus at least one cell[161] up to all cells of this cell assembly), is also involved in the representation of *other* patterns (see Fig. 3.10). In other words, two or more patterns, e.g. the words 'coffee' in the sense of 'cup with coffee' and 'coffee' in the sense of 'pot with coffee', are represented simultaneously by one and the same (overall) cell assembly. Thus, it is no longer possible to physically separate two or more mental objects in their representations, but only in the different cell activity configurations of the respective (overall) cell assembly.

The structural correspondence between the object to be represented and the representational neural resources is that the object is transferred to an object vector. The statistical correlations of the object vectors are then "extracted" from the synapse

---

The Finnish engineer and neuroinformatician T. Kohonen (1984) aptly describes this: "In distributed memories, every memory element or fragment of memory medium holds traces from many stored items, i.e., the representations are superimposed on each other. On the other hand, every piece of stored information is spread over a large area."

The terms "superposition" and "superimposition" are subject to a differentiated definition in van Gelder 1991a.

[161] In this case, one speaks only of "weakly distributed representation".
See e.g. van Gelder 1992a, 1990b.

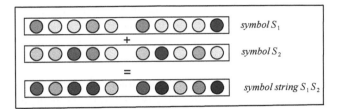

Figure 3.10: Schematic representation of the representation type "fully distributed" or "strongly distributed" as vector addition of two vectors with respectively ten active and distributed vector components. The gray scales indicate the different degrees of neuronal activity, and the superposition principle is illustrated by the addition of the respective gray scales of the vector components (inspired by Smolensky and Legendre 2006a).

vectors of the hidden neurons during a (training) series of distributed transformations into object representations. This is done in such a way that a (dis-)similarity relation between the synapse vectors exists due to the internal configuration of the vector components. This relation can be interpreted graphically within the "Potential Landscape" analogy, (see chap. 3.2.3.), as a (dis-)similarity[162] of the topological localization of the synapse vectors in the dynamic system state space. This precise localization is based on an exact, numerical, distance metric, e.g. the "Euclidean distance"[163], which is defined as:

$$d(x_i, x_j) = \|x_i - x_j\| = \sqrt{\sum_{k=1}^{m}(x_{ik} - x_{jk})^2}. \qquad (3.10)$$

For example, synapse vectors which are structurally similar (with regard to the internal configuration of their vector components), take up "adjacent" coordinates in the dynamic system state space.

In analogy to an (optical) hologram[164], an information item[165] to be stored as object vector components is thus "distributed" by comparing these components with each synapse vector of the neurons. This distribution occurs such that its object vector components simultaneously become the "computational part" of the activation,

---

[162]Sometimes the scalar product is also used to determine the (dis-)similarity of an information item. See e.g. Zell 2003, Cha 2007.

[163]Concerning the term "Euclidean distance", see e.g. Haykin 1999.
An alternative numerical distance metric is the "Hamming distance".
See e.g. Scherer 1997, Robinson 2003.

[164]According to van Gelder (1991a), based on K.S. Lashley's concept of "neural equipotentiality", a representation must satisfy the principle of equipotentialy in order to have a holographic function. This principle of equipotentiality is described in van Gelder 1999b.
Concerning the hologram analogy, see also Horgan and Tienson 1992a, van Gelder 1989.
Concerning the critique of the term "holographic representation", see e.g. Feldman and Shastri 2003.
On the criticism of the use of the term "holistic representation", see e.g. van Gelder 1991a.

[165]By a so-called "information item" or "information atom", one can understand, for example, a "cell" or a "pixel" of a letter to be represented.

and the propagation function of each neuron. In a fully distributed transformation function, the object vector components of the respective information item are simultaneously the "computational part" of the respective synapse vectors of each neuron of an assembly. Kohonen (1984) describes this as follows:

"(...) the spatial distributedness of memory traces, the central characteristic of holograms, may mean either of the following two facts: (i) Elements in a data set are spread by a transformation over a memory area, but different data sets are always stored in separate areas. (ii) Several data sets are superposed on the same medium in a distributed form."

3.2.3   CONNECTIONISTIC ENERGY FUNCTION AND POTENTIAL LANDSCAPE-METAPHOR

The system dynamics of an artificial neural network is described by interpreting a processing unit (or an array of processing units) as a dimension in a coordinate system, so that a "multi-dimensional system state space" is spanned. Using the transformation functions, i.e. the activation and propagation functions (including the respective learning algorithms that cause adjustment of the connection weights between the processing units), it is now possible to describe the transition from one activation state to a new activation state. This transition is represented by a numerical vector with the respective vector coordinates. A temporal sequence of activation states generates a path movement ("trajectory") from a coordinate point through the state space. In this case, the convergent or divergent (non-linear) dynamic system behavior (presented in the form of self-stabilizing, resonant "attractors" with respective "attractor basins") has an informative and representational function.[166] The degree of convergence or divergence of adjacent trajectories in the phase space, i.e. their stability behaviour, is indicated by the "Lyapunov exponent"[167] (named after the Russian mathematician and physicist, Aleksandr M. Lyapunov).

These sequences of internal system states can be illustrated as an n-dimensional "potential landscape" or "mountain landscape",[168] with "mountain ranges", "mountain peaks" and "mountain valleys". Each of these orbits of coordinate points can be interpreted as a specific dynamic piece of information of the artificial neural network (see Fig. 3.11) (Arbib 2003, Dorffner 1991). In analogy to the potential energy of a dynamic system in physics, each coordinate point in the system state space is assigned a function value by means of the transformation function. This value can be considered as the "total cost" of the artificial neural network to reach a certain system state. Within the framework of the classical "gradient descent method" (see chap. 3.2.5.3) the system tends to minimize the "cost" optimally, i.e. the negative gradient of the cost function tends towards its steepest descent (Kralemann 2006,

---

[166] See e.g. Stonier 1997: "If the message is able to resonate with some part of the internal information environment (the context) it will have meaning for the system; if not, it will be ignored."

[167] On the term "Lyapunov exponent", see e.g. Robinson 2012, Peitgen et al. 1994, Argyris et al. 1995, Metzler 1998, Katok and Hasselblatt 1995, Brin and Stuck 2002, Robinson 2004, Guckenheimer and Holmes 1990, Robinson 1999/2009, Leven et al. 1994, Ott 2002.

[168] For better illustration, a 2- or 3-dimensional mountain landscape is used. See e.g. Dorffner 1991.

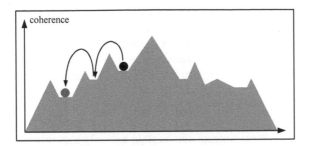

Figure 3.11: Schematic representation of the cross-section of an energy (or potential) landscape. The attainment of a (relatively) stable system state can be illustrated by means of a rolling ball in a mountain landscape, which tries to reach the deepest possible valley basin. First, the ball is located in a local (energy) minimum (black ball). Using the appropriate parameter settings in the activation and learning functions of a network, it can be achieved that the system jumps from one solution to another with varying degrees of probability. Geometrically speaking, this ideally allows the ball to move from a local to a global (energy) minimum (grey ball). This can be illustrated by taking into account that the relevant parameter settings control the so-called "computational temperature" of the system. This temperature can be imagined as the measure up to which the whole landscape is set into oscillation. This allows the ball, at a high temperature and with an increased degree of probability, to overcome an energy barrier in the shape of a mountain to reach the next lower energy level. During the learning phase, after the system has learned the respective input patterns, the temperature is gradually reduced. As a result, this slow cooling of the system increases the probability of not being "pulled out" again in an (optimal) minimum (following Köhle 1990).

Dorffner 1991, Nielson 2015). In other words, the path of a coordinate point moves as fast as possible, and always downhill, towards its steepest descent in state space. It will therefore end at least at a local minimum, and, at best at a global minimum. The "cost value" of a coordinate point in the potential landscape corresponds to the degree of activation of a system state (in (artificial) "energy" or – with a reversed sign – the so-called "harmony" [see chap. 10.2]) of the dynamic system, according to the "Lyapunov function"[169] in mathematical stability theory. The mathematical definition of the Lyapunov function can be desrcibed as follows (Königsberger 2002):

A Lyapunov function at a critical point x_0 of a vector field $v : \Omega \to \mathbb{R}^n$ is a $\mathscr{C}^1$-function $L : \Omega \to \mathbb{R}$ with the two properties:

(i) L has an isolated minimum in x_0 with $L(x_0) = 0$;

(ii) the derivation $\partial_v L$ of L along the field v takes only values ≤ 0 or values ≥ 0.

Thus, an artificial neural network always strives to take the global minimum of the "energy function" (Cottrell 2003) by means of the gradient descent method. This

---

[169]For detailed information, see e.g. Cohen and Grossberg 1983.
For an introduction, see e.g. Khalil 2002, Jetschke 1989, Hirsch and Smale 1974, Brin and Stuck 2002. See also Neelakanta and De Groff 1994, Unbehauen 2002, Kosko 1992, Petitot 2011. A Lyapunov function for the "Hopfield network" (see chap. 3.2.4.3) is specified in chap. 3.2.5.5.

corresponds to reaching a (relatively) stable system state with maximum coherence in terms of error reduction (see chap. 3.2.5.2, 3.2.5.4, 10.2). This can be regarded as a "quality assessment procedure" for determining the extent to which the connection weights have been successfully adapted to the input patterns presented.[170] A mountain valley basin thus stands for a group of converging trajectories, i.e. an attractor. This can thus be interpreted as a cognitive "representation" of an internal system concept in the broader sense (with reference to the data vectors entered), and corresponds, for example, to a classical symbol-based semantic concept. In contrast to this, an internal system concept can contain not only a conceptual, but also a pictorial representation and can – in contrast to a symbol – also reflect all transition or intermediate states of neighbouring mountain valley basins.

3.2.4 BASIC MODELS IN CONNECTIONISM

In the following sections, six basic networks are presented; these correspond to four basic classes of architectural models in connectionism with related cognitive functions.[171]

3.2.4.1 Perceptron by F. Rosenblatt

The "Perceptron"[172], originally developed by the American psychologist, Frank Rosenblatt, as a two-layer network for visual pattern recognition, is an abstract scheme of the visual perception process. As an extended multi-layered network, it belongs to the class of "(multilayer) Feedforward Architectures". This means that the flow of information processing only moves forward from the input neurons to the output neurons via the hidden neurons (which process the information by changing their connection weights). Thus, the activities of a layer's neurons can influence only the activation of the next layer's neurons (see Fig. 3.12).

---

[170]Concerning the proof of convergence that a Hopfield network achieves a stable final state with a lower total energy from any network state, assuming an asynchronous computation rule, see e.g. Rojas 1996.
Concerning the proof of convergence for a recurrent, fully interconnected network in general, see e.g. Kralemann 2006.

[171]For a more detailed overview of the different classes of architectural models in connectionism, see e.g. Zell 2003, Haykin 1999, Rey and Wender 2011, Haun 1998.
See also, Thomas and McClelland 2008.

[172]For fundamental information, see e.g. Rosenblatt 1958/1988.
See also, Minsky and Papert 1969/1988.
For an introduction, see e.g. Haykin 1999, Zell 2003, Rojas 1996, Köhle 1990, Graupe 2008, Müller et al. 1995, Haun 1998.
See also, Ritter et al. 1992, Kasabov 1998.
For a beginner' guide, see Bermúdez 2014.

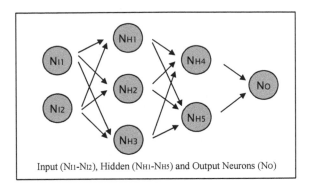

Figure 3.12: Schematic diagram of a multilayer feed-forward architecture (following Zell 2003).

3.2.4.2   Simple Recurrent Network by J.L. Elman

The "Simple Recurrent-Network (SRN)"[173], developed by the American linguist Jeffrey L. Elman, is an abstract scheme of dynamic working memory belonging to the class of "(Partial) Recurrent Architectures". In comparison to the Feedforward Architectures, the SRN is characterized by an additional recursive (i.e. feedback) information processing flow from the respective hidden neuron to a "context neuron" (see Fig. 3.13: shown as grey arrows). These context neurons store the activations of the respective hidden neurons (which contain the information about the preceding input pattern) as an exact "copy".[174] As soon as the hidden neurons process the next input pattern, they also receive the activation of the context neurons with information about the previous input pattern. This can be used to establish a temporal relationship between the individual patterns and, over time, to encode an internal abstract representation of dynamic information in the hidden neurons.

3.2.4.3   Hopfield Network by J.J. Hopfield and Linear Associator Model by J.A. Anderson

The "Hopfield Network"[175], developed by the American physicist John J. Hopfield, is an abstract scheme of the dynamic auto-associative long-term memory, belonging to the class of "(Total) Recurrent Architectures" (see Fig. 3.14).

---

[173]For fundamental information, see e.g. Elman 1990.
For an introduction, see e.g. Rey and Wender 2011, Haykin 1999.
See also, Thomas and McClelland 2008, Kasabov 1998, Bechtel and Abrahamsen 2002.

[174]The context neurons have the identity function as an activation function.

[175]For fundamental information, see e.g. Hopfield 1982/1988.
For an introduction, see e.g. Zell 2003, Rojas 1996, Haykin 1999, Graupe 2008, Müller et al. 1995, Köhle 1990, Scherer 1997, Ermentrout and Terman 2010, Haun 1998.
See also, Cottrell 2003, Ritter et al. 1992, Kasabov 1998.

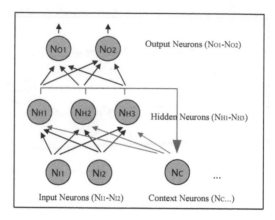

Figure 3.13: Schematic diagram of a Simple Recurrent Network (following Rey and Wender 2011).

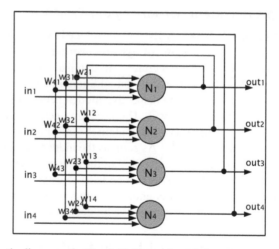

Figure 3.14: Schematic diagram of a Hopfield Network with four neurons, each of which is connected to all other neurons but not to itself (following Zell 2003).

The "Linear Associator Model"[176], developed by the American physiologist, neuroscientist and cognitive scientist James A. Anderson, represents an abstract scheme of a dynamic hetero-associative long-term memory (see Fig. 3.15). It consists of a layer with input neurons and another with output neurons. These layers are associated with each other via connection weights $w_{11}...w_{LK}$, so that, for example, memory patterns can be stored on the basis of Hebb's learning rule by adapting the connection weights to given stimuli.

---

[176]For fundamental information, see e.g. Anderson 1972, Hinton and Anderson 1981.
For detailed information, see e.g. McClelland et al. 1986.
For an introduction, see e.g. Rojas 1996, Rey and Wender 2011, Bothe 1998, Smith Churchland and Sejnowski 1992.

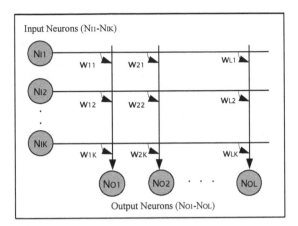

Figure 3.15: Schematic diagram of a Linear Associator Model (following Smith Churchland and Sejnowski 1992).

3.2.4.4   Self-Organizing (Feature) Map by T. Kohonen[177]

The "Self-Organizing (Feature) Map (SO(F)M)"[178] by the Finnish engineer Teuvo Kohonen, also known as "Kohonen Map," uses a self-organized learning algorithm within the framework of unsupervised competitive learning. In its basic form ("The Basic SOM" (Kohonen 2001)), it generates a similarity graph from input data within an unsupervised classification of data, with topology and distribution preserving mapping properties. The Kohonen map transforms the nonlinear statistical relationships between high-dimensional data into simple geometric relationships of low-dimensional pixel arrays (usually a regular two-dimensional grid of nodes) (Kohonen 2001). T. Kohonen himself usually recommends choosing a hexagonal grid over a square grid structure, and a rectangular grid over a square grid shape "for better visual inspection" (Zell 2003).

The self-organizing feature map thus typically consists of a two-dimensional topological configuration of formal neurons (see Fig. 3.16). Each formal neuron i represents a unit of computation to which an n-dimensional "synapse vector" m_i (or "reference vector") is matched, and the numerical vector components are randomly assigned ("initialization"). All neurons of the input layer are connected in parallel to all neurons of the competitive layer (also denoted the Kohonen layer) via these synapse vectors (as variable weight vectors). This means that all competitive neurons receive the same input signals – n-dimensional vectors – from the input vector

---

[177]This chapter is a largely adapted and partly revised version of chap. 1 of my B.Sc. Thesis (Studienarbeit) in computer science. See Maurer 2004/2009.

[178]For fundamental information, see Kohonen 1982c/1988b, 1982a, 1982b.
For detailed information, see e.g. Kohonen 2001, 1995, 1988a.
For an introduction, see e.g. Kohonen 2002, 1998.
For an introduction, see also e.g. Zell 2003, Bothe 1998, Haykin 1999, Rojas 1996, Rey and Wender 2011, Scherer 1997, Knieling 2007.
See also, Ritter et al. 1992, Kasabov 1998, Van Hulle 2000, Maurer 2016.

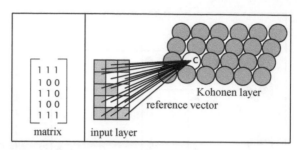

$$\begin{bmatrix} 1 & 1 & 1 \\ 1 & 0 & 0 \\ 1 & 1 & 0 \\ 1 & 0 & 0 \\ 1 & 1 & 1 \end{bmatrix}$$

matrix   input layer

Kohonen layer
reference vector

Figure 3.16: Schematic diagram of the network architecture of a Kohonen map. The Kohonen layer works in the context of the "winner function" following the principle of the "Winner-Takes-All (WTA)," which means that, in relation to each given input vector only one neuron of the Kohonen layer, shown here in white, can win. The connections from each input neuron of the input layer, (represented as a cell of the input layer), to the winning neuron are also illustrated. The input consists of the letter 'E' as an activity pattern consisting of 3×5 input neurons. In the graphic segment on the left, the corresponding 3×5 dimensional input vector is indicated in matrix notation, whereby a dark (light) drawn input neuron corresponds to a vector component of 'one' ('zero'). The synapse or reference vector of the winner neuron would come nearest to the configuration of the components of the input vector in comparison to the other neurons of the Kohonen layer. The winner neuron would try to adjust itself to this input vector with its 3×5 dimensional synapse or reference vector, so that the configuration of its reference vector components would also correspond to the given matrix during the training (based on Spitzer 2000, see also Kohonen 1982c).

space V. From this vector space V, a random input vector $x = [\xi_1, \xi_2, ..., \xi_n]^T \in \mathbb{R}^n$ is selected in accordance with the "probability density function" $w(x)$[179]; this is compared with all reference vectors $m_i = [\mu_{i1}, \mu_{i2}, ..., \mu_{in}]^T \in \mathbb{R}^n$ ("choice of stimulus"). The response (i.e. "excitation") of the individual competitive neurons to a given input signal varies. It is determined by the similarity between the input vector x and the respective reference vector m_i, in relation to an appropriate distance measure (usually the Euclidean distance characterized by $\| \cdot \|$ [chap. 3.2.2, 3.2.5.1]). The more similar the input vector is to the corresponding reference vector, the stronger the excitation of the related neuron. Thus, if an arbitrary input pattern is presented, each

---

[179]If a continuous random variable X is given, i.e. the values ξ assumed by X are continuously distributed, w is referred to as "probability density function" and $w(\xi)$ as the probability density of the random variable, which has to satisfy the following general properties:

(1) $\forall \xi : w(\xi) \geq 0,$

(2) $W \{a \leq X \leq b\} = \int_a^b w(\xi)d\xi,$

(3) $\int_{-\infty}^{+\infty} w(\xi)d\xi = 1.$

This means that $w(\xi)d\xi$ describes the probability W that the random variable X takes on a value in the interval $[a, b]$.

See e.g. Applebaum 1996, Schwabl 2006, Ritter et al. 1992, Scherer 1997, Cover and Thomas 2006. See also, Haken 1983, Stegmüller 1973, Eliasmith and Anderson 2003.

neuron of the Kohonen layer receives a (vector) copy of this pattern which is modified by the different synaptic weights. This means that the neuron whose synapse vector best matches the input vector will be the most excited (i.e. will "win"). The "Best Matching Unit (BMU)," denoted also as the "winner neuron" c or "location of the response", is defined by the minimal Euclidean difference between the input vector $x(t)$ and the corresponding reference vectors $m_i(t)$ in the "Winner-Takes-All (WTA) function"[180]:

$$c = \arg\min_i \{\|x(t) - m_i(t)\|\}. \tag{3.11}$$

Finally, after the neuron with the best matching reference vector ("response") has been determined, this "matching" is increased for this neuron and its topological "neighbors". This involves adapting the reference vector and its neighboring vectors in the direction of the actual input vector by a fraction of the total difference. In other words, learning occurs because the matching is not complete. The synapse vector of the BMU is now slightly shifted towards the input vector. To a smaller extent, the synapse vectors of the neurons within the BMUs "neighborhood" are also shifted toward the input vector. As a result, the input patterns which are similar to those represented by the BMU are represented with a higher degree of probability in the neighborhood of the BMU. This is defined by the time-varying "learning-rate factor"[181] $\alpha(t)$ and the "neighborhood function"[182] h_{ci} (also named "neighborhood kernel" or "distance function") (Kohonen 2001, Zell 2003):

$$m_i(t+1) = m_i(t) + \alpha(t)\, h_{ci}(t)[x(t) - m_i(t)]. \tag{3.12}$$

The normalized Gaussian[183] (density) function $h_{ci,gauss}(t)$ is typically used as the neighborhood function, and the variance $\sigma(t)$ defines the width of the neighborhood core (Kohonen 2001, Zell 2003):

$$h_{ci,gauss}(t) = \frac{1}{\sigma(t)\sqrt{2\pi}} \cdot \exp\left(\frac{-\|r_c - r_i\|^2}{2\sigma^2(t)}\right), \tag{3.13}$$

where r_c and r_i denote the vectors of the position of neuron c and neuron i in the neuron lattice.

---

[180] A basic description of the winner and neighbourhood function can be found in Kohonen 2001, Zell 2003.
The compressed SOM algorithm can be found most clearly in Ritter et al. 1992, Rojas 1996, Scherer 1997, Braun et al. 1996, and Fritzke 1992.
For detailed discussion, see Van Hulle 2000.
A physiological interpretation of the SOM algorithm, especially the "Winner-Takes-All (WTA) function" and the "neighborhood function", offered by Kohonen 1993 and Kohonen 2001.

[181] The "learning-rate factor" $\alpha(t)$ is usually a monotonically falling function. See Kohonen 2001. See also e.g. Zell 2003.

[182] The "distance or neighborhood function" h_{ci} is usually a monotonically falling function. See Kohonen 2001. See also e.g. Zell 2003. See also fn. 180.

[183] Named after the mathematician, astronomer, geodesist and physicist Carl Friedrich Gauss. For general information on the "Gaussian distribution", see e.g. Jaynes 2010.

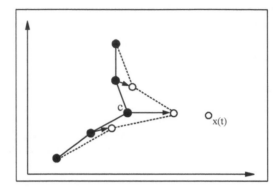

Figure 3.17: Schematic diagram of the learning scheme of a Kohonen map. The (geometrically interpreted) motion of the synapse vectors (black dots) of the winning neuron (c) and its two neighbours directed towards the input vector x(t) (white dots) is shown, illustrated by the arrows. The synapse vectors here are 2-dimensional for clarity. The synapse vector of the winner neuron is most strongly adjusted, illustrated by the length of the arrows. The synapse vectors of its two neighbors are also adjusted within the neighborhood function directed towards the input vector x(t), but somewhat less strongly. After adjusting the synapse weights, the new synapse vectors (white dots) which are interconnected with the dashed lines, are obtained (based on Bogdan 2017 and Zell 2003).

In other words, the BMU excites other neurons within a specific environment and inhibits more distant neurons according to the "principle of lateral inhibition" (Bear et al. 2016). This means that the BMU (which is most similar to the input vector of all reference vectors of the Kohonen layer) and some neurons in its environment are still approximated to the input pattern by a certain amount ("adaptation step") (see Fig. 3.17).

The set of all points from the input vector space V that have the same location as the response c now form a polygon F_c, the "Voronoi polygon." All the Voronoi polygons form a partitioning of the input space, the "Voronoi tesselation" (Haykin 1999, Bothe 1998, Knieling 2007). The aim of the Kohonen algorithm is to find an assignment of the reference vectors m_i such that the mapping resulting from input vector space V to the topological structure A has the following two properties: First, it is "topology preserving; that is, similar input vectors should be mapped to either neighboring neurons or the same formal neurons in structure A, so that neighboring elements in structure A also have similar reference vectors. Second, it has "distribution preservation: that is, the areas of the input space V with a high probability density $w(x)$ should be mapped to correspondingly large areas in structure A, so that the relative density of the reference vectors in A either approximates or adapts to the probability density $w(x)$ (Fritzke 1992). In summary, the neurons of the Kohonen layer can adjust their synapse weights by self-organization in such a manner that a topographical feature map is formed. This means that certain features of the input pattern are mapped in a regular manner onto a certain network location, such that similar input patterns are represented close together and input patterns that are often mapped are represented in a larger area.

Numerous variants of architecture types have been developed from the Standard SOM[184], e.g. so-called "Growing SOMs", "Hierarchical SOMs", "Tree-Structured SOMs", "Growing Hierarchical SOMs", "ASSOM" and others.

The self-organizing feature map has a multitude of applications (Kohonen 2001, 2002), especially in language processing (Kohonen 2001, Anderson 1999, Köhle 1990), e.g. H. Ritter's and T. Kohonen's semantic maps (Ritter and Kohonen 1989, Haykin 1999).

Finally, a software package, the "SOM_PAK", is offered for the implementation of the SOM algorithm (Kohonen 2001; see also, the webpage https://www.cis.hut.fi/research/som-research/nnrc-programs.shtml).

3.2.4.5 Adaptive Resonance Theory by S. Grossberg and G.A. Carpenter

The "Adaptive Resonance Theory (ART)",[185] put forward by the American mathematicians and neuroinformaticians Steven Grossberg and Gail A. Carpenter, also uses a self-organized learning algorithm within the framework of unsupervised competitive learning. They have developed an entire class of highly plausible models (neurobiologically and cognitive psychologically speaking), designed to solve the "stability plasticity dilemma"[186] of artificial neural networks. This dilemma, also known as the classification problem, is to account for how vectorial information (as a sequence of input patterns to be learned) is independently integrated into a (synchronous) statistical prototype, such that the already learned associations of the network can be adapted toward new input patterns ("plasticity") *without* causing these old associations to be modified too much ("catastrophic forgetting" (Grossberg and Versace 2008)). This ensures the preservation of the patterns once learned ("stability"). In other words, the classification problem leads to the fundamental question: "How can new associations be learned in a neural network without forgetting old associations?" (Zell 2003).

For this reason, all ART models that simulate human learning behavior try to solve the stability-plasticity dilemma by aiming to prevent very strong modifications of previously learned connection weights. Consequently, a specific new training pattern cannot cover or destroy an already stored prototypical category, although it can create a new prototypical category within only a single training cycle.

---

[184]See e.g. Kohonen 2001.
A detailed introduction and overview of the various architecture types of Kohonen maps can be found in Maurer 2004/2009 and Maurer et al. 2007.

[185]For foundational papers, see e.g. Grossberg 1976a, b, c, 1988, Carpenter and Grossberg 1987a, b, 1988.
For a more extensive discussion, see e.g. Carpenter and Grossberg 1990a.
For an introduction, see e.g. Carpenter and Grossberg 1990b, 2003, 2002, Carpenter 2011.
For a brief discussion, see e.g. Zell 2003, Graupe 2008, Rey and Wender 2011, Scherer 1997.
See also, Bothe 1998, Tanaka and Weitzenfeld 2002, Sapojnikova 2004, Kasabov 1998, Zabel 2005.

[186]For foundational papers, see e.g. Cohen and Grossberg 1983, Carpenter and Grossberg 1987a, b, Grossberg 1987, 1980.
For a brief discussion, see e.g. Rey and Wender 2011, Bothe 1998, Zell 2003, Haykin 1999.
See also, Abraham and Robins 2005, Yegnanarayana 1994, Tucker 2001, Norman et al. 2005.

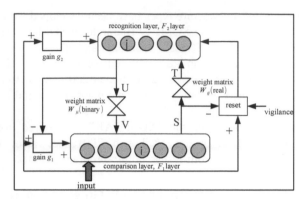

Figure 3.18: Schematic diagram of an ART-1 architecture (based on Zell 2003; see also, Carpenter and Grossberg 1987a).

The architecture and algorithm of the ART-1 network, the first version of the ART model class, is described below, followed by a brief description of the other versions: ART-2, ART-2a, ART-3, ARTMAP and FUZZY ART[187].

An ART-1 network[188] (see Fig. 3.18), which is (only) suitable for learning binary input vectors, consists of two layers of neurons. These neurons are arranged in a "comparison layer" F_1 (which serves as an input layer), and a "recognition layer" F_2 (which contains the classification neurons). The two layers are connected bidirectionally via weight matrices, and the data transfer between the two layers is controlled using a nonlinear control strategy. The F_1 comparison layer can be regarded as a short term memory (STM), whilst the F_2 recognition layer can be regarded as a long term memory (LTM).[189] The F_1 layer is connected to the F_2 layer via a real-valued bottom-up weight matrix W_{ij}, while the F_2 layer is connected to the F_1 layer via a binary-valued top-down weight matrix W_{ij}. A component for synchronization control is also added. This consists of g_1 and g_2 neurons called "gain (factor)", which synchronize the network. Furthermore, a component for orientation control has been added which allows for the size setting of a prototype class and the deactivation of classification neurons of the F_2 layer. This component operates by means of a "vigilance parameter" ρ, which is adjusted by the developer ("reset").

---

[187] An overview of the typology of ART architectures can be found, for example, in Sapojnikova 2004, Zabel 2005.

[188] For fundamental papers, see e.g. Grossberg 1976a, b, c, Carpenter and Grossberg 1987a, where, essentially, the functioning of the network is described.
For a detailed discussion, see e.g. Carpenter and Grossberg 1990a.
For an introduction, see e.g. Carpenter and Grossberg 2003, 1990b, Carpenter 2011.
For a brief discussion, see e.g. Zell 2003, Graupe 2008, with two examples and the programming code in Java, Rojas 1996, Köhle 1990, Bothe 1998, with an example, Tanaka and Weitzenfeld 2002, with an example and the programming code.
See also, Sapojnikova 2004, Zabel 2005.

[189] See e.g. Carpenter and Grossberg 1987a.

After the values of the two weight matrices and the vigilance parameter are set, the functioning of an ART-1 network consists of four phases[190]:

1. In the "recognition (phase)", an input vector I is read into the F_1 layer and passed on as a copy (vector S). Next, for each classification neuron j in the F_2 layer, the scalar product is computed as a similarity measure between its weight vector (or reference vector) W_j and S. The aim is to determine the neuron with the highest network input t_j whose scalar product is the largest (the winner neuron J), i.e. which is the most strongly activated. Therefore, only this single neuron, whose weight vector is most similar to the input vector, fires, so that

$$t_j = net_j = \langle S|W_j \rangle \text{ with } W_j = \sum_i W_{ij} \qquad (3.14)$$

and

$$u_j = \begin{cases} 1 & \text{if } t_J = \max\{t_j : j = 1...k\} \\ 0 & \text{else} \end{cases} . \qquad (3.15)$$

This means that a single component, u_J of vector U, is set to '1' and all other components are set to '0'. Until this step, the procedure is similar to competitive learning, as described in the self-organizing map by the Finnish engineer Teuvo Kohonen: A hypothetical prototype class is generated with the winner neuron. Therefore for the selection process of a vectorial prototype, the network "assumes" that the input vector that has been entered has sufficient similarity to this vectorial prototype, which is interpreted as establishing a classification hypothesis (Carpenter et al. 1991a, d, Grossberg and Versace 2008).

2. In the "comparison (phase)" this assumption is confirmed by a comparison. First, the hypothetical prototype W_j (vector V), which is the weighted sum of the outputs of the F_2 layer, is computed back to the F_1 layer. This allows each neuron i in the F_1 layer to receive a binary signal v_i, which is equal to the value of w_{Ji}:

$$v_i = \sum_j u_j w_{ji} = w_{Ji}. \qquad (3.16)$$

Since a neuron has now been activated in the F_2 layer, the neuron g_1 has the activation value '0'. This means that the only neurons active in the F_1 layer are those which receive the binary activation signal '1' from *both* the input vector I and the vector V[191]. Thus, the F_1 layer's newly generated output, vector S,

---

[190]See e.g. Carpenter and Grosssberg 1987a, which basically describes how the network functions. The description is essentially based on the presentation in Zell 2003, Tanaka and Weitzenfeld 2002, Zabel 2005.
A clear diagram of the ART algorithm can be found, for example, in Moore 1989, Zabel 2005, Graupe 2008.
An introductory presentation of the neuronal and synaptic dynamics, using the first-order nonlinear differential equations used by G. A. Carpenter and St. Grossberg, can be found in Sapojnikova 2004.
For a fundamental discussion, see e.g. Carpenter and Grossberg 1987a, Cohen and Grossberg 1983, Grossberg 1968a, b, 1970, 1972.

[191]For detailed discussion with reference to the 2/3 rule of the comparison layer F_1, see e.g. Carpenter and Grossberg 1987a.

should have a high number of vector components with the activation signal '1'. The decision as to whether the input pattern in question actually belongs to the class is made by determing whether the input pattern vector I is sufficiently similar to the newly generated output vector S of the F_1 layer:

$$\frac{|S|}{|I|} = \frac{|W_j \wedge I|}{|I|} \oplus \rho \qquad (3.17)$$

(Carpenter and Grossberg 1987a, 1987b, Carpenter et al. 1991a, 1991d, Rojas 1996, Zabel 2005).

The "vigilance parameter" $\rho \in [0,1]$, to be set by the developer, defines the degree of similarity between the vector of the input pattern X and the respective weight vector w_j of the neurons of the F_2 layer, computed by means of the angle between the input vector X and the weight vector W.

$$\frac{X^T W}{|X||W|} \approx \cos(\alpha), \text{ with } |X| = \sum_i x_i. \qquad (3.18)$$

The angle between the two vectors X and W is α. In practical applications, values for ρ in the range $0.7 < \rho < 0.99$ are often used.

3. As a result, the following alternatives are now available during the "search (phase)". If the similarity between the input vector and the prototype vector falls below the vigilance parameter already mentioned, the match between the input vector I and the newly generated output vector S is not sufficiently large. This means that the classification hypothesis could not be verified. In this scenario, this hypothetical prototype class (with the corresponding winner neuron in the F_2 layer) is blocked by the "(STM) reset (system)" (Carpenter and Grossberg 1987a). In a new comparison phase, a new winner neuron – the next most similar one – is determined and returned to the F_1 layer. This iterative process is carried out until one of the following two scenarios occur:

3.1 If none of the stored prototype classes and F_2 winner neurons match the input pattern sufficiently, (i.e. all F_1 neurons are blocked), then a previously predefined inactive F_2 neuron will activate. Its weight vector W_j is set so that it corresponds to the input vector. By dynamically generating a new class with the input vector as a prototype, the information spectrum of the network can be extended without greatly masking or deleting the previously stored weight vectors of the prototype classes. The previously mentioned stability-plasticity dilemma is therefore solved because it would not force each input pattern into an already existing prototype class (as in pure competitive learning).

3.2 If, however, there is sufficient matching between the F_2 winner neuron in one of the stored prototype classes and the input pattern, i.e. if the similarity exceeds the threshold of the vigilance parameter, then the ART-1 network for the respective input vector is in "(adaptive) resonance" (Carpenter et al. 1991b). The network passes into a corresponding training cycle, whereby the binary and the real-valued weight vector W_J (i.e. the weight vectors which belong to the winner neuron J of the F_2 layer), are adapted to the input vector, as in pure competition learning. This increases the similarity. Once an associated pattern is no longer assigned to a new prototype class, the input pattern is assigned to the corresponding prototype class. This also contributes to solving the stability-plasticity dilemma (Moore 1989).

4. In the context of the "weight adaptation phase", (the "training") ART networks distinguish between "slow training" (or "slow learning") and "fast training" (or "fast learning"). The former is applied if the pattern to be learned resembles a previously stored one, and the latter is applied if the pattern to be learned is completely unknown. Only for fast learning are the input vectors applied over a sufficiently long period of time for the real-valued bottom-up and binary top-down weight vectors to reach their asymptotic, stable values. The real-valued bottom-up weight vector W_j is set to the normalized values of the vector S:

$$w_{iJ} = \frac{Ls_i}{L - 1 + \sum_k s_k} \qquad (3.19)$$

and the binary top-down weight vector W_j is adapted to the vector S:

$$w_{Ji} = s_i \qquad (3.20)$$

(Carpenter and Grossberg 1987a, Zell 2003, Tanaka and Weitzenfeld 2002).

Finally, it should be mentioned that Carpenter and Grosssberg have proven a number of theorems about the ART-1 network on various topics of stability in the search and weight adaptation phase (Carpenter and Grossberg 1987a, Zell 2003, Tanaka and Weitzenfeld 2002, Bothe 1998).

An extension of ART-1 is the ART-2 network (Carpenter and Grossberg 1987b, Zell 2003, Bothe 1998, Sapojnikova 2004) and, in comparison, the simplified ART-2A network (Carpenter et al. 1991b, Zell 2003) (which is designed to accelerate the convergence of ART-2). These networks classify the sequences of input vectors with continuous, real-value components.

A further development of ART-2 is the ART-3 network (Carpenter and Grossberg 1990c, Zell 2003), which additionally models certain chemical processes of synapses using differential equations. For example, the amount, the accumulation, the release, and the degradation of neurotransmitters.

A Fuzzy-ART network (Carpenter et al. 1991a, 1991c, Zell 2003, Bothe 1998, Zabel 2005, Sapojnikova 2004) represents a combination of "fuzzy logic" (Zadeh 1965, Zimmermann 1994) with an ART-1 network. This produces a dynamic associative memory which extends the ART-1 algorithm working with binary input vectors in such a way that real-value input vectors can also be processed. This is done by replacing the intersection operator $\cap$ in the F_1 comparison layer of the ART-1 network, within the framework of the 2/3 rule by the MIN operator $\wedge$ of the fuzzy (set) theory.

The types of ART network mentioned previously have made an adaptive classification of input vectors in the context of unsupervised learning. In contrast, the ARTMAP network classifies[192] input vectors with a supervised learning method, by

---

[192]For an essential paper, see e.g. Carpenter et al. 1991d.

representing a combination of two ART-1, ART-2, ART-3, or Fuzzy-ART networks. This enables an exact classification of the class affiliation of input patterns using an input vector and an output vector associated therewith.

In order to solve the stability-plasticity dilemma, the "ART-Kohonen Neural Network (ART-KNN)" (according to B.-S. Yang, T. Han and Y.- S. Kim (2004)) also tried to combine the learning algorithm of Kohonen's SOM with the ART.

Based on their theory of adaptive resonance described above, S. Grosssberg et al.[193] have postulated that the cortical code (and thus also a neuronal matching process (Grossberg and Versace 2008)) can be modeled using resonant states (resonant standing waves[194]). This is caused by synchronous (phase) oscillations (in the gamma range of 20-70 Hz) of the participating cooperating neuronal assemblies within the framework of bottom-up and top-down feedback loops.

This approach was further developed into the "Synchronous Matching Adaptive Resonance Theory (SMART)" (Grossberg and Versace 2008). This analyses how the brain is able to perform different levels of thalamocortical and corticocortical information processing in such a way that reciprocal topdown and bottom-up corticocortical and thalamocortical adaptive filters work together. The connection between learning, attention, expectation, resonance and synchronicity can be shown with this analysis. Grossberg (2017) summarizes his Adaptive Resonance Theory and the basic concept of adaptive resonance as follows:

"An [adaptive] resonance is a dynamical state during which neuronal firings across a brain network are amplified and synchronized as they interact via reciprocal excitatory feedback signals during a matching process that occurs between bottom-up and top-down pathways. Often, the activities of these synchronized cells oscillate in phase with one another. Resonating cell activities also focus attention upon a subset of cells, thereby clarifying how the brain can become conscious of attended events. It is called an adaptive resonance because the resonant state can trigger learning within the adaptive weights, or long-term memory (LTM) traces that exist at the synapses of these pathways. ART explains how an adaptive resonance, when it occurs in different specialized anatomies that receive different types of environmental and brain inputs, can give rise to different conscious qualia as emergent, or interactive, properties of specialized networks of neurons. In particular, ART proposes how the brain resonances mirror parametric properties of conscious experiences of seeing, hearing, and feeling, and of knowing what these experiences are".

For an introduction, see e.g. Carpenter and Grossberg 2003.
For a brief discussion, see e.g. Zell 2003, Bothe 1998, Zabel 2005, Sapojnikova 2004.

[193] An overview can be found in Grossberg and Somers, 1991, with references to further literature, where the following cooperative coupling mechanisms between neuron activities are investigated: "Cooperative Bipole Coupling", "Adaptive Filter Coupling", "Nearest Neighbor Coupling" and "Random Connection Coupling".
See also e.g. Grossberg 1997, Carpenter and Grossberg 1991.

[194] See Grossberg and Somers 1991, where the authors emphasize that under certain conditions, this mathematical concept can be replaced by that of the attractor.
See also with regard to the related "Cohen Grosssberg Theorem" Cohen and Grossberg 1983.
For an introduction, see e.g. Haykin 1999, Zell 2003, Yegnanarayana 1994.

3.2.4.6 Classical Architectures in Connectionism

The most important classical architectures developed between the mid-1980s and mid-1990s in (early) connectionism are briefly listed below (Thomas and McClelland 2008, Plate 1994):

(1) J.B. Pollak's "Recursive Auto-Associative Memory (RAAM)" (Pollack 1990),
(2) G.E. Hinton's "Reduced Descriptions" (Hinton 1990),
(3) G.E. Hinton's, T.J. Sejnowski's and D.H. Ackley "Boltzman Machine" (Ackley et al. 1985),
(4) D.S. Touretzky's and G.E. Hinton's "Distributed Connectionist Production System (DCPS)" (Touretzky and Hinton 1988),
(5) D.S. Touretzky's "BoltzCONS system" (Touretzky 1986) and D.S. Touretzky's and S. Geva's "DUCS system" (Touretzky and Geva 1987),
(6) T.J. Sejnowski's and C. Rosenberg's "NETtalk" (Sejnowski and Rosenberg 1986),
(7) D.E. Rumelhart's and J.L. McClelland's "Past Tense Learning Model" (Rumelhart and McClelland 1986b),
(8) J.L. McClelland's and J.L. Elman's "TRACE model" (McClelland and Elman 1986),
(9) M. Derthick's "μKLONE" (Derthick 1990), and
(10) M.I. Jordan's "Connectionist Sequential Machine" (Jordan 1986).

3.2.5 METHODS AND METHODICAL PRINCIPLES IN CONNECTIONISM

This section presents the methods and methodical principles used in (early) connectionism to analyse data and information, most of which are available in vectorial form[195]. These methods are also applied in theoretical neuroarchitectures in the context of integrative (synchronization) mechanisms against the background of classification, optimization and learning problems.

3.2.5.1 Multivariate Cluster Analysis[196]

The "Multivariate Cluster Analysis (MCA)"[197] is a heuristic method for the systematic classification of objects of a given set based on the (dis-)similarity of their characteristic values. The set of objects to be classified is called $I = \{I_1, ..., I_N\}$. The initial data for a cluster analysis usually form the characteristic values of p characteristics $x' = (x_1, ..., x_p)$ measured on the objects, where the characteristic attributes can

---

[195] A very good introduction can be found, for example, in Pospeschill 2004.

[196] Chapter 3.2.5.1 is a largely adapted version of chapter 6.30 of my M.A. Thesis. See Maurer 2006/2009.

[197] For "multivariate cluster analysis" in statistics, see e.g. Everitt et al. 2001, Bacher et al. 2010, Gore, Jr. 2000, Kaufmann and Pape 1996, Hair et al. 2010, Backhaus et al. 2008, Bortz 1999, Marinell 1995, Litz 2000, Rinne 2000.
For "multivariate cluster analysis" in neuroinformatics and connectionism, see e.g. Brause 1995, Clark 1990, 2001, Bracholdt 2009.
For the geometric interpretation of multivariate cluster analysis, see e.g. Hair et al. 2010.

be real numbers, for example; the characteristic values thus obtained are summarized in an $N \times p$ data matrix:

$$
X = \begin{pmatrix} x_1' \\ \ldots \\ x_N' \end{pmatrix} = \begin{pmatrix} x_{11} & \ldots & x_{1p} \\ \ldots & \ldots & \ldots \\ x_{N1} & \ldots & x_{Np}. \end{pmatrix} \tag{3.21}
$$

Most methods form the classes in such a way that each object is a member of exactly one of g classes or clusters $C_1, ..., C_g$, so that such a disjoint class decomposition is called a "partition" $\mathfrak{C}$. (Kaufmann and Pape 1996).

In the present case, there are a set of data vectors that are understood as multivariate distributed random variables. The objects are combined in the form of vectors[198] in a multidimensional vector space according to their (dis-)similarity to an (often unknown) number of homogeneous groups, called "clusters".[199] This means that a group of vectors which have a minimum distance among themselves or in relation to a computed centroid are pooled. This distance is given as a metric (see Fig. 3.20), e.g. the "Euclidean distance"[200], which is generally defined as follows (see Fig. 3.19):

$$
d(x_i, x_j) = \|x_i - x_j\| = \sqrt{\sum_{k=1}^{m} (x_{ik} - x_{jk})^2}. \tag{3.22}
$$

The decisive factors for the result of a cluster analysis are therefore: (1) the choice of a proximity measure, i.e. a statistical (dis-)similarity measure (e.g. given in distance metrics), and (2) the choice of grouping procedures (given as fusion and partitioning algorithms[201]), with which one wants to achieve an optimal separation or fusion of the clusters. By combining several adjacent clusters into a new higher level cluster, a cluster hierarchy is formed whose tree structure is usually represented in a "dendrogram"[202] (see Fig. 3.21). A multivariate distribution exists when there is a common probability distribution of several statistical variables that must be correlated to each other.

---

[198]For the definition of a vector, see the introduction e.g. in Nolting 2016a, Fischer and Kaul 2011. With reference to connectionism, see e.g. Jordan 1986, Smolensky 1986c.

[199]In neuroinformatics one speaks of a "cluster" in the context of a "multivariate cluster analysis". This involves the determination of concentrations or accumulations of distributed vectors as points or point clouds in a multidimensional vector space, where the distance between the points within a cluster is smaller than the distance to points of other clusters.
See e.g. Brause 1995, Clark 1990, Calvo Garzón 2003, Shea 2007.

[200]For the term "Euclidean distance", see e.g. Haykin 1999, Kavouras and Kokla 2007. Another widely used distance measure for a metric variable structure is the "Minkowski metric". See e.g. Backhaus et al. 2008.

[201]Hierarchical grouping methods include, for example, the "Ward-Method", the "Single-Linkage-Method" and the "Complete-Linkage-Method".
See Hair et al. 2010, Backhaus et al. 2008, Bortz 1999.

[202]A "dendrogram" is a graphical representation of a classification process (in the context of "Multivaria(n)te Cluster Analysis (MCA]") in the form of a "tree graph." This tree graph illustrates the hierarchical structure of the individual clusters to each other by combining the cluster objects, step by step, in a hierarchical procedure, according to their distance relations.
See, for example, Hair et al. 2010, Bortz 1999.

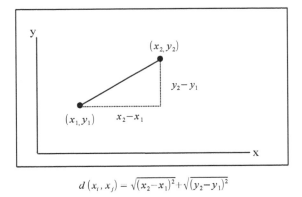

$$d\left(x_i, x_j\right) = \sqrt{\left(x_2 - x_1\right)^2} + \sqrt{\left(y_2 - y_1\right)^2}$$

Figure 3.19: Geometric interpretation of the concept of "Euclidean distance": Assuming that two 2-dimensional points are given in a coordinate system with the coordinates (x_1, y_1) and (x_2, y_2), the Euclidean distance between these two points is the length of the hypothenuse of a right-angled triangle, and is computed using the formula shown in the figure according to the Pythagorean Theorem (following Hair et al. 2010).

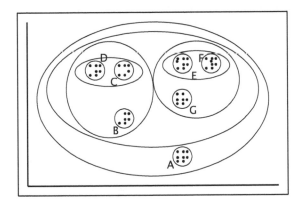

Figure 3.20: Schematic diagram of a cluster hierarchy (following Hair et al. 2010).

According to the American philosopher of science William Bechtel (1994), the holistic analysis of cluster analysis can reveal the structured classification of data properties and relationships. Thus, using real sensory data, a connectionist system could be understood as an "embodiment" of Fodor's "Representational Theory of Mind (RThM)". However, in this weak sense, the "intentional representations" of a connectionist system do not take the form of propositions or propositional attitudes, as these are typically understood in folk psychology. Nevertheless, according to Bechtel (1994) with reference to Bechtel and Abrahamsen (1993) (with reference to W.G. Lycan [1991] and D.C. Dennett [1978]) one can assume that mental representations and processes (including propositional attitudes) supervene on the "internal subpersonal operations". In contrast to the eliminativist positions of W. Ramsey, S.P. Stich and J. Garon (1990) as well as P.M. Churchland (1989), the connectionist

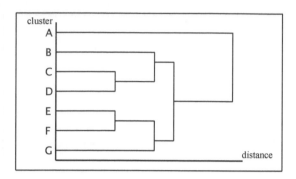

Figure 3.21: Schematic diagram of a dendrogram (following Hair et al. 2010).

paradigm (e.g. P. Smolensky's subsymbolic position) is compatible with the application of the intentional language used in folk psychology.

3.2.5.2   Parallel (Soft) Constraint Satisfaction Modeling[203]

The traditional mathematical methods[204] employed in Artificial Intelligence[205] (in relation to the so-called "Constraint Satisfaction Problem (CSP)"[206]) guarantee a consistent value assignment to the variables of a constraint network[207]. In contrast, in connectionism, mainly stochastic techniques are used within the context of problems of constraint optimization (Dechter and Rossi 2003, Guesgen and Hertzberg 1992). This is the case, for example, with the "Hopfield Network," or the "Boltzmann[208] machine"[209] with its learning method adapted to "Simulated Annealing" (Guesgen and Hertzberg 1992), which works with coherence standards instead of consistency

---

[203]This chapter 3.2.5.2 is a partially revised version of chapter 5.621 of my M.A. Thesis. See Maurer 2006/2009.

[204]For example, in logic programming, see e.g. Dechter and Rossi 2003.

[205]See e.g. Dechter 1999, Regier 2003, Dechter and Rossi 2003, Guesgen 2000, Guesgen and Hertzberg 1992.
See also Smith Churchland and Sejnowski 1992.

[206]For the exact definition of the term "constraint," see e.g. Lecoutre 2009.
A "constraint satisfaction problem (CSP)", consisting of a set of constraints or boundary conditions for a set of variables with their value ranges, is the task of finding combinations of assignments of values to variables that meet all conditions in terms of relations. These conditions are defined by subsets of variables, for which a multitude of (systematic) algorithms have been designed.
See e.g. Dechter and Rossi 2003, Guesgen 2000, Guesgen and Hertzberg 1992, Schmid and Kindsmüller 1996.

[207]For fundamental information, see e.g. Lecoutre 2009. For an exact definition of the term "Constraint Network", see e.g. Lecoutre 2009.

[208]Named after the Austrian physicist and philosopher, Ludwig Boltzmann.

[209]See e.g. Hinton and Sejnowski 1986, Hinton 1989.
See also, Guesgen and Hertzberg 1992, Guesgen 2000, Cottrell 2003.
For the recurrent network model of the "Boltzmann machine", see e.g. Zell 2003: In order to solve the problem of "Hopfield networks", which "often stabilize in a local minimum instead of in the desired global minimum", the Boltzmann machine uses "statistical methods in which the neurons change their

standards (see Box 3.2.5.2). The positive and negative relations between the variables are modeled using (non-linear) excitatory and inhibitory technical synapses (Simon and Holyoak 2002).

Box 3.2.5.2 Consistency vs. Coherence:

In mathematics and (mathematical) logic, the term "consistence" refers to the characteristic of an axiom system, e.g. a logical calculus, if there are no proven contradictions ("consistency"). In contrast, the concept of (stochastic) "coherence" (in the context of the theory of artificial neural networks, which knows no "hard" contradictions) is more likely to be understood in terms of "soft" constraint satisfaction (as far as possible), for example, when a value assignment to the variables which correspond to the neuronal vectors has a solution to the "Constraint Satisfaction Problem (CSP)" for a constraint net.

See e.g. Thagard 2000, 1989, Holyoak and Thagard 1989, Thagard and Verbeurgt 1998, Rumelhart et al. 1986c.

For an introduction to the mathematical and logical definition of consistency, see e.g. Bucher 1998, Guesgen 2000.

See also Kralemann 2006: "Solving coherence problems thus proves to be a highly feedback process of mutually presupposing relative conditions that structurally corresponds to the problem of solving a complex system of differential equations. Here, a set of functions is searched, whereby the only available information exists in relations between these functions and their derivatives. Whenever one wants to evaluate such a relation for the determination of one of these functions directly, one must already know the other functions, whose knowledge could be deduced, however, among other things only from the knowledge of those functions which one seeks to determine at the moment."

According to the American linguist and cognitive scientist Paul Smolensky[210] (in the context of a connectionist or sub-symbolic structural theory of cognition[211]), the computational processes in an artificial neural network can thus be interpreted as an optimization problem in the sense of "Parallel (Soft) Constraint Satisfaction Modeling"[212]. As already mentioned (see chap. 3.2.2, 3.2.3), a multidimensional system

---

state (...) randomly according to a probability distribution".
See also, Müller et al. 1995.

[210] See e.g. Smolensky 1988a.
Within the framework of the "Integrated Connectionist/Symbolic Cognitive Architecture (ICS)", P. Smolensky (1995) takes up the "Parallel Soft Constraint Satisfaction" model in conjunction with his "Harmony Theory", which is described in more detail in chap. 6.13 (3) and 10.2.

[211] For the term "subsymbol", see the explanations in chap. 6.1.1 and 3.2.2.

[212] For fundamental information, see e.g. Rumelhart et al. 1986c.
For an introduction, see e.g. Touretzky 2003, Guesgen and Hertzberg 1992.
See also, Bechtel and Abrahamsen 2002, Horgan and Tienson 1994a, Simon and Holyoak 2002, Thagard 2005.
See also, Read et al. 1997, who emphasize the similarities between the Parallel Constraint Satisfaction processes and the "Gestalt principles" of the "Gestalt psychology" of the twenties and thirties of the 20th century according to the psychologists Max Wertheimer, Wolfgang Köhler and Kurt Koffka.

state space is spanned using the architecture of an artificial neural network. The network connections and their weights represent the relationship between the differently weighted feature dimensions, and an input pattern is mapped to a point in this system state space given by a "distance metric" (see chap. 3.2.2, 3.2.5.1). The connections (given as a connection matrix) between the processing units can be understood as reciprocal "(soft) constraints" (Smolensky 1988a), which result from the structural properties of the input vectors and from the existing constraints. An artificial neural network is now – under certain conditions – striving to minimize its "energy function" (see chap. 3.2.3). That means that during the network training, in general, it is aiming to reach a state in which a high number of constraints are fulfilled as well as possible. The higher the number of fulfilled constraints, the lower the (artificial) "energy" of an artificial neural network (or the higher the "harmony") (Smolensky 1988a; see chap. 10.2). It is defined according to the general connectionist algorithm in terms of the "Lyapunov function" (see chap. 3.2.3):

$$E(t) = \sum_i \sum_j w_{ij} a_i(t) a_j(t), \tag{3.23}$$

$E(t)$ is the energy of the system at time t, w_{ij} the weight of the connection between the neurons i and j, $a_i(t)$, and $a_j(t)$ are the activation of the neuron $i(j)$ at time t (Rumelhart et al. 1986c, Thagard and Verbeurgt 1998, Read et al. 1997; see chap. 3.2.3).

The combination of elementary concepts towards more complex concepts within the framework of connectionist coherence algorithms can thus be identified with the computational process by which a network converges to the point which simultaneously fulfils as many constraints as possible (in the context of the "gradient descent method" [Smolensky 1988a; see chap. 3.2.5.3]) (Thagard and Verbeurgt 1998; see chap. 3.2.3). This continues, at least, until a relatively stable local minimum ("local coherence") or global minimum ("global coherence", where all current constraints are simultaneously fulfilled) of the energy function is reached. Thus, these constraints are "soft" because they do not have to be exhaustively fulfilled (such as axioms in a calculus of symbolic logic). Rather, these constraints only need to be fulfilled to a certain degree, i.e. with a certain probability (depending on the weighted probability transitions in the overall network). In other words, certain probability statements remain in the sub-symbolic, neuronal activities.

According to the German psychologist and philosopher, Thomas Goschke and the German philosopher of science, Dirk Koppelberg (1990a) with reference to Smolensky (1988a), the functioning of an artificial neural network can be understood by interpreting the neurons as microhypotheses. In this way, the degree of activation of the neurons can be understood as the measure of "confirmation" of such microhypotheses. Thus, Smolensky[213] postulates that the connection matrix can implement

---

Some of the traditional models in connectionism are, for example, the "ACME Model" by Holyoak and Thagard 1989, the "ECHO Model" by Thagard 1989, and the "DECO Model" by Thagard and Millgram 1995.

For a clear introduction, see Goschke and Koppelberg 1990a, Dorffner 1991, Romba 2001.

[213] For "The Structure/Statistics Dilemma", see Smolensky 1988b.
See also Smolensky 1988a, 1989a.

subsymbolic, statistical inference procedures by encoding the statistical structure relations of the input vectors, thereby extracting the relevant statistical information (see chap. 3.2.4.4, 3.2.4.5). At the subconceptual level, a cooperative process of a large number of "microinferences" (or "microconstraints")[214] takes place. On the conceptual level this is referred to as a "macroinference" (or "macroconstraint") in the form of an adaptation mechanism (from cognitive neuropsychology and evolutionary biology). According to the German philosopher Manuela Lenzen (2002), these microinferences correspond to the connection strengths between the computational units which establish the improbable or probable interrelationships between the "microfeatures" (see chap. 3.2.2). These can be coded by means of the sub-symbolic neuronal activities (the "sub-symbols" [see chap. 6.1.1, 3.2.2]). In my opinion (Maurer 2006/2009), however, it should be noted that the subsymbols as neuron activities in combination with the activation and propagation functions also encode the microfeatures as "static representation data". Furthermore, they participate as "dynamic representation processes" in the constantly changing determination of connection weights, interpreted as microdecisions. In other words, a subsymbol combines memory and computation units at the same time.

3.2.5.3 (Stochastic) Gradient Descent Method

The classical "gradient descent method"[215] in mathematics, also known as "steepest descent method"[216], is a direct numerical optimization method with the iterative form

$$x^{k+1} = x^k + \alpha_k \cdot d^k. \tag{3.24}$$

The step size at point x^k is α_k, d^k is the descent direction at point x^k, $x^1 = x^s$ is the starting point to be set, and, if the descent direction is selected in the form $d = - \operatorname{grad} f(x)$, the negative gradient of the function points in the direction of its steepest descent. This means that the function values decrease in this direction, i.e. one tries to approximately compute a (local) minimum of a given target function $f(x) = f(x_1, x_2, ..., x_n)$.

In connectionism, the "gradient descent method"[217] ("gradient descent learning" [Dawson and Medler 2010]) computes the gradient of an "error function" (see chap. 3.2.3). This means that when applying the training pattern, one tries to minimize the average "Least-Mean-Square (LMS) error" (Widrow and Stearns 1985, Haykin 1999, Bothe 1998) of the connection weight vectors between the expected and actual

---

[214] See e.g. Smolensky and Legendre 2006a. Smolensky (1988a) also describes this as "microdecisions" or "macrodecisions".

[215] For an extensive introduction, see e.g. Rey and Wender 2011, Bonnans et al. 2003, Bhatti 2000, Snyman and Wilke 2018, Fletcher 1987, Benker 2003, Hirsch and Smale 1974.

[216] See e.g. Bonnans et al. 2003, Bhatti 2000, Snyman and Wilke 2018, Benker 2003.

[217] For an essential paper, see e.g. Widrow and Hoff Jr. 1960, Widrow and Stearns 1985, Rosenblatt 1962, Rumelhart et al. 1986a, Hinton 1989.
For a beginner's guide, see e.g. Zell 2003, Bothe 1998, Müller et al. 1995, Graupe 2008, Sutton and Barto 1998.
See the remarks in chap. 3.2.3.
For the "stochastic gradient descent methods", see e.g. Engel and van den Broeck 2001, Bothe 1998.

output for all training patterns.[218] This is done by changing all connection weight vectors ΔW by a fraction of the negative gradient of the error function $-\nabla E(W)$ with a (learning) factor η, also called step size (Zell 2003):

$$\Delta W = \eta \nabla E(W). \tag{3.26}$$

The "delta rule," also known as "Widrow-Hoff rule"[219], can be derived from this error minimization function[220,221]:

$$\Delta w_{ij} = \eta o_i \delta_j = \eta o_i(t_j - o_j), \tag{3.27}$$

where δ_j is the difference between the current output o_j and the expected output t_j, the "teaching input".

3.2.5.4 Statistical Mechanics Analysis

The analytical method of statistical mechanics[222] deals with the statistical and probabilistic analysis of many-particle systems (so-called "canonical ensembles" or

---

[218]The total error E of the error function is therefore computed as follows:

$$E = 0.5 \sum_j (t_j - o_j)^2, \tag{3.25}$$

where t_j is the teaching input and o_j the neuron output j.
See, for example, Zell 2003.

[219]Named after the American electrical engineers Bernard Widrow and Marcian E. Hoff.
The first example of a gradient descent learning rule is, according to Widrow and Hoff Jr. (1960), the "α-LMS-Algorithm", which was developed for training an "Adaptive Linear Neuron (Adaline)", later also named as "adaptive linear combiner element".
See also, Widrow and Stearns 1985.
For an introduction, see e.g. Bothe 1998, Graupe 2008.
See also, the explanations in chap. 3.2.1.

[220]And thus also the general mathematical form of the "Hebb('s) rule".
See the explanations in chap. 3.2.1.

[221]For fundamental information, see e.g. Stone 1986.
For an introduction, see e.g. Zell 2003, Bothe 1998.
The "delta (learning) rule" is generally only used in the context of supervised learning procedures with networks that can be trained via a single neuron layer, whose technical neurons are equipped with a deterministic, linear activation function, such as the "Perceptron" by Frank Rosenblatt.
For the "perceptron learning rule", see e.g. Müller et al. 1995.
For the "perceptron convergence theorem", see Rosenblatt 1962.
See e.g. Haykin 1999.
A generalization of the delta rule, the "backpropagation (learning) rule", is used in multi-layer networks whose technical neurons are equipped with a non-linear activation function.
For a basic information on the backpropagation algorithm, see e.g. Werbos 1974, Rumelhart et al. 1986a.
For an introduction see, for example, Zell 2003, Kasabov 1998.
See the explanations in chap. 3.2.1 and 3.2.4.1.

[222]The analytical method of statistical mechanics is used in statistical physics, especially in the subdiscipline of statistical thermodynamics, based on the work of J.C. Maxwell, L. Boltzmann and J.W. Gibbs.
For a brief discussion, see e.g. Nolting 2017b, Reichl 2009, Schwabl 2006, Gerthsen 1999.
For a beginner's guide, see e.g. Kugler and Turvey 1987.
See also, the remarks in chap. 5.1.

"Gibbs ensembles"[223]) and their microscopic system states. The concept of (statistical) entropy (as put forward by L. Boltzmann) is of fundamental importance here:

$$S = -k_B \ln w \tag{3.28}$$

or

$$S = -k_B \sum_i w_i \ln w_i.^{224} \tag{3.29}$$

This method has been applied to the analysis of recurrent (artificial) neural networks.[225] For example, it has been applied to the convergence analysis of neuronal dynamics with respect to stationary attractors or oscillatory orbits in the context of the "energy function" (see chap. 3.2.3). This is especially so in the case of the Hopfield model (and its application as an associative memory [Amit et al. 1987, Sompolinsky 1988, Gutfreund 1990, Bovier and Gayrard 1997; see chap. 3.2.3, 3.2.5.2.]) and the Willshaw model (Sompolinsky 1988 with reference to Willshaw et al. 1969). Furthermore, it has been applied to the analysis of neural dynamics using neuronal (probabilistic) wave functions (Neelakanta and De Groff 1994), in which the eigenstate of the neuronal wave represents the neuronal information. And finally, it has been applied to the information theoretical analysis of stochastic aspects of a neural system (Neelakanta and De Groff 1994).

3.2.5.5 Attractor Modeling

The neuronal dynamics of a (recurrent) neural network can be analyzed in the context of stochastic optimization problems using convergent processes in the form of attractors ("attractor modeling") (Wang 2008; see chap. 3.2.5.2). This allows human "content-addressable memory" to be modelled as "attractor networks".[226] In relation to the Hopfield network (see chap. 3.2.4.3), for example, the fixed points result from the corresponding "energy function" (see chap. 3.2.3, 3.2.5.4) or the "Lyapunov function" (see chap. 3.2.3):

$$E(t) = -0.5 \sum_i \sum_j w_{ij} o_i(t) o_j(t) - \sum_j e_j o_j(t), \tag{3.30}$$

---

[223] A "(canonical) ensemble" or "Gibbs ensemble", named after the American physicist Josiah W. Gibbs, is an observed (many-particle) system with a fixed number of elements and a predetermined volume that is integrated into a system surrounding it, e.g. a heat bath, with which energy is exchanged via the heat reservoir and is in thermal equilibrium with it.
For an introduction, see e.g. Nolting 2017b, Reichl 2009, Schwabl 2006, Gerthsen 1999.
For a beginner's guide, see e.g. Prigogine and Stengers 1993, 1981/1993.

[224] See the remarks in chap. 5.1.

[225] For a detailed discussion, see e.g. Coolen 2001a, b, Engel and Van den Broeck 2001.
For a brief discussion, see e.g. Müller et al. 1995.
For a detailed overview, see e.g. Neelakanta and De Groff 1994.
See also, e.g. Zippelius 1993, Clark 1988.

[226] For a groundbreaking discussion, see e.g. Amit 1989.
For an fundamental discussion, see e.g. Coolen 2001a, b, Gutfreund 1990.
For a brief discussion, see e.g. Cottrell 2003, 2016, Brunel and Nadal 1998.
See the remarks in chap. 3.2.5.4 and Kap. 3.2.7.

wherein $E(t)$ represents the energy of the Hopfield network at time t, w_{ij} the weight of the connection between the neurons i and j, $o_i(t)$ and $o_j(t)$ represent the output of the neuron $i(j)$ at time t. The variable e_j represents the external input into the neuron j (Amit 1989, Petitot 2011). This input is assumed to be constant during the time interval of the measurement.

3.2.6 CONNECTIONISM AND DYNAMICAL SYSTEMS THEORY

According to D. Marr's methodological analysis (see chap. 1.3), the mathematical model of an artificial neural network (in the context of the theory of [nonlinear] dynamic systems) is analyzed at the algorithmic level (Kosko 1992; see chap. 1.4, 2., 3.2.3). This is done by considering the activation and propagation functions, the learning rules (as transformation functions), and the activation values of the technical neurons or the connection weights of the technical synapses (as state vectors of an n-dimensional state space). These vectors can form stable and asymptotic system states in the form of attractors (with time as iteration index), by means of an internal self-organized system dynamics (see chap. 2.2, 7). A large number of authors in connectionism point this out, e.g. P. Smolensky (1988a), F. Pasemann (1995), J.F. Elman (1998, 2005, Elman et al. 1998), Cosmelli et al. (2007), W. Tabor (2009), M.S.C. Thomas et al. (2009), J.L. McClelland et al. (2010), J. Petitot (2011), and C. von der Malsburg (2018). Attempts are increasingly being made to merge the connectionist models with the approach of dynamic systems theory. These attempts come, not only from neuroinformatics and connectionism (see chap. 3.2.4.4, 3.2.4.5, 6, 7, 8, 10), but also recently from developmental psychology (Spencer et al. 2009c, McClelland and Vallabha 2009, Schöner 2009). For example, this has been attempted by the American development psychologists, Esther Thelen and Linda B. Smith, since the 1990s (through their "Dynamic Systems Approach"[227]), and the subsequent "Dynamic Field Approach"[228] of the American psychologist, John P. Spencer and the German neuroinformatician, Gregor Schöner (see chap. 11.2.1). Furthermore, an approximation of dynamic systems theory and connectionism is carried out via "Evolutionary Robotics" (Nolfi and Floreano 2001, Schlesinger 2009, Rohde 2013) and "Developmental Robotics" (Lungarella et al. 2003, Weng et al. 2001, Schlesinger 2009) in connection with the mathematical method of "Evolutionary Computation (EC)" (Wiles and Hallinan 2003, Schlesinger 2004). For an example, see the work of the American developmental psychologist, Matthew Schlesinger.[229]

---

[227]For a grounbreaking paper, see e.g. Thelen and Smith 1993.
For a fundamental paper, see e.g. Thelen and Bates 2003, Thelen 1995, Smith and Samuelson 2003.
For an introduction, see e.g. Thelen and Smith 2006, Wicki 2010, Petermann et al. 2004.
For a beginner's guide, see e.g. Bermúdez 2014.

[228]For an fundamental discussion, see e.g. Spencer and Schöner 2003, Spencer et al. 2009a, b, Johnson et al. 2009.
For an introduction, see e.g. Schöner 2009, 2008, Calvo Garzón 2008.

[229]For an detailed discussion, see e.g. Schlesinger and Parisi 2001, Schlesinger 2003, 2004.
For an introduction, see e.g. Schlesinger 2009, Schlesinger and Parisi 2007.

3.2.7 POSITIVE MOTIVATION FOR CONNECTIONISM

The main appeal of the connectionist paradigm lies in its "neural plausibility" (or "biological and psychological plausibility").[230] Its "inductive" and case-related information processing of artificial neural networks corresponds, in particular, much more closely with the learning behavior of the human brain than a "deductive", rule-based or rule-driven information processing model. In other words, there is an undeniably high structural and functional equivalence between the performances of certain connectionist architectural models and human cognition.

According to prevailing opinion in the literature[231], this argument is presented as an essential justification for connectionism, and underpinned with the following main positive features of artificial neural networks[232]:

1. Dynamical, self-organizing and adaptive learning ability:
   A connectionist network functions without an external global control function[233] (with the exception of a predefined set of input data and the targeted provision of output data as part of supervised learning [see chap. 3.2.1]). This is in contrast to the classic symbolic AI systems. In comparison to these, the connectionist network offers the advantageous ability to adapt one's own system behavior variably and flexibly to the changing presentation of data structures. In addition, unsupervised learning (see chap. 3.2.1) enables independent learning of a task and an appropriate deduction of regular behaviour ("self-organization") (see chap. 2.3, 3.2, 4.4, 3.2.4.5). In other words, a network "learns from experience".

2. High degree of graceful degradation:
   A connectionist model, like humans, can deal with "noisy", incomplete, inaccurate, conflicting and otherwise disturbed or faulty data ("resistance to noise" [McClelland et al. 1986]). This is in contrast with symbolic AI systems, which require clear, complete and error-free data input. Alternatively, a connectionist model can compensate for the failure of individual processing units by means of a continuous performance degradation. That is, the model can still provide useful results by means of gradual compensation ("graceful degradation" [McClelland et al. 1986]).

---

[230]For a detailed discussion, see e.g. Thomas and McClelland 2008, Bechtel and Abrahamsen 2002, 1991, Dorffner 1997.
For an introduction, see e.g. Thagard 2005.
With a restriction, see e.g. Thomas and McClelland 2008, Bechtel and Abrahamsen 2002, Clark 2001, Berkeley 1997.

[231]See Barnden and Chady 2003, Bechtel and Abrahamsen 1991, Horgan and Tienson 1994a, Dorffner 1991, 1997, Helm 1991, Keller 1990.
A very good summary, which is followed in essence, can be found in Romba 2001.

[232]Only the most important main features are listed here; for an exhaustive discussion, reference is made to the literature in chap. 3.2.9.
Furthermore, the feature of the so-called "Parallel Soft Constraint Satisfaction" is discussed in detail in chap. 3.2.5.2.

[233]However, the system parameters, such as the learning rate, and the network architecture of an artificial neural network still have to be adjusted "externally".

3. Distributed ("holistic") and active information representation, with massively parallel information processing:

   In the symbolic AI systems, an active component (the program) accesses a passive representation (the data). In contrast, connectionistic models have an active representation that is directly involved in the information processing procedure. The overall activation pattern of the network is changing continuously and in parallel due to the simultaneous and mutual influence of the network units via weighted and directed connections in which "knowledge" is stored in distributed form (McClelland et al. 1986, Romba 2001, Dorffner 1991). The entire network is the knowledge structure or information structure (McClelland et al. 1986). This is why it achieves a low susceptibility to interference in the event of a failure of individual processing units, and it is actively involved in data interpretation.

4. Associative, classifying and generalizing information storage with "hypothesis formation" and "hypothesis testing":

   Symbolic AI systems store and call up information in an address-oriented manner. In contrast, the information in a connectionist model is stored content-relatedly ("content-addressable memory" [McClelland et al. 1986, Bechtel and Abrahamsen 1991], "content-based access" [Barnden and Chady 2003]) or associatively ("associative access"). It therefore acquires the ability of "mapping" a given input pattern to a corresponding output pattern, whereby the input and output patterns to be generated are either identical ("auto-association") or different ("hetero-association"). The latter are used for the simulation of categorization, generalization and inference performances, as well as for "hypothesis formation" and "hypothesis testing" ("default assignment", "spontaneous generalization"). The former are used for pattern recognition, pattern completion ("completion task"), and error correction (McClelland et al. 1986).

3.2.8   CRITICISM OF CONNECTIONISM

In the context of the "symbolism vs. connectionism debate", there has now also been fierce criticism of connectionism and the models of connectionist artificial intelligence by the Symbolists.[234] For this reason, the most important arguments are only briefly mentioned here:

1. the insufficient explanation of cognition, due to the lack of a combinatorial syntax and semantics of mental representations and structure-sensitive processes in connectionist models,
2. the difficult "controllability" of complex artificial neural networks due to their lack of transparency,

---

[234] For an overview of the topic, see e.g. Eliasmith and Bechtel 2003, Mangold 1996, Clark 2001, Berkeley 1997, Quinlan 1991, Romba 2001.
See also, Levelt 1991, Strube 1990, McCloskey 1991.
For a detailed discussion, see e.g. Maurer 2006/2009.

3. the slowness of most common connectionist learning methods,
4. insufficient performance in the realization of logical sequential inferences,
5. the restriction of connectionist models to narrowly defined cognitive performances, and the pre-selection of data material already prepared within the scope of a task well defined by the experimenter,
6. the lack of size of the connectionist network architectures and its abstract distance to biological neural networks,
7. the inability of artificial neural networks to learn certain data or the superimposition of already learned patterns during the new learning process ("catastrophic forgetting" [French 2003]), and
8. the limited generalization performance of connectionist models.

4 Integrative Synchronization Mechanisms and Models in the Cognitive Neurosciences

The first part of this chapter provides a brief overview of the experimental methods and techniques in the cognitive neurosciences (chap. 4.1). The methodological principles and schemes of neural coding are then discussed (chap. 4.2), in particular, the schemes of temporal and population coding on which the temporal synchronization hypothesis is based. According to this hypothesis, precise temporal correlations between the impulses of neurons and stimulus-dependent temporal synchronizations of the coherent activity of neuronal populations contribute to solving the general binding problem. After the general binding problem has been explained (chap. 4.3), the most important empirical-experimental models in perception and cognitive neuropsychology, in medical neurophysiology and in cognitive neurobiology are presented, focusing in paticular on dynamic binding models. This means, that those approaches that assume temporal integrative synchronization mechanisms for solving the binding problem (by means of the temporal synchronization of neuronal phase activity of a population of neurons) are presented. This is based on the dynamic, self-organizing processes in the corresponding neural networks. Finally, feature binding in visual perception by means of the integrative neural synchronization mechanisms is discussed in more detail. This is done with reference to the Binding-by-Synchrony Hypothesis put forward by W. Singer, A.K. Engel and P. König et al. This hypothesis thematizes the binding problem with reference to visual information processing in the context of integrative synchronization mechanisms in visual scene analysis (chap. 4.4).

4.1 EXPERIMENTAL METHODS AND TECHNIQUES IN THE COGNITIVE NEUROSCIENCES

A variety of experimental methods and techniques have been developed, since the 1970s, to obtain empirical data on the structure and functioning of the neuronal system. It is therefore beneficial to provide a brief introductory overview of these[235]:

(1) The methods of experimental "electrophysiology"[236] (on animals) in medical neurophysiology describe the electrical activity of neurons by using (micro-)-electrodes to derive the action potentials from individual neurons, mostly extracellular ("single-cell recording").[237] Another option is the simultaneous detection of the summed and averaged, extracellularly registered signals from multiple neurons in the form of "Local Field Potentials (LFP)"[238] ("multiunit recording").[239]

(2) The methods of "clinical electrophysiology"[240] in neurology are "Electroencephalography (EEG)", "Electroneurography (ENG)", "Electromyography (EMG)", "Magnetoencephalography (MEG)" and the techniques of EEG- and MEG data analysis, the "Event-Related Potential (ERP)".

(3) The most important methods of "neuroimaging"[241] are the "Computed/Computerized Tomography (CT)", "(functional) Magnetic Resonance Imaging ((f)MRI)", "Positron Emission Tomography (PET)" and "Magnetic Resonance Spectroscopy (MRS)".

(4) The most important of the (magnetic and electrical) stimulation methods ("brain stimulation techniques")[242] is "Transcranial Magnetic Stimulation (TMS)".

4.2 METHODICAL PRINCIPLES AND SCHEMATA OF THE NEURONAL CODING IN THE COGNITIVE NEUROSCIENCES

Starting from the electrical activity of a neuron (an "action potential", or in simple terms, "spike") (see chap. 3.2.1), or a sequence of action potentials ("(neuronal) spike

---

[235]The overview is primarily oriented towards Gazzaniga et al. 2018, Purves et al. 2013, Kolb and Whishaw 2015, Pinel et al. 2018, Büchel et al. 2012, Mareschal et al. 2007.

[236]For an introduction, see e.g. Jäncke 2017, Gazzaniga et al. 2018, Purves et al. 2013, Büchel et al. 2012, Pinel et al. 2018.
For a detailed discussion, see e.g. Abeles 1994.

[237]See e.g. Gazzaniga et al. 2018, Kolb and Whishaw 2015, Bear et al. 2016, Kandel et al. 2013, Büchel et al. 2012, Breedlove et al. 2017.

[238]For a detailed discussion, see Csicsvari et al. 2003, Katzner et al. 2009, Engel et al. 1990a.
For an introduction, see e.g. Quian Quiroga and Panzeri 2009.

[239]See e.g. Gazzaniga et al. 2018.
For a detailed overview of the statistical methods of neural data analysis of action potential sequences, so-called "spike trains", see e.g. Brown et al. 2004.
See also the remarks in chap. 4.2.

[240]For an introduction, see e.g. Jäncke 2017, Kolb and Whishaw 2015, Gazzaniga et al. 2018, Purves et al. 2013, Büchel et al. 2012, Pinel et al. 2018, Bressler 2003.

[241]For an introduction, see e.g. Jäncke 2017, Büchel et al. 2012, Gazzaniga et al. 2018, Purves et al. 2013, Kolb and Whishaw 2015, Pinel et al. 2018.

[242]For an introduction, see e.g. Gazzaniga et al. 2018, Büchel et al. 2012, Purves et al. 2013, Kolb and Whishaw 2015, Pinel et al. 2018.

train"), one of the fundamental questions in cognitive neuroscience is that of "neuronal coding"[243]: Which "(neuronal) code" should be used to represent and transform the neuronal information in the neuronal system? This includes the associated mathematical analysis within the framework of "theoretical and computational neuroscience" (Dayan and Abbott 2001, Rieke et al. 1997, Gerstner and Kistler 2002), e.g. statistical, probabilistic and stochastic methods (Brown et al. 2004, Abeles 1994, Rieke et al. 1997). There is an ongoing debate[244] in the neurosciences about which methodical coding scheme is preferable. The discussion initially focused on the traditional scheme, under which the relevant information is contained in the mean fire rate of a neuron. In the last two decades, however, mounting empirical evidence seems to suggest that precise temporal correlations between neuron impulses, and stimulus-dependent synchronizations of the activity of neuronal populations also contribute to neuronal information being adequately structured or encoded. The different schemes and strategies of neuronal coding will be discussed here.

4.2.1 (EN-)CODING ANALYSIS VS. DECODING ANALYSIS

First of all, it should be noted that there are two complementary perspectives from which to approach neural coding (Trappenberg 2010, Brown et al. 2004, Eliasmith 2009). One can approach neural coding from the analysis of the "encoding process" (Dayan and Abbott 2001, Rieke et al. 1997). This describes the response of one or more neurons as a function of certain physical environment variables, the "stimulus", using the generation of neural action potentials (Dayan and Abbott 2001, Brown et al. 2004). Alternatively, one can approach neural coding from the analysis of the "decoding process" (Dayan and Abbott 2001, Rieke et al. 1997). This describes the (estimated) reconstruction of the originally coded stimulus (or specific aspects thereof) from a sequence of action potentials using decoding algorithms (at least, in principle).

4.2.2 SCHEME 1: FREQUENCY CODING

The classical (statistical) coding strategy is to assume that the relevant information, i.e. the degree of intensity of a stimulus or signal, is contained in the (mean) firing rate of a neuron ("[mean] firing rate coding").[245] The definition of the mean fire rate

---

[243]For the term "spike", see e.g. Abeles 1994.
For the terms "spike" and "(neur(-on-)al) spike train" see e.g. Shadlen 2003, Gerstner and Kistler 2002.
For a fundamental discussion, see e.g. Perkel and Bullock 1968b, a.
For an introduction, see e.g. Dayan and Abbott 2001.
See also Gerstner and Kistler 2002, Rieke et al. 1997, Purves et al. 2013.
For a historical overview, see e.g. Rieke et al. 1997, pp. 2-13.

[244]For an introduction, see e.g. Shadlen 2003, von der Malsburg 2001, Sougné 2003, Eliasmith 2009.
See also Gerstner and Kistler 2002, Rieke et al. 1997.
For a detailed discussion, see e.g. Bialek et al. 1991, Abeles 1994, Shadlen and Newsome 1994, Hopfield 1995, Softky 1995, Friston 1997, Oram et al. 1999, Stein et al. 2005.

[245]For a fundamental discussion, see e.g. Adrian and Zotterman 1926, Hubel and Wiesel 1959.
For an introduction, see e.g. Gabbiani 2003, Shadlen 2003, Kandel et al. 2013.
See also Gerstner and Kistler 2002, Rieke et al. 1997.

ν is thus obtained (Gerstner and Kistler 2002):

$$\nu = \frac{n_{sp}(T)}{T}, \tag{4.1}$$

where T describes a time interval in which the number of action potentials or spikes n_{sp} of a neuron are counted.

This mean is based on the number of counted spikes in a certain time interval, usually 100 milliseconds ("spike-count rate coding") (Gerstner and Kistler 2002). This means that the information is basically coded by the frequency of a neuron ("frequency coding") (Hölscher 2009). The same stimulation can be repeated several times, and then recorded in a "Peri-Stimulus-Time Histogram (PSTH)"[246] ("spike-density rate coding" or "time-dependent firing rate coding") (Gerstner and Kistler 2002). The identity of a stimulus is encoded by the position of the neurons in the cortex ("place coding"), and by very specific projection tracts or by "labeled lines" ("labeled-line coding") towards these positions (Shadlen 2003, Bear et al. 2016, Hölscher 2009, Singer et al. 1997).

4.2.3 SCHEME 2: TEMPORAL CODING

For several decades, there has been mounting evidence that rapidly alternating changes in the temporal sequence of action potentials are important for coding certain aspects of neuronal information ("temporal (en-)coding").[247] Such evidence includes, for example, a certain temporal pattern of the intervals between the individual action potentials ("spike bar code" or "interspike interval code") (Shadlen 2003, Stein et al. 2005), the temporal change of the fire rate in a sequence of action potentials ("rate waveform code") (Shadlen 2003), and the temporal occurrence of a certain action potential after the presentation of a new stimulus ("delay coding") (Gerstner and Kistler 2002, Kostal et al. 2007) or in relation to a periodic signal, e.g. an oscillation ("phase coding") (Gerstner and Kistler 2002, Hölscher 2009, Montemurro et al. 2008).

In addition, there is increasing evidence to suggest that precise temporal correlations between the impulses of neurons (Abeles 1994, Lestienne 1996) and stimulus-dependent temporal synchronizations of the coherent activity of neuronal populations, the "assemblies", contribute to solving the (general) binding problem using the

---

For a critique of the concept of "(mean) firing rate coding", see e.g. Bialek et al. 1991, Abeles 1994, Shadlen and Newsome 1994, Hopfield 1995, Softky 1995, Oram et al. 1999, Stein et al. 2005, von der Malsburg 2001.
In the case of dynamic signals that change over time, however, information is encoded using the (instantaneous) fire rate of a neuron that changes over time ("time-varying rate coding" or "instantaneous rate coding"). This coding scheme should already be understood as "temporal coding".
See e.g. Shadlen 2003, Gabbiani 2003.
See also the remarks in chap. 4.2.3.

[246]Concerning the "(Joint) Peri-Stimulus-Time Histogram ((J)PSTH)", see e.g. Brown et al. 2004.

[247]For an introduction, see e.g. Bear et al. 2016, Dayan and Abbott 2001.
See also, Gerstner and Kistler 2002, Rieke et al. 1997, Hölscher 2009.
For a detailed discussion, see e.g. Abeles 1994, Shadlen and Newsome 1998, Stein et al. 2005, Theunissen and Miller 1995.

"Binding-By-Synchrony (BBS) Hypothesis" (which is discussed in detail in chapters 4.3. and 4.4).

4.2.4   SCHEME 3: POPULATION CODING

In contrast to the classical frequency coding strategy, which was initially developed using measurements of neural activity on individual neurons only ("single-cell coding"), the "(ensemble) population coding"[248] states that stimulus information is encoded using the joint activities of an entire group of neurons. An individual neuron in the population prefers to selectively respond to a specific stimulus feature, but the statistical activity distribution functions of the individual neurons overlap. Thus, not necessarily all, but only a limited number of neurons respond to a certain stimulus feature.

(1) In experiments on rhesus monkeys, A.P. Georgopoulos et al.[249] have shown that each neuron in the motor cortex seems to encode a preferred movement direction of an arm, but the coding of this direction is weakly selective. A certain direction of movement can only be determined by the joint activity of a neuron population, and an arm's direction of movement can be predicted during decoding using the "(neuronal) population vector" (Georgopoulos et al. 1988, 1983, 1986, 1989). This is achieved by multiplying the fire rates of the neurons in the motor cortex by their preferred direction of movement and then vectorially summing the data over the corresponding population of motor neurons ("population rate coding") (Pipa 2006).

(2) In contrast, for S.J. Thorpe et al.[250], the temporal ranking of the activity of each individual neuron is decisive for information coding. By basing the asynchronous activities of a neuron population with respect to the time of stimulus presentation, the neuron is assigned a higher rank as a function of its activation ("population rank coding") (Pipa 2006), which first generates an action potential relative to the others in the population.

(3) In addition, as already mentioned (see chap. 4.2.3), there is increasing evidence suggesting that stimulus-dependent temporal synchronizations of the coherent activity of neuronal populations solve the (general) binding problem in the context of the "Binding-By-Synchrony (BBS) Hypothesis" (see chap. 4.4).

---

[248]For fundamental information, see e.g. Hebb (1949), who, in 1949, had already formulated the hypothesis that the neurons join together to form cell assemblies, which are to be regarded as functional units of neuronal information processing.
For an introduction, see e.g. Pouget and Latham 2003, who mainly discuss information-theoretical decoding techniques; Dayan and Abbott 2001, Bear et al. 2016.
See also, Gerstner and Kistler 2002, Hölscher 2009, Quian Quiroga and Panzeri 2009, Pipa 2006.
For a historical overview of population coding, see e.g. McIlwain 2001.

[249]For fundamental information, see e.g. Georgopoulos et al. 1982, 1983, 1986, 1988, 1989.
For an introduction, see e.g. Amirikian and Georgopolous 2003, Bear et al. 2016, Gazzaniga et al. 2018, Eliasmith 2009.
See also, Dilger 2003/2004, Gerstner and Kistler 2002, Rieke et al. 1997.

[250]See e.g. Gautrais and Thorpe 1998, Delorme et al. 2001, Van Rullen and Thorpe 2001, Van Rullen et al. 2005.

Following classical coding strategy with regard to the representation of relations of properties of perceptual objects ("combination coding"), "conjunction-specific (binding) neurons" (also called "elaborate cells") at higher processing levels receive convergent signal inputs of neurons at lower processing levels in different constellations (Singer 1999b, Reid and Alonso 1995, Chapman et al. 1991, Jagadeesh et al. 1993, Tanaka et al. 1991). Thus, feature binding is achieved by means of temporal signal convergence in the context of hard-wired projection tracts ("labeled-line coding") (see chap. 4.2.2). In contrast to this, based on D.O. Hebb (1949), a parallel coding strategy, according to which recurrently and reciprocally linked overlapping cell groups guarantee a dynamic and context-dependent association of neurons (Bear et al. 2016) is postulated. This creates functionally coherent assemblies[251] on the basis of their synchronous activity.[252]

(4) However, if a definite assignment of two or more perceptual objects, which are presented simultaneously, has to be made in the context of the binding problem, the classical coding strategy of "(Local)[253] Conjunctive (En-)Coding"[254] is (still) applied in a large number of cases. According to this, a single neuron that does not overlap with other neurons represents every possible combination or conjunction of information elements, such as objects and object features. However, this is usually very inefficient (Plate 2003a, Köhle 1990).

(5) A higher degree of efficiency is achieved with the coding strategy of "Coarse Coding"[255]. Here, each neuron of an assembly is represented by a circular region, with radius r (which indicates its receptive field [see chap. 4.4.2]). A point in the k-dimensional data set is represented by a plurality of overlapping regions n, where an increase in the radius of the regions increases the accuracy a of the coding:

$$a \propto nr^{k-1}. \tag{4.2}$$

4.2.5   APPENDIX: SPARSE CODING

An extremely important characteristic of the analysis of the neural code is to determine the proportion of neurons active in a population at a certain time ("activity ratio") (Földiák 2003). This is called "Sparse Coding"[256], if an information element

---

[251] See e.g. Palm 1990, 1982, Gerstein et al. 1989, von der Malsburg 1986, Braitenberg 1978. The advantages of "assembly coding" are discussed in detail in Sakurai 1999.

[252] See e.g. Singer 2003a, 1999b, Singer et al. 1997, Phillips and Singer 1997. See also, Maye and Engel 2012, Engel 1996a. For an introduction, see e.g. Peters and Payne 2002.

[253] This technique can also be applied to distributed representations.

[254] For an detailed discussion, see e.g. Hinton et al. 1986. For an introduction, see e.g. Plate 2003a, Köhle 1990.

[255] For an detailed discussion, see e.g. Hinton et al. 1986. For an introduction, see e.g. Plate 2003a, Köhle 1990. See also, Maye 2002.

[256] For an introduction, see e.g. Földiák 2003, Plate 2003a, Dayan and Abbott 2001. See also, Rieke et al. 1997, Trappenberg 2010.

is represented by a relatively small (sub-)set of (strongly) activated neurons. That is, if the neural representation shows a low degree of density (Plate 2003a), e.g. "local codes" (see chap. 3.2.2) or "dense distributed or 'holographic' codes." (Földiák 2003; see chap. 6.2).

4.3 GENERAL BINDING PROBLEM AND INTEGRATIVE NEURONAL SYNCHRONIZATION MECHANISMS IN THE COGNITIVE NEUROSCIENCES

The "(general) binding problem"[257] comprises a class of perceptual and cognitive problems in neurophysiology, perception psychology, cognitive (neuro-)psychology, and cognitive neurobiology. A neurocognitive system, e.g. the human brain or a theoretical model thereof[258], has to encode or represent conjunctions of informational components either within the framework of static binding models[259] or dynamic binding models (Singer 1999b; see chap. 4.4) (see Box 4.3).

The (general) binding problem arises in the most basic perceptual representations ("perceptual binding problems") such as a visual object ("feature binding"), up to the most complex cognitive representations ("cognitive binding problems"), such as a compositional symbol structure ("variable binding").[260] The immense combinatorial problems associated require efficient, dynamic and integrative binding mechanisms. These mechanisms describe how the neuronal information processes that simultaneously occur in spatially separated (sub-)cortical areas are coordinated and bound together to produce coherent perceptual and cognitive (symbolic) representations and appropriate motor activity. One candidate for solving this general binding problem is the assumption of temporal integrative synchronization mechanisms. This means that one of the coordinating mechanisms seems to be the temporal synchronization of neuronal (phase) activity

---

See the remarks in chap. 3.2.2.

[257]For an introduction, see e.g. Burwick 2014, Feldman 2013, Hardcastle 1998, Sougné 2003, Singer 1999a, von der Malsburg 2001, Hummel 1999, Holcombe 2010, Maurer 2016.
For an overview, see e.g. von der Malsburg 1999, Treisman 1996, 1999, Engel 1996a, Herrmann 2002, Bennett and Hacker 2008.
For a beginner's guide, see e.g. Engel 2012, Engel and König 1998, Engel and König 1996, Engel et al. 1993, Schechter 1996, Roskies 1999, Goebel 1994.
For detailed information, see Maurer 2014a, 2016, 2018.

[258]For the theoretical models in connectionism and the binding problem, see the remarks in chap. 6-10.

[259]See e.g. Hubel and Wiesel 1965, with their higher-order hyper-complex cells, Barlow 1972, with his "cardinal cells" or Riesenhuber and Poggio 1999a with their "simple hierarchical feed-forward architecture", consisting of "simple cells", "complex cells", "composite feature cells", "complex composite cells" and "view-tuned cells" as a model of translation-invariant object recognition.
See in detail the explanations in chap. 4.2, 4.4.

[260]For an introduction, see e.g. Roskies 1999, Fuster 2003, Singer 2009, Treisman 1998, Maye and Werning 2007, Roskies 1999, Engel 1996a, Sougné 2003, Hummel 1999, von der Malsburg 1995b.
See also, Bechtel and Abrahamsen 1991.
See the remarks in chap. 6.

of a population of neurons, based on dynamic, self-organizing processes in the corresponding neuronal networks.[261]

Box 4.3   Neural Binding Strategies:

There are two complementary binding strategies in neural coding theory. On the one hand, there is the strategy that the neuronal activities are bound together via the progressive convergence of axonal projection tracts to the next highest information processing layers. For example, using "(hyper-)complex cells" in the primary visual area V1, in the secondary visual area V2 and in Brodmann area 19 (V3) ("binding by convergence", "binding by conjunction cells" or "static binding"). On the other hand, there is the strategy that the information about a more flexible combination of features is contained in the dynamic-temporal configuration of the response properties of a group of distributed neuron populations ("dynamic binding").
See e.g. Singer 1999b, 2002e. See also e.g. Tacca 2010, Maye 2002. See the remarks in chap. 4.2 and 4.4.

---

(1) In neuroinformatics, the German neuroinformatician Christoph von der Malsburg's "correlation theory of brain function"[262] had already suggested in the 1970s and 1980s, that "synaptic modulation" depends on the correlated activity of pre- and post-synaptic neurons (von der Malsburg 1981). This means that if different neurons encoding the simultaneous occurrence of a signal feature are synchronously coactivated over a period of a few milliseconds[263], the weighted coupling of the synapses between these neurons is amplified. This leads to the formation of an assembly of these neurons, called a "correlate" via self-reinforcing, positive feedback mechanisms. In this way, the binding problem can be solved with temporal correlation of the synchronous activity of various neurons on the basis of self-organization in an artificial topological network.[264]

---

[261] See e.g. Engel et al. 1992, Singer 1993, 1990, von der Malsburg 1981, 1986.
See also, Abeles 1991, 1982a, Gerstein et al. 1989, Palm 1982, 1990, Braitenberg 1978, Grossberg 1980, Edelman 1987.
For an overview of the phenomenon of synchronization in neuronal systems, see e.g. Pikovsky et al. 2001.
For general information on the topic of the physiological rhythmic process, see e.g. Glass 2001.

[262] For an essential paper, see von der Malsburg 1981.
For a brief discussion, see e.g. von der Malsburg 2001, Maye and Engel 2012, Maye 2002.
The correlation theory by von der Malsburg is applied in a study on the so-called "Cocktail Party Effect".
See von der Malsburg and Schneider 1986.

[263] These synaptic modifications, taking place in very short periods of time on the time scale of a short-term memory, can then be converted into a long-lasting weight change at the synapses in the sense of Hebb's synaptic plasticity ("[refined] synaptic plasticity"), which would correspond to a long-term memory.
See von der Malsburg 1981.

[264] See e.g. von der Malsburg 1981, in which he emphasizes the analogy to other self-organizing system models, e.g. that of H. Haken's synergetics.
For a more extensive discussion, see e.g. von der Malsburg 2003a.
See also, von der Malsburg 1973, 1990, 1995c, 2002b, von der Malsburg and Willshaw 1976, von der Malsburg and Singer 1988, Wiskott and von der Malsburg 1999, Triesch and von der Malsburg 2001.

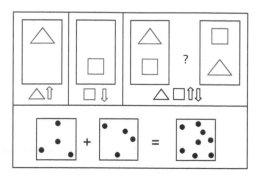

Figure 4.1: Schematic representation of the "superposition catastrophe"[265] in the sense of F. Rosenblatt: For simplicity, this assumes a visual perception system whose neural network consists of four neurons. In this network, two neurons recognize a certain object, e.g. a triangle or a square. The other two neurons can indicate the position of the object in question, e.g. if it is in the upper or lower half of the image. If only *one* object is shown, a clear assignment can be made, e.g. '(triangle, top)' or '(rectangle, bottom)', while a binding problem occurs if two objects are presented simultaneously (following von der Malsburg 1999 with reference to Rosenblatt 1962).

In the meantime, as von der Malsburg describes in his review paper (1999; 1995b), the temporal synchronisation mechanism has been successfully applied to a multitude of binding problems. For instance, it has been successfully applied to the following topics: "(...) logical reasoning, figure-ground segregation in the visual, auditory and olfactory modalities, and in invariant object recognition" (von der Malsburg 2001) avoiding, in particular, the "superposition catastrophe"[265] according to F. Rosenblatt (see Fig. 4.1).

For self-organization in neural systems, see e.g. Willshaw 2006.

See also the remarks in chap. 2.3.

The structure of the network is described in von der Malsburg 1981.

[265]The general binding problem with respect to perception can be adequately solved only if the "superposition catastrophe" (see F. Rosenblatt (1962)) is avoided (see Fig. 4.1). The fundamental difficulty is to (co-)activate two sensory objects presented at the same time, each of which is encoded or represented in the same mental operation by a set of neurons (in the meaning of an assembly). However, this coactivation must not lead to a intermixing pattern superposition in information coding by the two neuron populations. This would not allow the information related to a particular object component to be adequately filtered out of a sensory compound, e.g. a visual scene, which would be necessary for this compound to be analyzed into its object components. In other words, the information of the set assignment in relation to the two given, simultaneously activated sets of neurons would be lost.

In the example of Fig. 4.1, the assignment of the two objects to their respective positions would be unclear, since the simultaneous (co-)activation of '(triangle, square, top, bottom)' could be interpreted as either the assignment '(triangle, top)' and '(square, bottom)', or vice versa '(triangle, bottom)' and '(square, top)' (shown in the upper half of the figure). For the sake of simplicity, assuming that the activity of an assembly of two neurons could encode a particular object or the respective position of the object in question, one would have four active neurons for the respective combinations of assignment, e.g. '(triangle, above)' or '(rectangle below)'. However, their set membership would be lost if two objects were to occur simultaneously, since the two subassemblies (consisting of a total of eight simultaneously (co-)active neurons), would now superpose each other. Thus the information of the assembly with its internal (proposition) structure, e.g. 'The triangle is above', would also be lost (shown in the lower half of the figure) (von der

C. von der Malsburg has further developed his signal correlation theory with the "Dynamic Link Architecture (DLA)", which will be discussed in chap. 6.4.

(2) Since the 1980s, the British-American psychologist Anne M. Treisman, with her highly influential "Feature Integration Theory (FIT) of (Visual) Attention" [266], has addressed the binding problem in the process of visual perception (though she herself is rather sceptical about (phase) synchronization mechanisms). She sought to answer the question: How are the separately coded features of an object combined into a coherent object representation?

In her theory, it is assumed that at least two information processing steps are necessary for the analysis of a visual scene. In a fast, preattentive process (which operates independently of attention), the different visual object features are processed locally and in parallel, and detected in the context of dimension-specific feature maps (Treisman 1988, 1986, Treisman and Gelade 1980). Then, in a slow and attentive process, the different visual object features are serially integrated into a single object by directing attention ("focal attention") to a location on the master map ("master map of locations") (Treisman and Gelade 1980, Treisman 1988, 1986). This binds the object features registered in the individual feature maps to the appropriate location, although the focus of attention can only be directed to a small area ("spotlight theory").[267] If stored knowledge or a directed attention is missing, the features of different objects are combined at random, so that "illusory conjunctions"[268] can arise. The experimental evidence is based on the paradigm of "visual search" in perceptual psychology (Treisman and Gelade 1980, Treisman 1998), in which subjects are given the task of deciding as quickly as possible whether or not a target stimulus is present in amongst a set of "distractors"[269]. The target stimulus differs either by a simple feature or by a combination of features.

(3) From the early 1990s, the English physicist and biologist, Francis Crick and the American physicist and theoretical neuroscientist, Christoph Koch[270] proposed a model of neuronal synchronization as a temporal integration mechanism

---

Malsburg 1999 with reference to Rosenblatt 1962).

[266]For a foundational information, see e.g. Treisman and Gelade 1980, Treisman 1986, 1988, 1993, 1996 (with various modifications of the theory), 1998, 1999, 2006, Treisman and Sato 1990.
For an introduction, see Burwick 2014.
See also, the remarks in chap. 4.4.7.
For critical information, see e.g. Wolfe 1998, with his "Guided Search Theory (GST)" and Duncan and Humphreys 1989, 1992 with their "Attentional Engagement Theory (AET)".

[267]See e.g. Treisman and Gelade 1980, which refers to Posner et al. 1980, which in turn was based on Norman 1968.

[268]See e.g. Treisman and Gelade 1980 with reference to Treisman 1977.
For a detailed discussion, see e.g. Treisman and Schmidt 1982, Treisman 1998.
For a critical discussion, see e.g. von der Malsburg 1999, Wolfe and Cave 1999.

[269]In experimental psychology, the term "distractor" refers to a supposedly correct, but actually wrong alternative answer to a certain stimulus in the context of a multiple choice task, derived from the English verb "to distract".
See e.g. Stapf 2009.

[270]For a fundamental discussion, see e.g. Crick and Koch 1990, which refers to the empirical results from neurophysiology, e.g. W. Singer et al., W.J. Freeman and R. Eckhorn et al. (see chap. 4.3 [4.2]), the

to solve the binding problem in neurobiology and computational neuroscience. They then applied this model to the discussion of the "Neural Correlates of (visual) Consciousness (NCC)" ("Neuronal Coalitions Theory"). According to this discussion, sensory information can only enter consciousness if a perceived object is encoded in such a way that the neurons activated by the object are bound together to a temporal group (an "assembly"[271]). This is done by means of a coherent semi-synchronous oscillation in the range of 40-70 Hz, which activates a short-term working memory.

(4) From the second half of the 1980s, experimental data had been collected in neurophysiology and neurobiology, focusing on the synchronous activity of neurons:

(4.1) The research group led by the German neurophysiologist Wolf Singer, the German neurophysiologist Andreas K. Engel and the German physicist and neurophysiologist Peter König developed the "Binding-By-Synchrony (BBS) Hypothesis", together with their colleagues (C.M. Gray, P. Fries, A.K. Kreiter, P.R. Roelfsema, S. Neuenschwander and M. Brecht). Temporal correlations occurring precisely in the range of ten to twenty milliseconds between the impulses of neurons and stimulus-dependent temporal synchronizations of the coherent activity of neuronal populations, called "assemblies" [251], contribute to solving the (general) binding problem. This is discussed in detail in chap. 4.4.

(4.2) The research group led by the German physicist and neurophysiologist, Reinhard Eckhorn[272] has also observed a synchronously correlated oscillatory activity of neurons in the context of a "Binding-By-Synchronization Hypothesis" and a "Linking-By-Synchronization Hypothesis" by examining the visual cortex of cats using multi-microelectrodes (Eckhorn et al. 2001, 1992) (see chap. 4.1 (1), 4.4.3). This is with respect to orientation preferences between different visual areas within a hemisphere, e.g. between areas 17, 18 and 19 in cats, or between the two hemispheres (Eckhorn et al. 1992).

(4.3) With evoked EEG potentials in humans, the French neurobiologist, Catherine Tallon-Baudry[273] has found an increased synchronous activity of induced neuronal oscillations in the gamma band (24-60 Hz) and beta band (15-20 Hz)

---

experimental findings from perception psychology, e.g. in A. Treisman (see chap. 4.3 [2]), and based on the model of C. von der Malsburg from neuroinformatics (see chap. 4.3 [1]).

In Crick and Koch 2003, the authors dispute, however, that the synchronous oscillations of neurons are a sufficient condition for a neuronal correlate of consciousness: "We no longer think that synchronized firing, such as the so-called 40 Hz oscillations, is a sufficient condition for the NCC."

See also Tononi and Koch 2008.

For a synchronization (network) model (so-called "Coincidence Network") see e.g. Koch and Schuster 1992.

For a beginner's guide, see e.g. Schuster 2007.

[271] See Crick and Koch 2003, which speak of "coalitions of neurons".
See the explanations in chap. 4.2.4.

[272] See e.g. Eckhorn et al. 1988, 1989, 1992, 2001, 2007, Frien et al. 1994.
For an introduction, see e.g. Hardcastle 1998, Buzsáki 2006.

[273] See e.g. Tallon et al. 1995, Tallon-Baudry et al. 1996, 1997, 1998, 1999, Tallon-Baudry 2003.

within the framework of coherent object representations, e.g. of a dalmation. Thus, this synchronization of neuronal oscillations can be a mechanism to encode a particular object as a whole.

(4.4) The French veterinarian and theoretical neuroscientist Gilles Laurent[274] has proven precise neuronal synchronization phenomena in the olfactory system. This is done, for example, by using fast "Local Field Potential (LFP)" oscillations" in the frequency range of 20-30 Hz in honeybees, grasshoppers and zebrafish, as well as in the dynamic pigmentation of octopuses.

(4.5) With EEG and EMG recordings in humans, together with an MRI analysis of the data, the Dutch biophysicist Ad Aertsen[275] has shown dynamic synchronization processes in the beta band (16-28 Hz) between the cortical motor areas and muscular activity.

(4.6) The research group led by the American neurophysiologist and neuropharmacologist, Roger D. Traub[276] has demonstrated synchronizations of induced gammafrequency field potential oscillations with recordings using microelectrodes on hippocampal slice preparations of the CA1 region in rats (Traub et al. 1996). These long-range gamma oscillations in the frequency range of about 40-50 Hz and beta oscillations in the frequency range of about 20-30 Hz have been confirmed on a theoretical model (Traub et al. 1996, Bibbig et al. 2001, 2002). Furthermore, neuronal synchronization mechanisms have also been detected in the auditory cortex of rats (Ainsworth et al. 2011).

(4.7) The Germans, Simon Nikolas Jacob (physician), Daniel H. Hähnke (biologist), and Andreas Nieder (neurobiologist) have demonstrated that multiple visual quantities held in working memory can be separated by frequency-specific oscillatory synchrony in the primate prefrontal and parietal cortex (Jacob et al. 2018). By reading out spikes at distinct phases of parietal theta oscillations, multiple memorized numbers of visual items (numerosity) can be differentiated and protected from distractors.

For an introduction, see Tallon-Baudry and Bertand 2003.
See also, Tallon-Baudry 2004, 2009.

[274] See e.g. Laurent and Davidowitz 1994, Laurent 1996, 2002, MacLeod and Laurent 1996, Stopfer et al. 1997, Perez-Orive et al. 2002, Friedrich et al. 2004, Cassenaer and Laurent 2007, Laan et al. 2014.
For an introduction, see e.g. Buzsáki 2006.
See the explanations in chap. 4.4.4.

[275] See Feige et al. 2000.
For the macaques, see also Riehle et al. 1997.
See also Rodriguez-Molina et al. 2007.
For the theoretical (attractor) model of the neural synchronization phenomenon based on the "Synfire Chain (SFC) Model" by M. Abeles, see e.g. Diesmann et al. 1999, 2001, Mehring et al. 2003, Kumar et al. 2008.
For the "Synfire Chain (SFC) Model" by M. Abeles, see the remarks in chap. 9.5.
For the theoretical model of the neural synchronization phenomenon of the visual cortex in cats, see Kremkow et al. 2007.
For an introduction to the temporal synchronization phenomenon in the (visual) cortex, see Aertsen and Arndt 1993, Rotter and Aertsen 1998.

[276] See e.g. Whittington et al. 1995, 2001, Traub et al. 1996, 1999, 2001, Bibbig et al. 2002.
For an introduction, see e.g. Buzsáki 2006.
For an introduction to the temporal synchronization phenomenon, see Ainsworth et al. 2012.

(4.8) Recently, the American neuroscientists, Robert M. G. Reinhart and John A. Nguyen, have shown that a non-invasive transcranial alternating-current stimulation (tACS) improves working memory performance in older adults. This stimulation improves working memory performance by modulating the theta phase synchronization between prefrontal and temporal areas, which is coupled with the amplitude of gamma rhythms (Reinhart and Nguyen 2019). This is a specific form of cross-frequency coupling (Engel et al. 2013b, Maye et al. 2019) called theta (48 Hz) gamma (> 25 Hz) phase-amplitude coupling (PAC).

(4.9) The Spanish computer scientist and mathematician Alex Arenas, together with the Cuban theoretical physicist Yamir Moreno and the Spanish physicist Gómez-Gardeñes, describe the process of transient and global synchronization using the Kuramoto model of phase-coupled oscillators assigned to cortical areas in the cerebral cat cortex (Gómez-Gardeñes et al. 2010). Each cortical area is modeled as a phase oscillator with an independent internal frequency, and the coupling between these areas is modeled using Kuramoto nonlinear coupling. It is shown that a complex structure of a few, highly connected cortical areas drives the dynamic organization of the system. This complex structure, the so-called "rich-club" phenomenon in the corticocortical network (Colizza et al. 2006), plays a key role in the synchronization organization transition, that goes from a modular decentralized coherence to a centralized synchronized regime.

4.4 EXCURSION: INTEGRATION OF NEURONAL INFORMATION IN VISUAL PERCEPTION BY MEANS OF THE BINDING-BY-SYNCHRONY HYPOTHESIS BY W. SINGER ET AL.[277]

The binding problem of visual information processing is thematized in this section. This is done with "Binding-By-Synchrony (BBS) Hypothesis" of W. Singers, A.K. Engel and P. König's et al. in the context of the integrative mechanisms in visual scene analysis. It is for this reason that the neuroanatomical architecture of the visual system is briefly outlined in advance, primarily with respect to humans and primates (see Fig. 4.2).[278]

4.4.1 NEUROANATOMICAL ARCHITECTURE OF THE VISUAL SYSTEM

The processing of visual information begins with the retina, which contains photoreceptors that convert electromagnetic light energy into neuronal activity ("phototransduction"). In doing so, extensive image processing is already being carried out. The information from the photoreceptors then flows to the retinal ganglion cells via the bipolar cells, whose bundled axons form the optic nerves of the two eyes. After the optic nerves have merged and crossed in the optic chiasm, they project the neuronal information (in the form of action potentials) into the first switching station of the visual pathway, the lateral geniculate nucleus (CGL) in the dorsal thala-

---

[277]The line of thought in the chapter is mainly oriented towards Engel 2012, as well as Engel 2005, Engel and König 1998, and Engel 1996b.

[278]For an introduction, mainly with reference to humans, see e.g. Jäncke 2017, Bear et al. 2016, Kandel et al. 2013, Rösler 2011, Gazzaniga et al. 2018, Reid and Usrey 2008, Purves et al. 2013, Pinel et al. 2018. For an introduction, mainly with reference to mammals, see e.g. Kirschfeld 2001, Hoffmann and Wehrhahn 2001, Breedlove et al. 2017.

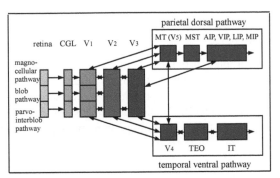

Figure 4.2: Schematic, simplified illustration of the three parallel information processing pathways of the visual system in humans and primates: the magnocellular pathway, the blob pathway and the parvo-interblob pathway. These pathways begin at the retina, continue via the lateral geniculate nucleus (LGN) to the primary (V1), secondary (V2), and tertiary (V3) visual cortex, and then lead to the two large pathways of cortical visual processing, the dorsal pathway and the ventral pathway with the corresponding cortical (association) areas (see the text). (following Kandel et al. 2013, Gazzaniga et al. 2018, Bear et al. 2016 and Rösler 2011).

mus ("retinofugal projection"). In this case, the sensory information is not processed by a single, hierarchically organized system, but by means of (at least) three parallel, functionally separated major pathways of visual information processing. These pathways specialize in processing neural information about (1) the shape and depth ("parvo-interblob pathway"), (2) the color ("blob pathway"), and (3) the movement and depth of visual objects ("magnocellular pathway"). The information transmitted in the three separate pathways must then be re-integrated into a single perceptual image. The axons of the neurons of the CGL now project further into the primary visual cortex V1, also called striate cortex. This cortex contains a complete map of the retina due to the retinotopic structure of the projections ("retinotopic organization"). The striary cortex is built up from a multitude of functional, cortical modules (the hypercolumns), which consist of ocular dominance, orientation columns, and "blobs". Each of these can completely analyze a very specific point within the visual field. From there, the neural information is further processed and distributed over a multitude of feedback processing pathways over various specialized areas in V2 and V3. This means that there are then two large pathways of cortical, visual processing with different visual functions, which require that neural information flows into one of the following two pathways. On one hand, the neural information flows into the dorsal pathway, which "seems to be responsible for the analysis of visual movement and the visual control of movements" (Bear et al. 2016). The neural information also flows into the ventral pathway, which "should be involved in the conscious perception of the visual world and the recognition of objects" (Bear et al. 2016). In other words, "the dorsal pathway is decisive for the perception of 'where' objects are, the ventral pathway for the perception of 'what' the objects are" (Pinel et al. 2018). The following cortex areas are assigned to the dorsal path: the middle temporal area (V5), the medial superior temporal (MST) area and other areas in the parietal cortex (the anterior intraparietal (AIP) area, the ventral intraparietal (VIP) area, the lateral intraparietal (LIP) area, and the medial intraparietal (MIP) area). In contrast, the area V4, the temporal-occipital (TEO) area and the inferior-temporal (IT) area are assigned to the ventral pathway.

4.4.2 GENERAL BINDING PROBLEM IN THE COGNITIVE NEUROSCIENCES

The (general) binding problem is to identify mechanisms that integrate neuronal signals and information processes such that sensory information can be "bound", i.e. integrated, into coherent perceptual impressions. According to the German neurophysiologist, Andreas K. Engel (2012), there are at least three subproblems that arise from neurophysiology, cognitive neurobiology, perceptual psychology and cognitive neuropsychology:

1. The problem of intramodal perceptive integration: How can the integration of neuron impulses within a single sensory system or modality (e.g. visual perception) produce unified perceptual impressions?
2. The problem of intermodal integration: How is the integration of neuronal impulses, which have been pre-processed in different sensory systems, achieved such as to be summarized into unified perceptual impressions?
3. The problem of sensorimotor integration: How are neuronal impulses of sensory information processing integrated with motor information processing such that the sensory system can coordinate with the motor system?

4.4.3 SENSORY (CONTOUR-)SEGMENTATION IN THE VISUAL SCENE ANALYSIS

The first subproblem of intramodal perceptive integration focuses on the "sensory segmentation problem" or "scene analysis" (von der Malsburg 1999, Engel 1996b, Singer 2002b): to determine which neurophysiological integration mechanisms of (object) feature binding and psychological Gestalt formation (see 4.4.3 (3)) are active in perception. This determines which elementary object features and object areas must be combined, i.e. "bound", for adequate analysis and representation of a visual situation.

(1) The classical model of "single-cell coding"[279] is based on the "single-cell doctrine" of the British neurophysiologist Horace Barlow[280], which was developed with the serial computer metaphor prevalent in neurobiology in the 1960s and 1970s (Engel and König 1998). The model is characterized by its assumtion that highly specific binding neurons ("cardinal cells", or "grandmother cells"[281]) are the neurophysiological correlate of psychological Gestalt formation (see 4.4.3 (3)). According to this, not only elementary object attributes, but also complex object attributes and objects should be encoded by the increase in the fire rate of individual or very few neurons. This means

---

[279] For an overview, see e.g. Engel and König 1998, 1996.
For a beginner's guide, see e.g. Singer 2002c, d, a, 2005.

[280] See Barlow 1972.
For an introduction, see e.g. Buzsáki 2006, Bennett and Hacker 2008.

[281] See Gross 2002.
For an introduction, see e.g. Sougné 2003.
See also, von der Malsburg 2001, who calls these neurons "combination-coding units".

that the neuronal signals to be bound are merged via the convergent connection structure of the visual system into "binding units", called "conjunction(-specific) units", within the framework of a static binding model. These units can thus generate highly specific response properties at the highest level of the information processing hierarchy ("binding by convergence" or "binding by conjunction cells", also known under the coding principle of "labeled-line coding").[282]

(2) The central problem of this static model is that a "combinatorial explosion" would occur with respect to the number of required representational elements, since with the number of identifiable features (and therefore the number of possible feature combinations) would also "explode" (Perlovsky 1998, Sejnowski 1986, Singer and Gray 1995). A sufficiently large number of specialized neurons would have to be available for this, many of which would also have to remain "in reserve" for new constellations of features. This would be contrary to the economy principle in evolutionary biology.[283] Furthermore, no experimental evidence was found for the aforementioned grandmother cells apart from facial recognition (e.g. Desimone et al. 1984, Desimone and Ungerlieder 1989, Gross et al. 1972 or Logothetis et al. 1995, Riesenhuber and Poggio 1999a found that individual neurons could certainly fire on a certain portrait) and numerosities (e.g. Nieder et al. 2002, Nieder 2013, 2016 found that "number neurons" respond selectively to a specific number of items).[284]

(3) Since the 1980s, in contrast, the connectionist model of population coding[285] (the "assembly model"[286]) has been developed in neurophysiological perception theory. The model is characterized by the assumption that elementary object attributes and complex objects are represented in the visual cortex by

---

[282]See e.g. Singer 2003a, 1999b.
For an introduction, see e.g. Maye 2002.
See the remarks in chap. 4.2.2.

[283]For a detailed information on a general criticism of single-cell coding, see e.g. Singer 2003a, Engel and König 1996, 1998, Engel 1996a.
For an introduction, see e.g. Singer 2002d, a, 2005.

[284]See also the rejection of the "resurrection" of the "Grandmother-Cell" Coding in the sense of Bowers (2009, 2010), by Plaut and McClelland (2010).
See Quian Quiroga et al. 2008, Quian Quiroga and Kreiman 2010.
See also, the remarks in chap. 4.2.5.

[285]For detailed information, see e.g. Singer 2003a, 1999a, b.
For an introduction, see e.g. Engel 2012, 1996b, 2005, Engel and König 1998, 1996.
For a beginner's guide, see e.g. Singer 2002b, c, d, a, 2003b, 2005, Engel and Singer 1997, Engel et al. 1993.
In some cases, the term "assembly coding" is also used, e.g.in Singer 1999a.
See also the remarks in chap. 4.2.4.

[286]See e.g. Engel 2012, Singer 1999a.
The English term "(cell) assembly" or "(cell) assemblies", derived from "to assemble," goes back to the Canadian psychologist, Donald O. Hebb (1949).
According to Engel and König (1998), the term "assembly" in neurophysiology refers to "a population of dynamically interacting neurons that instantiate an object representation *as a whole*".
For detailed information, see e.g. Palm 1982, 1990, Braitenberg 1978, Gerstein et al. 1989, Edelman 1987.

populations of synchronously active neurons (the "assemblies"). According
to the "Binding-By-Synchrony (BBS) Hypothesis"[287] (from the German neurophysiologists Wolf Singer and Andreas K. Engel and the German physicist
and neurophysiologist Peter König et al.), these cell assemblies have to be regarded as the basic units of information processing in the cortex. This means
they represent a basic descriptive and functional category in the cognitive neurobiology and medical neurophysiology (Engel and König 1998). According
to A.K. Engel and P. König[288], the new accompanying connectionist paradigm
of perception emphasizes that neural network structures are to be understood
as resulting from self-organization processes. Thus, the dynamic (i.e. temporal) network features of sensory systems must be taken into account (Hummel
1999). As a result, W. Singer[289] and his former colleagues at the Max Planck
Institute for Brain Research in Frankfurt am Main, in particular A.K. Engel
and P. König, proposed a temporal integration mechanism[290] to solve the visual integration problem. They proposed the "Binding-By-Synchrony (BBS)
Hypothesis" (Engel 2012). These hypotheses hold that sensory neurons activated by the same object are bound by a temporal (phase) synchronization[291]

---

[287]For fundamental information, see e.g. Gray and Singer 1989, Gray et al. 1989, Engel et al. 1990a,
b, 2001, Singer 1990, 1993, 1996, Singer et al. 1990, 1997, Singer and Gray 1995, König et al. 1995b,
Engel and Singer 2001.
For an introduction, see e.g. Burwick 2014, Singer 2004, 2003a, 1995, 1999a, b, d, 2001, Engel 2009,
Tallon-Baudry and Bertand 2003, Hummel 1999, von der Malsburg 2001, Nelson 1995.
For an overview, see e.g. Gray et al. 1992, Singer 1994a, b, 1996, 2000, Gray 1994, Freiwald et al. 2001,
Buzsáki et al. 2013, Tallon-Baudry 2009, Stanley 2013, Benchenane et al. 2011, Brette 2012.
For a review, see e.g. Huyck and Passmore 2011.
For a beginner's guide, see e.g. Singer 1999c, Engel 1996b, 2005, Engel and Singer 1997.

[288]This new connectionist paradigm of perception in neurobiology can be explained, according to Engel
and König (1998), on five aspects:
(1) Parallel and distributed processing,
(2) Self-organisation and plasticity,
(3) Context-dependence of neuronal responses,
(4) Assemblies as basic functional units, and
(5) Dynamics of neural processing.

[289]According to Singer (2002c), six "basic postulates" can be stated for experimental testing of the
binding hypothesis: "First, the representation of perceptual objects happens not only explicitly by highly
specific neurons, but also implicitly by dynamically associated ensembles of cells. Second, this dynamic
association takes place through a self-organizing process based on internal interactions mediated by
second-class connections. Third, the rules (the Gestalt rules) for the preferred association of certain nerve
groups are determined by the architecture of the network of associative connections. Fourthly, this architecture is partly genetically determined and partly transformed by experience. Fifth, successful grouping
of cells into ensembles is expressed in the synchronization of the discharge activity of the respective
neurons. Sixth, on the basis of these specific synchronization patterns, ensembles become separable and
identifiable as units."

[290]The approach that the binding problem could be solved through a temporal integration mechanism
goes back to von der Malsburg (1981), Abeles (1982a) and Milner (1974).
See Buzsáki et al. (2013) on the concept of neurophysiological, rhythmic oscillations in biological evolution in general.
See e.g. Metzinger (1995) on the reception in (neuro-)philosophy.

[291]For information on the term "phase synchronization", see the explanations in chap. 4.4 (4.4).

of their electrical impulses to populations of neurons ("cell assemblies"). The connection of an object or a fact is thus encoded by means of these temporal correlations between neurons (impulses) of an assembly. This allows for the construction of a coherent percept, e.g. by making an appropriate assignment of contours to a specific object within "visual scene analysis" (Wang 2003, Engel et al. 1991c, Singer 2002b). In other words, the synchronous activity of those neurons that belong to the same cell assembly is responsible for the holistic (Gestalt) structure[292] of visual perceptual impressions in the sense of "Gestalt psychology" of the 1920s and 1930s, according to the German psychologists Max Wertheimer, Wolfgang Köhler and Kurt Koffka.[293]

In addition, the BBS Hypothesis state that no such temporal correlations may occur between those neurons encoding *different* elementary object features or complex objects. This would clearly determine which subset of active neurons belongs to the same assembly, and this desynchronization of different cell assemblies would therefore support the separate further processing of unrelated neuronal information. This processing could enable segmentation processes in visual scene analysis. For example, it could enable the differentiation of a figure from the background ("figure-ground separation")[294], or the differentiation of objects as the basic operations of any pattern recognition process (Engel and König 1996).

(4) It has been shown[295] by means of "cross correlation analysis"[296] (especially in cats and monkeys) that the neurons in cortical and subcortical areas of the visual system can precisely synchronize their action potentials in the range of ten to twenty milliseconds. This synchronization leads to a dynamic grouping mechanism, and thereby lays the foundation for the sequential analysis and representation of highly different constellations of neurons using a flexible recombination of neuron impulses. However, the individual neurons react,

---

For a general introduction, see e.g. Varela et al. 2001, Walter and Müller 2012.

See also König et al. 1995b, Womelsdorf et al. 2007, Nikolić et al. 2013.

See e.g. Başar-Eroğlu et al. (2003) with an overview of the problem of phase binding in connection with the gamma band.

[292] A schematic representation of the elementary "Gestalt criteria" of a visual scene, on the basis of which the laws of perceptual integration mechanisms on the psychological level can be described, is given in Engel 2012, 1996b.

See also Singer 2002c, a, Engel and König 1998.

[293] The most important "Gestalt criteria" or "Gestalt laws" are the law of (1) continuity, (2) proximity, (3) similarity, (4) common fate, (5) closure, (6) good continuation, (7) symmetry and (8) good form.

For an introduction, see e.g. Purves et al. 2013, Kandel et al. 2013.

See also, Bennett and Hacker 2008.

[294] For a more extensive discussion, see Wang 2003.

For a beginner's guide, see e.g. Singer 2002b, c, Engel 1996b.

[295] For detailed information on the experiments, see e.g. Singer 2003a, 1999a, b, 1993, 1995, Engel et al. 1992, König et al. 1995a, Singer and Gray 1995, Engel 1996a, Maye and Engel 2012, Maye 2002.

For an introduction on the experiments, see e.g. Engel 2012, 2005, 1996b, Engel and König 1996, 1998, Engel et al. 1998.

For a beginner's guide, see e.g. Singer 2002a, b, c, 1997.

[296] See the explanations in chap. 4.4.3 (4.4).

relatively unselectively, to a broad spectrum of different object features. Thus, a single neuron can be an element of several populations at different times. It can therefore participate in the representation of many different object features, which is why the neuronal populations can overlap to a high degree (Singer 2002a). This means that a description of a specific object feature can only be obtained if all of the response properties of a population of neurons that respond to that feature are evaluated together. It follows that, with a limited number of neurons, an almost unlimited number of (dynamic) populations can be generated which differ from each other only by the respective configuration and degree of activation of the neurons. As a result, an almost unlimited number of object features can be represented. Furthermore, the synchronization strategy solves the superposition problem[297] by making the signature of the synchronous neural signals more effectively identify as belonging together for the subsequent information processing structures.

The following subsections present different types of experiments that focus on the BBS Hypothesis:

(4.1) In a multitude of experiments on animals (e.g. cats, mice, monkeys, pigeons and turtles) [298] it has been proven that the neurons in the visual cortex can synchronize their action potentials with a precision of a few milliseconds. Such neurons can thus be grouped into assemblies. This is true, not only within individual cortical columns and areas (e.g. the primary visual area V1 [Frien et al. 1994, Salin and Bullier 1995]), but also between the different visual areas within a hemisphere. For example, individual assemblies can be constituted by neurons across areas 17, 18 and 19 in cats (Eckhorn et al. 1988, 1992, Engel et al. 1991a, Nelson et al. 1992), area 17 and area PMLS[299] (Engel et al. 1991a), areas V1 and V2 (Engel 2012), and even between primary visual areas in the two cerebral hemispheres (Engel et al. 1991b, Eckhorn et al. 1992). The relevant synchronization processes are predominantly observed in a certain frequency band (the "gamma(γ)-band"[300]), i.e. in the frequency ranging

---

[297] See e.g. Singer 1999a, b, von der Malsburg 1999, 1994, Singer et al. 1997, von der Malsburg and Schneider 1986.
See the remarks in chap. 4.3 (1).

[298] In the case of cats, see e.g. Eckhorn et al. 1988, Gray and Singer 1989, Engel et al. 1990a, Brosch et al. 1995.
For an overview, see e.g. Singer 2002e.
In the case of mice, see e.g. Engel 2012.
In the case of monkeys, the evidence was found in the (extra-)striate cortex. See e.g. Ts'o and Gilbert 1988, Kreiter and Singer 1992.
In the case of pigeons, see e.g. Neuenschwander et al. 1996.
In the case of turtles, see e.g. Prechtl 1994.

[299] The abbreviation "PMLS" stands for the cortical area "posteromedial lateral suprasylvian area".

[300] See e.g. Fries et al. 2007.
One also speaks of "gamma-oscillations" or "40-Hz oscillations".
See e.g. Engel 2009.
A general overview of "neural oscillations" can be found in Buzsáki and Freeman 2015, Wang 2003.
See also Buzsáki 2006, Herrmann 2002.

between 30-70 Hz.[301] A typical experiment to demonstrate this would be to derive neural signals from several sensory neurons in the same column within areas 17 and 18 of a cat's visual cortex using multiple microelectrodes, while moving a light stimulus in a certain direction at a constant speed. For example, a light bar gliding through the receptive fields[302] of motion-sensitive neurons with similar directional preference (Gray and Singer 1989, Engel et al. 1990a, Gray et al. 1989) (see Fig. 4.3).

The vast majority of the tests were carried out on anaesthetised laboratory animals. Highly similar synchronisation phenomena have also been demonstrated in awake animals, however; for example, awake monkeys and cats (Kreiter and Singer 1992, 1996, Roelfsema et al. 1995).

Furthermore, there is experimental evidence that this neuronal synchronization can also be observed between cortical and subcortical visual structures. For example, this synchronization can be observed between the retina, thalamus and primary visual cortex (Neuenschwander and Singer 1996, Castelo-Branco et al. 1998), and between the PMLS and the superior colliculus and cortical areas 18 (Brecht and Engel 1996, Brecht et al. 1998). Furthermore, the results of EEG studies showed that similarly precise synchronization phenomena occur in visual cortical areas in humans (Tallon et al. 1995, Herrmann et al. 2004, Freiwald et al. 2001).

(4.2) In addition, a multitude of experimental evidence[303] has shown that these temporal synchronization processes in the visual cortex are actually modulated by the configuration of the presented stimuli. This means that the neuronal impulses are only synchronously active if the neurons are activated by the same object (e.g. by moving a continuous light bar over its respective receptive fields). However, if the neurons are activated with two opposed light bars, the temporal coupling decreases or even completely disappears, proving that the temporal correlation depends on the configuration of certain stimulus parameters, such as continuity or coherence of movement (see Fig. 4.3).

---

[301] The bandwidth of the gamma band is defined differently by various authors, so that other values can also be found, e.g. in the range from 30-100 Hz.

[302] The "(classical) Receptive Field (cRF)" of a (visual) neuron, e.g. a ganglion cell, is used in cognitive neuroscience or neurophysiology to describe the region of a sensory organ, e.g. the retina, in which a change in the activation of a sensory neuron can be caused by (visual) stimulation with a small stimulus, e.g. light.
For a fundamental information, see e.g. Hubel and Wiesel 1959 with referece to Hartline 1949.
For a detailed information, see e.g. Palmer 1999.
For an introduction, see e.g. Kandel et al. 2013, Purves et al. 2013, Bear et al. 2016, Rösler 2011, Pinel et al. 2018.
See also, Smith Churchland 2002, Gerstner and Kistler 2002.

[303] For intercolumnar correlations in cats, see e.g. Gray et al. 1989.
For intra areal correlations of the primary visual area 17 in the cat, see e.g. Gray and Singer 1989, Engel et al. 1991c, Freiwald et al. 1995.
For intra areal correlations, see e.g. Engel et al. 1991a, Eckhorn et al. 1988.
For correlations in awake animals, see e.g. Kreiter and Singer 1996, Kayser et al. 2003.
For an detailed overview, see e.g. Engel et al. 1992.

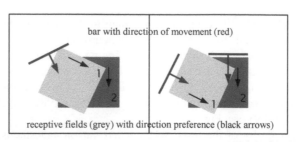

Figure 4.3: Schematic illustration of the bar experiment: The neuronal signals of two groups of neurons with different directional preferences, indicated by the arrows (black) in the respective receptive field (grey squares) 1 and 2, are derived using several microelectrodes. (1) A continuous light bar with constant speed (left graphic segment) is moved in a certain direction (red arrow). It glides through the receptive fields 1 and 2 of the motion-sensitive neurons of the two neuron populations with similar directional preferences. This results in the neuronal impulses of the two neuron groups being synchronously active, since the neurons are activated by the same object and its direction of movement is approximately in the middle of the respective direction preferences of the neurons. (2) However, if the neurons are activated with two opposing bars (right graphic segment), the synchronization of the neuronal signals decreases, since each of the two light bars activates in each case, only the neuron group whose preferred direction preference corresponds to the direction of movement of the respective light bar, indicated by the parallel arrows (red and black) (following Kreiter and Singer 1996 and Singer 1999b).

(4.3) The experiments discussed so far only demonstrate that temporal binding can occur in the visual perception system via these synchronization processes; however, they "do not yet prove that the neuronal correlations have [a] causal relevance". That is, they do not yet show that a neuronal synchronization process correlates "with behaviorally measurable perceptual performances". In other words, they do not yet show that the temporal correlations between the neuronal impulses are "a necessary condition for the formation [of] coherent perceptual impressions" (Engel 2012, Engel and König 1996). In a series of experiments on cats with malpositioned eyes (e.g. cats with a convergent squint [Roelfsema et al. 1994], a so-called "strabismic amblyopia") some indications for the required functional relevance of the observed synchronization phenomena could be collected. While the neurons which are preferably activated by the intact eye show a normal synchronization performance, the neurons which are preferably innervated by the amblyopic eye show a significantly reduced synchronization performance. It follows that this selective disturbance of the intracortical synchronization is functionally relevant for the perceptual disturbances occurring in cats with convergent squint.

This correlation between functional deficit and disturbed neuronal synchronization has also been demonstrated in a neurophysiological (correlation) study (König et al. 1993). This study was accompanied by a neuroanatomical study in cats with divergent strabismus (Löwel and Singer 1992). The neuronal synchronization which is particularly disturbed is that of the cortical neurons which receive their information from sensory neurons in both eyes.

This is in contrast with normal synchronization performance, which occurs (only) in cortical neurons dominated by the same (healthy) eye.

Another highly significant correlation between cortical synchronization and perceptive function arises from experiments on "binocular rivalry" in awake cats.[304] The synchronization of cortical neurons in the visual areas 17 and 18 varies, depending on whether they represent the dominant or the suppressed stimulus. This means that the synchronization effect increases for those neurons that represent the perceived pattern by being activated by the eye dominating perception. In contrast, the synchronization effect decreases between the neurons encoding the suppressed pattern.

In conclusion, these neurophysiological results strongly suggest that "the construction of a coherent object representation and the emergence of a perceptive impression is only possible if the relevant neuronal populations are sufficiently synchronized" (Engel 2012), though, as yet, there is no direct evidence for this (see chap. 4.4.8).

(4.4) The statistical method used here, the "cross-correlation analysis"[305] (see Fig. 4.4), typically serves to determine the temporal relationship of events at different locations. An event can, for example, be the generation of an action potential, the generation of a local field potential[306], or the variation of the mean fire rate of a neuron or a neuron population. This means that the time that the events occur is crucial.

For discrete signal sequences, i.e. a sequence of action potentials, the cross correlation can be described using the correlation product of two signals or signal sequences $S_1(t), S_2(t)$:

$$C(\tau) = \sum_{-\infty}^{\infty} S_1(t) \cdot S_2(t+\tau), \qquad (4.3)$$

in which τ is the "delay" of the signals relative to each other. The degree of correlation can then be specified using the (cross) correlation coefficient

$$r_{s_1,s_2} = \frac{\sum_{i=1}^{N}(S_{1i}(t) - \bar{s}_1)(S_{2i}(t+\tau) - \bar{s}_2)}{\sqrt{\sum_{i=1}^{N}(S_{1i}(t) - \bar{s}_1)^2 \cdot \sum_{i=1}^{N}(S_{2i}(t+\tau) - \bar{s}_2)^2}} \qquad (4.4)$$

---

[304] See e.g. Fries et al. 1997, 2002, Engel et al. 1999a.
See also Genç et al. 2015.
For an overview, see e.g. Engel 2012, 2005, Singer 2003a.

[305] For detailed information, see e.g. Brody 1999, Aertsen and Gerstein 1985, König 1994.
For an introduction, see e.g. Brown et al. 2004, Abeles 1994, Unbehauen 2002, Maye 2002, Salari and Maye 2008, Fickel 2007.
For a beginner's guide, see e.g. Goebel 1994.

[306] A detailed description of (recording) methods and data processing analysis which measure a "Local Field Potential (LFP) using multi-electrodes can be found, for example, in Engel et al. 1990a.

[307] The signal can be an "action potential" of a neuron or a "Local Field Potential (LFP)" of a neuron population.
See e.g. Engel et al. 1990a.

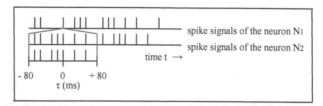

Figure 4.4: Schematic diagram of a cross correlation analysis: The cross correlogram of two spike trains $S_1(t)$, $S_2(t)$ computes the probability that a signal[307] of neuron N2 occurs in a time interval τ, with respect to a certain time t_i of the occurrence of a signal (here: red) of the (reference) neuron N1. This means that for each spike that occurs at time t_i in signal $S_1(t)$, a correlation window (here: blue) is defined, which contains a certain number of time segments, so-called "bins", and those spikes of signal $S_2(t)$ that occur within the time interval $\tau = t_i \pm 80$ ms are counted ("bin count"). After the procedure has been carried out for all n spikes of signal $S_1(t)$, the results are summed up and recorded in a cross correlation histogram (see Fig. 4.5) (following Engel et al. 1990a, Salari and Maye 2008, Fickel 2007).

for discrete time signal sequences $S_{1(1...N)}$ and $S_{2(1...N)}$ with mean values $\bar{s}_1 = \frac{1}{N}\sum_i^N s_{1i}$ and $\bar{s}_2 = \frac{1}{N}\sum_i^N s_{2i}$ and discrete time points $i = 1...N$.

In contrast, if the mean fire rates $F_1(t)$ and $F_2(t)$ of two neurons (populations) are considered, the cross correlation function $K(\Delta t)$ describes the (cross) correlation between these two (time) functions, depending on the relative time shift Δt:

$$K(\Delta t) = corr(F_1(t), F_2(t + \Delta t)) = $$
$$\frac{\int (F_1(t) - \langle f_1 \rangle)(F_2(t + \Delta t) - \langle f_2 \rangle)\, dt}{\sqrt{\int (F_1(t) - \langle f_1 \rangle)^2\, dt \cdot \int (F_2(t + \Delta t) - \langle f_2 \rangle)^2\, dt}} \quad (4.5)$$

with the expected values $\langle f_1 \rangle$ and $\langle f_2 \rangle$ based on the general cross correlation function with two continuous functions $F_1(t), F_2(t)$:

$$K(\Delta t) = \int_{-\infty}^{\infty} F_1(t) \cdot F_2(t + \Delta t)\, dt. \quad (4.6)$$

A (phase) synchronization of the signal sequences happens if the (cross) correlation coefficient, which takes the value $0 < r_{s_1, s_2} \leq 1$, is as close as possible to '1'. In the case of oscillation functions, (phase) synchronization of the signal sequences takes place if the time delay (referred to here as "phase lag" or "phase difference" (see Box 4.4.3) is close to '0'.

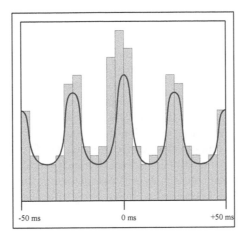

-50 ms   0 ms   +50 ms

Figure 4.5: Schematic diagram of a cross correlation histogram: If spikes occur very frequently in signal $S_2(t)$ in the range around τ_{0ms} of the correlation window of a signal $S_1(t)$ in the cross correlogram, then a peak appears in the correlation histogram, indicating a synchronization of the signals. Otherwise, the resulting cross correlation remains flat. Finally, the data of the correlogram is approximated using a Gabor function (here: red) so that an oscillation occurs (following Engel et al. 1990a, Salari and Maye 2008).

The data is transferred to a cross correlation histogram, e.g. to a "(Joint) Peri-Stimulus Time Histogram ((J)PSTH)"[308] or to a "Field Potential Histogram (FPH)"[309] (see Fig. 4.5).

(5) The extension of the BBS Hypothesis (that precise temporal coherence, in the form of phase synchronization of oscillations in neural assemblies, serves to encode relations) by the German neurophysiologist Pascal Fries[310], is known as the "Communication Through Coherence (CTC) Hypothesis". The original

---

[308]For a detailed description of (recording) methods and data processing analysis, see e.g. Engel et al. 1990a, Nase et al. 2003.
For a general in-depth analysis, see e.g. Aertsen et al. 1989, 1991, Gerstein et al. 1989, Aertsen and Braitenberg 1992.
For an introduction, see e.g. Brown et al. 2004 with multiple figures, Abeles 1994, Ziemke and Cardoso de Oliveira 1996.
An improved variant for determining the effective connectivity between two neurons is the "normalized Joint Peri-Stimulus Time Histogram (JPSTH)" by distinguishing between "rate coherence" und "event coherence".
See e.g. Neven and Aertsen 1992.

[309]For a detailed description of (recording) methods and data processing analysis, see e.g. Engel et al. 1990a.

[310]For detailed information, see e.g. Fries 2015, 2005.
For an introduction, see e.g. Burwick 2014.
The relationship between the BBS hypothesis and the CTC hypothesis is described by Fries (2005) as follows. "The CTC and the BBS hypotheses are fully compatible with each other, but they are also clearly distinct. Whereas the BBS hypothesis is primarily suggesting a representational code, the CTC hypothesis considers the mechanistic consequences of neuronal oscillations for neuronal communication. It suggests that at the heart of our cognitive dynamic is a dynamic communication structure and that the neuronal substrate is the flexible neuronal coherence pattern."

CTC Hypothesis states that two groups of neurons communicate, i.e. exchange information, most effectively when their excitability fluctuations are coherent, i.e. coordinated in time depending on neuronal (zero or non-zero phase) synchronization. This control by cortical coherence is a fundamental brain mechanism for large-scale, distant transmission of neuronal information. This hypothesis can be summarized as follows: "An activated neuronal group tends to engage in rhythmic synchronization. Rhythmic synchronization creates sequences of excitation and inhibition that focus both spike output and sensitivity to synaptic input to short temporal windows. The rhythmic modulation of postsynaptic excitability constitutes rhythmic modulations in synaptic input gain. Inputs that consistently arrive at moments of high input benefit from enhanced effective connectivity. Thus, strong effective connectivity requires rhythmic synchronization within pre- and postsynaptic groups and coherence between them, or, in short, communication requires coherence. In the absence of coherence, inputs arrive at random phases of the excitability cycle and will have a lower effective connectivity. A postsynaptic neuronal group receiving inputs from several different presynaptic groups responds primarily to the presynaptic group to which it is coherent. Thereby, selective communication is implemented through selective coherence" (Fries 2015).

This original CTC formulation has now been supplemented by a new formulation in two aspects (Fries 2015): First, if two communicating neuronal groups are bidirectionally coupled, the (gamma-band) coherence between neuronal groups in widely separated areas does not occur at zero phase, but with a systematic delay. Secondly, mathematical implementations of the new CTC formulation assume that postsynaptic excitability is modulated by rhythmic synchronization in such a way, that there is neither a sinusoidal oscillation nor a linear relation between phase and excitability.

Box 4.4.3 Phase Difference:

The term "phase difference" is defined, starting from neural signals $x(t)$ in the form of oscillation functions or dominant modes, by the general formula

$$\widetilde{x}(f,t) = at \exp\left(i(ft + \phi_x(t))\right), \qquad (4.7)$$

as the difference between the two phase terms

$$\phi_{xy}(t) = \left| n\phi_x(t) - m\phi_y(t) \right|. \qquad (4.8)$$

For an introduction, see e.g. Varela et al. 2001.

4.4.4 INTRAMODAL PERCEPTIVE INTEGRATION OF OTHER SENSORY SYSTEMS

Within the first subproblem of intramodal sensory integration, the BBS Hypothesis can now be applied to other sensory systems. In fact, precise neuronal synchronizations have now been detected in a series of experiments. For example, they have been found in the olfactory system (Laurent 1996), the auditory system (deCharms and Merzenich 1996, Bockhorst et al. 2018) and the somatosensory system (Murthy and Fetz 1992), "which in turn suggests that neuronal synchronization is generally significant for integrative processes" (Engel 2012).

4.4.5   INTERMODAL INTEGRATION OF SENSORY INFORMATION

As far as the second subproblem of intermodal sensory integration is concerned, initial experimental evidence for the synchronization hypothesis has been verified by several research groups in recent years.[311] Hipp et al. (2011) provided evidence for the existence of dynamic functional large-scale synchronized clusters underlying the crossmodal integration of auditory and visual information in humans. Wang et al. (2019) have analyzed the integration of sensory signals from different modalities (visuotactile pattern matching task) by a transient synchronization mechanism across the theta ($\sim$ 5 Hz), alpha ($\sim$ 10 Hz), and beta ($\sim$ 20 Hz) frequency bands. Within a task in which human participants (male and female) matched changes in amplitude of concurrent visual, auditory and tactile stimuli, Misselhorn et al. (2019) has shown that "coordinated sensory gamma oscillations play an important role for direct cross-modal interactions" and suggest that, "comparable to interactions within sensory streams, phase-coupled gamma oscillations might provide the functional scaffold for cross-modal communication."

4.4.6   SENSOMOTORIC INTEGRATION OF NEURONAL INFORMATION

As far as the third subproblem of sensorimotor integration is concerned, several research groups have empirically shown that neuronal synchronization occurs between the somatosensory and motor areas of the cerebral cortex. This has been found in cats (Roelfsema et al. 1995, MacKay 1997), monkeys (Murthy and Fetz 1992) and even humans (Farmer 1998), which indicates that the synchronization of neuronal impulses "could be essential for the selective coordination of sensory and motor behavioral aspects" (Engel 2012).

4.4.7   NEURONAL SYNCHRONIZATION AND VISUAL ATTENTION MECHANISMS

Many of the experiments already mentioned show that the neuronal synchronization processes occurring in the various sensory areas not only depend on the processing of external stimuli, but are also largely determined by system-internal dynamic factors (e.g. attention, memory or motivation). In particular, a majority of studies[312] carried out on awake monkeys show that the synchronization effects increased when

---

[311] For detailed information, see e.g. Wang et al. 2019, Friese et al. 2016, Göschl et al. 2015. For a review, see e.g. Engel et al. 2012, Senkowski et al. 2008.

[312] See e.g. Fries et al. 2001, Engel et al. 2001. For an overview, see e.g. Engel 2012, 2005. See also Wang 2003, Singer 1994a.

the neurons in the visual or somatosensory cortex encoded information about a stimulus which the animal had attentively observed or touched. In contrast, these effects decreased when the attention of the animal was directed to another stimulus. This indicates that attention and memory processes are accompanied by a modulation of neuronal synchronization effects in neurons involved in the processing of the same stimulus.

This could mean that the information encoded by means of synchronous assemblies in an earlier sensory area "with a high preference" is forwarded to other cortical centres (e.g. the sensory association cortex or the premotor cortex), where it is preferably processed further. This is "a functional principle that could be described as 'saliency by synchrony'" (Engel 2012). On the other hand, preparing the development of neural synchronization processes in earlier sensory areas could lead to synchronously structured activity in later cortical centres, even before a new stimulus is received and processed. These "temporal coupling patterns" could thus be suitable for "matching of neuronal predictions or expectations with reality". This results in a "selection" of those neuronal signals that contain information corresponding to the specific context of action via "a process of neuronal 'resonance'". This corresponds to a functional principle that can be described as "dynamic contextual prediction" (Engel 2012).

Furthermore, a large number of EEG and MEG studies on humans[313] suggest that the neuronal synchronization processes themselves are "of great importance" for increased vigilance [314] and the control of attention. Thus, these processes are also of great importance for the selection of neuronal signals (Engel 2005, Singer 1996). This underpins the assumption that "temporal binding is a precondition for conscious perception" (Engel 2005, Singer 1996). This has been empirically proven (e.g. on awake cats [Brecht et al. 1999, 2004]), where it has been shown that the neurons of the visual cortex synchronize with those in the subcortical structure of the superior colliculus. This determined the selection of targets for eye movements.

This comes close to the "Feature Integration Theory (FIT) of (Visual) Attention" proposed by the British-American psychologist, Anne M. Treisman (see chap. 4.3 [2]). This model states that the necessary binding between the different neuronal impulses is brought about by (visual) attention (though she herself is rather sceptical about the BBS Hypothesis) (Treisman 1996, 1999).

4.4.8   CRITICISM OF THE BINDING-BY-SYNCHRONY HYPOTHESIS

The Binding-By-Synchrony Hypothesis by W. Singer, A.K. Engel and P. König et al. has often been criticized in the literature[315]:

---

[313] See e.g. Schwender et al. 1994, Tallon-Baudry et al. 1997, Debener et al. 2003, Rodriguez et al. 1999.
For an overview, see e.g. Herrmann et al. 2004.

[314] For the term "vigilance", see e.g. Parasuraman 1986.

[315] See e.g. Shadlen and Newsome 1994.
See also, Phillips and Singer 1997.

(1) An overview of several theoretical arguments against the "temporal binding hypothesis"[316] has been compiled by the American neurobiologist and physician, Michael N. Shadlen and the experimental psychologist, J. Anthony Movshon (Shadlen and Movshon 1999, O'Reilly et al. 2003). The first argument is that the BBS Hypothesis does not describe the relevant computational algorithms which structure the neuronal signal impulses into a synchronous activity. Instead, this argument holds, it only describes the result of the binding computations as a representation of synchronous neuronal activity (Shadlen and Movshon 1999). A second argument concerns neuroanatomical data. According to previous investigations, the organization of the feedback projections from the higher cortical areas does not have the required precision and dynamically configurable connections. This means, for example, that object-based synchronization could occur between the object-constituting neurons in the temporal cortex and the neurons in the primary visual cortex (which encode the relevant elements of an object) (Shadlen and Movshon 1999 with reference to Salin and Bullier 1995). A third argument refers to the realistic construction of a cortical architecture, according to which a neuron in a cortical column is (in principle) already embedded in a network of neural signals with a high degree of convergence. Thus, in a time window of 5-10 milliseconds, the incoming impulses of neighbouring neurons are synchronous solely due to the cortical design. In other words, the resulting response behavior of the neurons is already synchronous due to these similar environmental conditions. Therefore, the synchronization phenomenon is of no particular importance unless a time window of only 3 milliseconds or less is considered. However, this has rarely been experimentally verified (Shadlen and Movshon 1999 with reference to Koch 1999 and von der Malsburg 1981).

(2) A further overview of significant arguments and counterarguments concerning the BBS Hypothesis has been compiled by A.K. Engel (2005). In addition to those mentioned above, he presents a fourth argument dealing with the objection of the American philosopher and cognitive scientist, Valerie G. Hardcastle.[317] This objection is that the correspondence (observed in experiments on binocular rivalry between the neuronal synchronization phenomenon and perceptual selection) does not constitute a causal relation, but that "at best there is a covariance between these phenomena." Thus the synchronous ac-

---

A detailed overview can be found, e.g. in the journal, Neuron Vol. 24, 1999, esp. in Shadlen and Movshon 1999, and in the journal, Consciousness and Cognition Vol. 8, 1999, esp. in Engel et al. 1999b, also in the anthology by Cleeremans 2003.

For an overview, see e.g. Engel 2005, Pareti and De Palma 2004, Goebel 1994.

See also, Maye 2002.

[316] See Shadlen and Movshon 1999, which refers to the above described research projects by W. Singer and R. Eckhorn and their research groups.

[317] See Hardcastle 1999, 1998, 1994.

See also Hardcastle 1997.

For other authors' criticism of the functional relevance of the synchronization phenomenon, see the Proceedings of the 3rd electronic seminar of the Association for the Scientific Study of Consciousness (ASSC 1997), on "Temporal Binding, Binocular Rivalry and Consciousness".

tivity under consideration, as a "neuronal correlate of consciousness" (Singer 2009), is not directly causally relevant for the emergence of consciousness, but is merely a "distal" causal factor of the same. Engel counters this objection by stating that it can only be invalidated (according to the standards of philosophy of science); one could selectively manipulate synchronization effects without impairing the other characteristics of visual processing (Engel 2005, Engel et al. 1999b, Fickel 2007). However, this is experimentally very difficult in mammals. Therefore, this is very little experimental evidence of this kind.[318] A fifth argument maintains that the synchronization hypothesis cannot explain why the described temporal binding is a necessary, but insufficient, condition for the emergence of self-conscious experience. Therefore, as Engel (2005) admits, the criteria concerned must be examined on the basis of a more comprehensive theory of consciousness, such as those offered by J. Newman and B.J. Baars or F. Crick and C. Koch (Newman and Baars 1993, Crick and Koch 2003, Koch 2004; see also Massimini and Tononi 2018). In this context, sensory information only leads to conscious perception if the neuronal activity is integrated into an explicit representation and the prefrontal cortex areas are actively involved in the flow of information over a sufficiently long period of time. A sixth argument deals with the objection of the German neurologist and clinical neuropsychologist, Martin Kurthen (1999). The objection is that the present neurophysiological data on binocular rivalry can, in principle, only refer to the subjective experience aspects of consciousness via indirect correlations. This is conveyed by a naturalistic theory of conscious behavior accessible from the third-person-perspective. The subjective experience aspects, however, describe access to the phenomenal states from the first-person-perspective of an individual. This objection is based on the "explanatory gap argument" from philosophy (see Box 4.4.8), introduced by the American philosopher, Joseph Levine (1983). Engel's response is twofold (Engel 2005, Engel et al. 1999b). Firstly, if private phenomenal facts can be analyzed relationally or functionally (Dennett 1990), a theory of "neuronal correlates of conscious behavior (...) could be largely coextensive with a theory of neuronal correlates of consciousness". And secondly, as Kurthen himself emphasizes, "neuro- and cognitive scientific research itself can and will lead in the long term to a change of the explanandum 'consciousness'," so that "under the influence of scientific research" these explanatory gaps "(will) appear less serious" (Kurthen 1999).

(3) Finally, the Binding-By-Synchrony Hypothesis has been criticized by a large number of authors on the basis of empirical evidence (Bartels 2009):

(3.1) According to Y. Dong et al. (2008), the "border ownership coding" is done by a simple increase of the mean fire rate in connection with a feedback attention modulation, and the found synchronous activity indicates only the member-

---

[318] See e.g. the already mentioned microstimulation experiment at the Colliculus superior by Brecht et al. 2004.
See the remarks in chap. 4.4.3 (4.1), 4.4.7.
See also, MacLeod and Laurent 1996.

ship to a special network (see also Fang et al. 2009, Qiu et al. 2007, Zhou et al. 2000),

(3.2) According to V.A.F. Lamme and H. Spekreijse (1998), an increased synchronous activity of neurons was found in the area V1 in primates when the orientation of the object line segments differed by 90° from those of the background, but this is understood as a reflection of the function of horizontal connections of a column. In accordance with this, P.R. Roelfsema, V.A. Lamme and H. Spekreijse suggest that a simultaneous increase in the frequency of V1 neurons in macaques will be measured (Roelfsema et al. 2004). This will be a neural correlate for visual attention, and thus (in accordance with Treisman's Feature-Integration Theory of (Visual) Attention) is responsible for feature binding ("Binding-By-Rate Enhancement Hypothesis"),

(3.3) A. Thiele and G. Stoner (2003) found that increased synchronous activity in the cortical area MT in macaques does not occur just in the case of coherent (check) structures of the stimulus. This also occurs in the case of non-coherent patterns,

(3.4) According to B.J.A. Palanca and G.C. DeAngelis (2005), in the cortical area MT in primates, a highly significant neural synchronicity can only be determined in neurons with overlapping, collinear receptive fields,

(3.5) M. Riesenhuber and T. Poggio's[319] "Hierarchical Model of Object Recognition" suggests (in the context of a "static binding model") that no oscillation or synchronization mechanisms are required. Based on a "simple hierarchical feed-forward architecture" (Riesenhuber and Poggio 1999a), consisting of a hierarchy of "simple cells", "complex cells", "composite feature cells", "complex composite cells" and "view-tuned cells", a nonlinear "MAX (pooling) function" determines the activity of a neuron as an active selection mechanism (Riesenhuber and Poggio 1999a). This favors the information of the stimulus that excites the respective neuron most, i.e. that generates the highest fire rate, so that the criterion of invariance is guaranteed. This seems to be proven by neurophysiological data (Riesenhuber and Poggio 1999a, which refer to Sato 1989).

(3.6) According to D. Hermes et al. (2014), synchronous oscillations are, in principle, not necessary for visual perception processing, since they often do not occur with certain stimuli (for criticism of this, see Brunet et al. 2014).

(3.7) B.V. Atallah and M. Scanziani (2009), S.P. Burns et al. (2010), S. Ray and J.H.R. Maunsell (2010), and X. Jia et al. (2013a, 2013b) argued that the synchronized oscillations cannot have a functional role because these oscillations (with variable frequencies sustained over short time intervals) and their synchronization (with varying phase relations) are incompatible with the idea that spike synchronization can be used to encode semantic relations (for a review

---

[319] See Riesenhuber and Poggio 1999b.
For fundamental information to the "Hierarchical Model of Object Recognition", see e.g. Riesenhuber and Poggio 1999a, Poggio and Edelman 1990.
For an introduction, see e.g. Riesenhuber and Poggio 1999b.

on this arguments, see Ray and Maunsell 2015, Palmigiano et al. 2017). Thus, there does not seem to be enough time for feature binding and the formation of object-specific neuronal assemblies in distributed coding regimes. However, recent experimental studies[320] "combining multisite recordings with time resolved analysis of coherent oscillations and spike synchronization in awake, behaviourally trained monkeys have confirmed the volatile features of synchronization phenomena: non-stationarity, frequency variability, short duration, rapid phase shifts and fast formation and dissolution of coherent states." This variability and non-stationarity of the complex cortical dynamics are therefore necessary properties for fast, flexible, versatile, and reliable processing, and finally.

(3.8) M. Vinck and C.A. Bosman (2016) seek the functional role of gamma-synchronizations in the context of efficient and predictive coding.[321] They have shown evidence that gamma-synchronizations arises in very specific circumstances requiring predictive integration of classical receptive field input and the information outside of the classical receptive field which is referred to as the "surround". The resulting gamma-synchronous dynamics are "likely critical for the emergence of sparse and highly informative firing rate representations that are effectively routed to the next brain area."

(3.9) The so-called "Transient Coding Hypothesis" by K. Friston (1997, 1995) investigates dynamic changes in correlations and covariations among *different* frequencies, not phase-synchronized correlations at the *same* frequencies as in the BBS Hypothesis, and can therefore be considered, according to Friston, as a more general form of coding. This Transient Code Hypothesis suggests that "interactions are mediated by the expression and induction of reproducible, highly structured spatiotemporal dynamics that endure over extended periods of time (i.e., neuronal transients). (...) In particular the frequency structure of a transient in one part of the brain may be very different from that in another, whereas in synchronous interactions the frequency structures of both will be the same (whether they are oscillatory or not). (...) Synchronization represents the direct, reciprocal exchange of signals between two populations, wherein the activity in one population has a direct effect on the activity of the second, such that the dynamics become entrained and mutually reinforcing. In transient coding the incoming activity from one population exerts a modulatory influence, not on the activity of units in the second, but on the interactions (e.g., synaptic or effective connectivity) among these units to change the dynamics intrinsic to the second population. In this model there is no necessary synchrony between the intrinsic dynamics that ensue and the temporal pattern of modulatory input (Friston 1997)."

---

[320]For a review, see e.g. Singer (2018).

[321]This is also emphasized by Jacob et al. 2018, referring to theta synchronizations. See chap. 4.3 (4.7)

Box 4.4.8   Explanatory Gap Argument:

The explanatory gap argument states that, viewed from an expistemic viewpoint, the phenomenal contents of consciousness experienced in a certain subjectively experienced manner (i.e. the mental properties and states, the so-called "qualia") which are therefore (only) accessible from the first-person perspective, cannot in principle (reductively) be explained by a complete scientific theory (e.g. a theory from neuroscience or cognitive science) which (only) can be described from the third-person-perspective. For an introduction, see e.g. Chalmers 1995.

4.4.9   EVALUATION

In summary, according to Singer et al.[322] neuronal information processing is characterized by two complementary coding mechanisms (or coding strategies) that solve the binding problem. On the one hand, elementary object features are analyzed using the classical coding strategy, according to which the average frequency of the action potentials of the active neurons increases. This increased neuronal activity makes it more likely that the information in question will be selected for subsequent joint processing by more effective summation of the synaptic potentials in the downstream neuronal structures. This leads to the formation of neurons with increasingly specific feature preferences (e.g. neurons in V1) via the class of ascending, excitatory pathways (e.g. the retinofugal projection), on the basis of repeated recombination and the selective convergence of input signals. On the other hand, there is a second and far more important class of connections, the cortico-cortical connections of the neocortex. By reciprocal coupling of the feature-sensitive neurons (and using the dynamic grouping mechanism of population coding), these connections are responsible for the flexible association of these spatially distributed neurons to functionally coherent and synchronously active assemblies. Very different complex constellations or configurations of percept components, e.g. in visual scenes, can then be analyzed and represented in succession within the same network.

Recently, a novel unifying framework for cortical processing has been proposed by Singer and Lazar (2016): The core statement is that the cortex is a dynamic, complex, and self-organizing system architecture that provides a high-dimensional state space "required for the storage of statistical priors (stand for "stored knowledge"; author's note), the fast integration with input signals and the representation of the results in a classifiable format." The recurrent neural networks generate nonlinear dynamics "in order to perform flexible and efficient computation". In the context of the various analyses of the correlation structure of cortical dynamics, this leads to a synthetic interpretation of both (1) low-dimensional states characterized by sustained, frequency-stable oscillations and synchronization of these oscillations with stable phase relations, and (2) high-dimensional states characterized by transient oscillations with complex and rapidly changing frequencies, e.g. brief bursts, and highly

---

[322] See e.g. Uhlhaas et al. 2009 with reference to Biederlack et al. 2006, Singer 1999b. See also Singer 2002c, a.

variable phase shifts. Thus, this variability and non-stationarity of the neural dynamics can best be modelled with artificial recurrent network architectures (as they have been developed in the approach of "reservoir" or "liquid computing" [see chap. 9.1, 9.3, 9.4]), or with delay coupled, recurrent, oscillator network architectures (Singer 2018) (see chap. 8).

The cortical dynamics within and between neuronal ensembles are further characterized as follows (Friederici and Singer 2015, Buzsáki et al. 2013): "Coherence of small, spatially restricted assemblies appears to be assured by synchronization of oscillatory activity in the gamma frequency range (30-80 Hz) (...), whereas coherence in large, spatially extended assemblies appears to be established by synchronization of oscillations in lower-frequency bands (beta, 15-30 Hz; theta, 4-8 Hz)."

Recently, the canonical, neuronal, (synchronization) mechanisms of the complex cognitive function of language processing have been increasingly investigated by the German neuropsychologist, Angela D. Friederici and Wolf Singer[323]: "At the neuronal level, complex cognitive processes appear to be implemented by the integration of a large number of local processes into multidimensional coherent global states or, in other words, by the hierarchical nesting of operations realized at different scales in densely interconnected subnetworks of variable size. These principles appear to hold for all cognitive subsystems (...). Highly stereotyped, automatic processes such as syntactic computation are achieved in devoted subnetworks, as shown by the findings of strictly local processing of the most basic syntactic computations," i.e. the basic operation of "Merge"[324] in the dorsal pathway connecting the left Brodmann area (BA) 44 (the pars opercularis Brocas area) and the posterior superior temporal gyrus (pSTG) that constitute the sentence-processing system. This is the neural substrate for the processing of syntactically complex sentences.

---

[323] See Friederici and Singer 2015.
For detailed information, see e.g. Chomsky 2013, Friederici and Gierhan (2013), Makuuchi et al. 2009. For a review, see Berwick et al. 2013.

[324] See e.g. Berwick et al. 2013: "Merge: in human language, the computational mechanism that constructs new syntactic objects Z (e.g., 'ate the apples') from already-constructed syntactic objects X ('ate'), Y ('the apples')."

5 Mathematical, Physical and Neuronal Entropy Based Information Theory

This chapter begins with a short introduction to the concept of thermodynamic entropy (chap. 5.1). Then, based on the mathematical definition of information, the concept of information entropy is introduced (chap. 5.2). Finally, the main features of the theory of (neg-)entropy-based information theory are briefly described, along with their implications for a theory of neuronal information in connectionism (chap. 5.4), e.g. with reference to Paul Smolensky's Harmony Theory (chap. 5.3).

5.1 THERMODYNAMICAL ENTROPY IN PHYSICAL CHEMISTRY

In the context of the "Second Law of Thermodynamics" (see chap. 2.3.1), the Austrian physicist and philosopher, Ludwig Boltzmann, uses the term "thermodynamic entropy" as a statistical measure of order to operationally measure "(dis-)order" in a thermodynamic system (see Box 5.1). Thus the phenomenological thermodynamics can be traced back to the description of the statistical mechanics of gas molecule configurations (Reichl 2009, Kondepudi 2008, Vemulapalli 2010, Moore 1998).

In Statistical Mechanics, the thermodynamic entropy S of a macrostate is defined as the logarithm of the thermodynamic probability w of a thermodynamic system to take up a certain microstate:

$$S = -k_B \ln w, \qquad (5.1)$$

in which k_B is the so-called "Boltzmann constant". Under the assumption that these are different microstates with the corresponding probabilities w_i, a more general expression is obtained:

$$S = -k_B \sum_i w_i \ln w_i. \qquad (5.2)$$

Box 5.1   Thermodynamic Entropy:

The term "thermodynamic entropy" originally comes from thermodynamics, where it was introduced in 1850 by the German physicist, Rudolf Clausius, to describe thermodynamic processes, and is related to the following equation

$$E = F + TS, \qquad (5.3)$$

in which E denotes the total energy of a closed multi-particle system, F the free energy, and T the absolute temperature. S describes the entropy as a measure (of order) for the part of the total energy that cannot be converted freely into a directed energy flow or into work. In a heat engine, for example, it is given off to the system environment as transformed heat.

For a detailed explanation, see e.g. Vemulapalli 2010, Reichl 2009, Kondepudi 2008, Moore 1998, Arndt 2001, Haken 2004.

For an introduction, see e.g. Prigogine 1980, Ebeling et al. 1998.

For a beginner's guide, see e.g. Prigogine and Stengers 1984, 1993, Jantsch 1979/1980, Floridi 2010, Stegmüller 1987.

5.2   (NEG-)ENTROPY BASED INFORMATION THEORY IN MATHEMATICS AND PHYSICS

Based on probability theory and statistics (i.e. based on the mathematical definition of syntactic information[325]), the foundation of "information theory"[326] was an attempt to establish a connection between C.E. Shannon's[327] syntactic-statistical information concept (from communications engineering[328]) and L. Boltzmann's sta-

---

[325]For a critique of the syntactic aspect of Shannon's concept of information, see Rechenberg 2003. For general criticism of the concept of information, see e.g. Janich 2006.

[326]For fundamental information, see e.g. Cover and Thomas 2006, Borda 2011, Arndt 2001, Mathar 1996, Pompe 2005, Bossert et al. 2002.

For detailed information, see e.g. Gray 2009, Ebeling et al. 1998, 1995, Ebeling 1989, Bremer and Cohnitz 2004, von Weizsäcker 1988, 1974.

For an introduction, see e.g. Stone 2015, Lyre 2002, Glaser 2006, Schweitzer 1997, Rechenberg 2003, Elstner 2010, Maurer 2014a.

For an overview, see e.g. Kornwachs and Jacoby 1996.

On the etymology of the concept of information, see e.g. Capurro 1978, 1996, 2000, Capurro and Hjørland 2003.

On the relationship between information theory and connectionism, see e.g. Haykin 1999, Rissanen 1996, Holthausen 1995.

On the critique of information theory, see e.g. Rechenberg 2003, Janich 2006.

On the applications of information theory in neuroscience and cognitive science, see e.g. Cover and Thomas 1999, Ghahramani 2003, Rauterberg 1989.

On the applications of information theory in psychology, see e.g. Glaser 2006.

On the applications of information theory in computer science, see e.g. Holthausen and Breidbach 1997, Jost et al. 1997.

[327]See Shannon 1948.

For an introduction, see e.g. Gallistel and King 2009, Floridi 2010.

[328]The mathematical quantification of the concept of information in communications engineering is based on the early work of the American electrical engineer, Ralph Hartley (1928) and the Swedish-

tistical interpretation of entropy (from thermodynamics) (Lyre 2002 with reference to Shannon 1948 and Boltzmann 1896). According to the German physicist and philosopher Carl Friedrich von Weizsäcker, this is done as follows[329]: Assuming the existence of an experimental alternative (i.e. a binary decision tree), one expects the occurrence of k mutually exclusive, possible events x_k if an alternative with the probability p_k is chosen. For each decision step, the probability for each of the two possibilities is $p = 0.5$[330], which is why $p = (0.5)^n = 2^{-n}$ for n steps. The "individual piece of information" I_k, which shall measure the "novelty value" of the event x_k (if x_k has taken place during the decision), is then defined by

$$I_k = -\operatorname{ld} p_k = n, \tag{5.4}$$

in which ld is the logarithm for the base 2. In relation to the character set $X = \{x_i, i = 1, ..., m\}$ with p_i as the probability of occurrence assigned to x_i, one gets the corresponding information content of a character x_i

$$I_i = -\operatorname{ld} p_i. \tag{5.5}$$

If one is interested in the average information content of a source of information, i.e. the expected value of the information content, one obtains the "information entropy" H[331] (from the American mathematician and electrical engineer, Claude E. Shannon, and the American mathematician, Warren Weaver [Shannon and Weaver 1949/1963, Shannon 1948]). This information entropy is a measure of the average uncertainty or indeterminacy of the prediction of syntactic information:

$$H = -\sum_{i=1}^{m} p_i \operatorname{ld} p_i, \tag{5.6}$$

whose structural isomorphism to L. Boltzmann's "thermodynamic entropy" is evident.

$$S = -k_B \sum_i w_i \ln w_i \tag{5.7}$$

in which k_B is the "Boltzmann constant" and w_i describes the probability of a thermodynamic system taking on a certain microstate.[332]

American physicist, Harry Nyquist (1924).

In addition, the American mathematician and cyberneticist, Norbert Wiener (1948/1961) made important contributions to mathematical-statistical information theory.

See, for example, Lyre 2002, Elstner 2010

[329] The explanations are mainly based on: von Weizsäcker 1988, 1974, Ebeling et al. 1998. See also, Rieke et al. 1997.

[330] In information theory, a binary decision is referred to as a bit (abbreviation for "binary digit"), which is the unit of the information content or information value with $I_0 = \operatorname{ld} 2$.

[331] For detailed information, see e.g. Jaynes 2010.

For an introduction, see e.g. Lyre 2002, Floridi 2010, Martinás 1999.

See also, Applebaum 1996, Haken 2004, Riedl 1975/1990, Rapoport 1986.

Shannon has assigned the Greek letter H ("Eta") to the information entropy.

[332] As Lyre (2002) points out, this caused Brillouin (1962) to postulate the content-related equality of

If $p(x)$ is the normalizable probability distribution for a set of m order parameters $x = \{x_i, i = 1, ..., m\}$ the Shannon entropy (H function) is defined by

$$H(x) = \langle -\ln p(x) \rangle = -\int p(x) \ln p(x) \, dx, \qquad (5.8)$$

so that the information entropy results from the mean indeterminacy of the probability density $p(x)$.[333]

In the case of a discrete (state) variable x, the Shannon entropy is defined as follows (Rioul 2018, Ebeling et al. 1998):

$$H(x) = -\sum_{i=1}^{m} p_i \ln p_i. \qquad (5.9)$$

5.3 STRUCTURAL ANALOGY TO THE HARMONY THEORY BY P. SMOLENSKY

According to the American linguist and cognitive scientist Paul Smolensky[334], this structural analogy to statistical physics also exists for his so-called "Harmony Theory" (see chap. 10.2) (within the framework of his "competence theorem"). This is the case if one obtains the following formulae[335], starting from the relationship between the harmony function and the probability theory $p \propto e^{H/T}$:

$$H \propto T \ln p \quad \text{or} \quad H \propto T \sum_{i=1}^{l} p_i \ln p_i. \qquad (5.10)$$

---

information and "negentropy," which von Weizsäcker (1988) criticizes by assuming a distinction between actual and potential information: "Information has been correlated with knowledge, entropy with unknowing, and consequently the information has been called negentropy. However, this is a conceptual or verbal ambiguity. Shannon's H is also equal to entropy by its algebraic sign. H is the expectancy value of the news content of an event that has not yet occurred, i.e. a measure of what I could know, but do not know at present. H is a measure of potential knowledge and thus a measure of a defined type of unknowing. This is also true of thermodynamic entropy. It is a measure of the number of microstates in the macrostate. It measures how much the person who knows the macrostate could still know if he also knew the microstate. (...) We call entropy (...) the *potential information* contained in the macrostate. It is the largest for the thermodynamic equilibrium state. (...) It contains the smallest amount of *actual information* about the microstates."

[333] See Shannon and Weaver 1949/1963.
For an introduction, see e.g. Ebeling et al. 1998, Pompe 2005.
See the remarks in chap. 3.2.4.4.

[334] Smolensky (1986a) describes this as "The 'Physics Analogy'" and writes: "In harmony theory, the concept of self-consistency plays the leading role. The theory extends the relationship that Shannon exploited between information and physical entropy: Computational self-consistency is related to physical energy, and computational randomness to physical temperature. The centrality of the consistency or harmony function mirrors that of the energy or Hamiltonian function in statistical physics. Insights from statistical physics, adapted to the cognitive systems of harmony theory, can be exploited to relate the micro- and macrolevel accounts of the computation. Theoretical concepts, theorems, and computational techniques are being pursued, towards the ultimate goal of a subsymbolic formulation of the theory of information processing." The Hamiltonian function is named after the Irish mathematician and physicist William Rowan Hamilton. For information on the Hamiltonian function, see e.g. Nolting 2016b.

[335] These formulas are not found in this form in P. Smolensky.

T is the so-called "computational temperature"[336]. The harmony H, following von Weizsäcker (1988), is the actual (structural) information of the sub-symbolic microstates I in the context of the "Parallel (Soft) Constraint Satisfaction Modeling". This is (already) known as "neg-entropy".,[337,338] In other words, H is to be interpreted as a measure of the mean certainty or determinacy of the prediction of sub-symbolic information, e.g. in the context of a completion task (see chap. 10.2). This is the information that best satisfies the constraints according to the harmony maximization theorem (see chap. 6.1 (3.1)), or as a measure of the number of existing sub-symbolic microstates with maximum self-consistency in the symbolic macrostate.

5.4   INFORMATION THEORETICAL ANALYSIS OF NEURONAL POPULATIONS IN COGNITIVE SCIENCE

Shannon's information entropy H can now be used to compute the (maximum) degree of information transfer in a neuronal population using a probability distribution (function).[339] Assuming that a stimulus s_i is given to a set S with a certain probability $p(s_i)$, then the information entropy $H(S)$ of the probability distribution $p(s_i)$ is defined for each stimulus s_i

$$H(x) = -\sum_i p(s_i) \log_2 p(s_i) \qquad (5.11)$$

(Borst and Theunissen 1999, Quian Quiroga and Panzeri 2009).

Thus, using the so-called "Bayes' theorem" (see Box 5.4) in the encoding process, the conditional information entropy

$$H(R|S) = -\sum_j p(s_j) \sum_i p(r_i|s_j) \log_2 p(r_i|s_j) \qquad (5.12)$$

measures the mean uncertainty or indeterminacy of the information transfer (Borst and Theunissen 1999). This remains in a neuronal (population) activity (so-called

---

[336]See e.g. Smolensky 1988a: "There is a system parameter called the computational temperature that governs the degree of randomness in the units' behavior, it goes to zero as the computation proceeds. (The process is *simulated annealing*, like in the Boltzmann machine (...))."
See also, Köhle 1990.

[337]As Schrödinger (1944/2012) has already pointed out, of the term "negentropy" or "negative entropy" the term "free energy" should be used.
See also, Ebeling et al. 1998.
For the term "free energy," see the explanations in chap. 10.3.
For an introduction, see e.g. Martinás 1999.
See also, Riedl 1975/1990, 1992, Rapoport 1986.

[338]This can be seen from the positive sign of the harmony function.

[339]For an introduction, see e.g. Borst and Theunissen 1999, Quian Quiroga and Panzeri 2009, related to the decoding process.
For detailed information, see also Rieke et al. 1997.
For an introduction, see also Baddeley 2008.
See also, the remarks in chap. 4.2.1.

"neural response" r_i) if the stimulus conditions s_j are known. For example, this enables the determination of the selective differentiation of neuronal populations (see the "Theory of Neural Group Selection"[340] by G.M. Edelman, O. Sporns and G. Tononi).

Box 5.4 Bayes' Theorem:

"Bayes' theorem", named after the English mathematician, statistician, philosopher and Presbyterian, Reverend Thomas Bayes, describes the conditional probability of an event, i.e. the probability of an event under the condition that another event has already occurred. In the case of an information transfer in a neural population, this conditional probability $p(r_i|s_j)$ is the probability of neural activity r_i given known stimulus conditions s_j. It is defined as:

$$p(r_i|s_j) = \frac{p(s_j|r_i) \cdot p(r_i)}{p(s_j)} \tag{5.13}$$

See e.g. Haslwanter 2016, Bortz 1999, Gallistel and King 2009.
See also, Haykin 2012, Griffiths et al. 2008.

---

[340]For detailed information, see e.g. Edelman 1987, Sporns 1994.
See also Sporns and Tononi 1994.
For an introduction, see e.g. Edelman and Tononi 2000.
See also, Siebert 1998.
See also, the explanations in chap. 10.1.

Part II

Cognitive Neuroarchitectures in Neuroinformatics, in Cognitive Science and in Computational Neuroscience

6 Systematic Class of Classical, Vector-Based Architecture Types

The systematic class of classical, vector-based types of neuroarchitectures comprises those connectionist models that attempt to solve the "variable binding"[341] problem by means of integrative synchronization mechanisms. For this purpose, vector and tensor constructions are used in the context of continuous mathematics. This means that the variable binding problem concerns a neurocognitive problem: How to correctly assign or "bind" a value or filler (as a semantic concept) to a variable (as a syntactic function or role).

Thus, the criteria of systematicity and compositionality for complex mental representations, which are guaranteed in the symbol structures of the Classical Symbol Theory in the context of discrete mathematics, are also preserved in the transformations into relevant vector-based constructions and mechanisms of the connectionist neuroarchitectures.

(1) The objection of the symbol theorists, e.g. the American philosopher, Jerry A. Fodor and the Canadian philosopher, Zenon W. Pylyshyn ("Fodor/Pylyshyn Challenge" (see chap. 6.1.2)), or the American linguist, Ray Jackendoff ("Jackendoff's Four Challenges for Cognitive Neuroscience")[342], states that connec-

---

[341] For detailed information, see, e.g. Maurer 2014a, Marcus et al. 2014a, b.
For an introduction, see Maurer 2016, 2018.
See the remarks in chap. 4.3.

[342] See Jackendoff 2002:

3.5 "Four challenges for cognitive neuroscience (...)

3.5.1 The massiveness of the binding problem
(...) The need for combining independent bits into a single coherent percept has been recognized in the theory of vision under the name of the *binding problem* (...).
(...)
However, the binding problem presented by linguistic structure is far more massive than this simple description. (...)

3.5.2 The problem of 2
(...)
The (...) problem occurs in conceptual structure when conceptualizing a relation involving two tokens of the same type (...) and in spatial structure when viewing or imagining two identical objects.
(...)

tionist accounts cannot create systematic and compositional mental representations, as they were designed in classical symbol theory with artificial neural networks.

In order to counter this criticism of connectionism, connectionist neuroarchitectures which have been labelled as the class of "Vector Symbol Architectures (VSA)"[343] have been developed (chap. 6.1, 6.2 and 6.3). This class contains the subclass of the "Convolution-Based Memory Models (CBMMs)" (Plate 2003b, a), also called "Holographic Memory Models"[344] (chap. 6.2 and 6.3). The Vector Symbolic Architectures include Smolensky's "Integrated Connectionist/Symbolic (ICS) Cognitive Architecture" (chap. 6.1), T.A. Plate's "Holographic Reduced Representations (HRRs)" (chap. 6.2) and C. Eliasmith's and T.C. Stewart's "Neural Engineering Framework (NEF)" (chap. 6.3). The following authors who have dealt with these VSA and CBMMs models and have partly developed alternative compression formulas of Smolensky's underlying tensor product, are also worth mentioning: Simon D. Levy (Levy 2010, 2007a, 2007b, Levy and Kirby 2006, Levy and Gayler 2008), Ross Gayler (Gayler 1998, 2003, 2006, Levy and Gayler 2008, Gayler and Wales 1998), Pentti Kanerva (Kanerva 2009, 1997, 1993, 1994, 1996, 1990, Sutton and Barto 1998), D.A. Rachkovskij and E.M. Kussul (2001). The CBMMs model type also includes B.B. Murdock's "Theory of Distributed Associative Memory (TODAM)" (Murdock 1982) and J. Metcalfe Eich's "Composite Holographic Associative Recall Model (CHARM)" (Metcalfe Eich 1982).

In contrast to conventional connectionist architectures, a VSA architecture can represent a part-whole relation. This is done by combining a semantic filler vector with a syntactic role vector via a variable binding operation (mathematically, a vector multiplication), in such a way that a semantic content is assigned

---

3.5.3 The problem of variables

(...)

(...) all combinatorial rules of language -- formation rules, derivational rules, and constraints – require typed variables. (...) But some further technical innovation is called for in neural network models, which will permit them to encode typed variables and the operation of instantiating them.
(...)

3.5.4 Binding in working memory vs. long-term memory

(...) contemporary neuroscience tends to see transient (short-term) connections among items in memory as instantiated either by spreading activation through synapses or by the 'binding' relation, often thought of in terms of firing synchrony. By contrast, lasting (longterm) connections are usually thought of as encoded in terms of strength of synaptic connections. However, the combinatoriality of language presents the problem that the very same relation may be encoded either in a transient structure or in one stored in memory".

A detailed refutation of Jackendoff's four challenges can be found in Gayler 2003, 2006.

[343] See e.g. Levy and Gayler 2008, Gayler 2003, 2006.
A comparison of the different models can be found, for example, in Eliasmith 2013, Plate 1997b, Gayler 1998.
See also, Werning 2012.

[344] See, for example, Plate 2003a: The reason is that (as in an optical hologram) the neural information on each informational element of a representational concept is distributed across the entire storage medium.
See the explanations in chap. 3.2.2.

to a syntactic position ("operation of binding") (Levy and Gayler 2008, Werning 2012). A more complex structure can be generated ("operation of merging [Werning 2012] or "operation of bundling [Levy and Gayler 2008]) via a merging or bundling operation (mathematically, a vector addition, i.e. a "superposition operation" [Plate 2003a]). These two recursively applicable VSA operations are used to generate the meaning of a complex term from the meanings of its syntactic component terms. Thus, a VSA architecture has a compositional semantic in which the semantic structure represents a homomorphic image of the syntactic structure of the language to be mapped.

(2) The systematic class of classical vector-based architecture types (Maurer 2014a) also includes those connectionist models that belong to "symbolic/structured connectionism" ("Learning and Inference with Schemas and Analogies (LISA) Model" by John E. Hummel and Keith J. Holyoak (1997, 2003), "SHRUTI Architectures" by Lokendra Shastri et al. (Ajjanagadde and Shastri 1989, Shastri and Ajjanagadde 1993, Mani and Shastri 1993, Shastri 1996, 1999, 2007)). These models use both local and distributed representational formats, or have a "hybrid architecture" ([Hybrid] "CONSYDERR Architecture" by Ron Sun [1995]). This means that such models consist of connectionistic and symbolic modules, or have an almost classic symbol system with a local representation format ("Neural Blackboard Architectures (NBAs)" by Frank van der Velde and Marc De Kamps (2006a, b, 2003). This also includes those connectionist architectures whose binding method only corresponds to the classical temporal synchronization mechanism in connectionism to a limited extent ("(Combinatorial Endowed) Hebbian-Competitive Network" by Robert F. Hadley and Michael B. Hayward (1995, 1997), whose binding method varies ("Dynamic Link Architecture [DLA]" by Christoph von der Malsburg [chap. 6.4]), or which deals with certain special cases ("INFERNET" by Jacques P. Sougné [1999]).

(3) Another connectionist neuroarchitecture, which is based on Jeffrey L. Elman's "Simple Recurrent Network (SRN)", which tries to solve the variable binding problem with a temporal synchronization mechanism, is Peter C.R. Lane and James B. Henderson's "Simple Synchrony Network (SSN)" (Lane and Henderson 1998).

6.1 INTEGRATED CONNECTIONIST/SYMBOLIC COGNITIVE ARCHITECTURE BY P. SMOLENSKY[345]

6.1.1 SUBSYMBOLIC PARADIGM

The "Subsymbolic Paradigm"[346] of the American linguist and cognitive scientist Paul Smolensky, who belonged to D.E. Rumelhart and J.L. McClelland's "PDP Re-

---

[345]This chapter is a largely adapted and partly revised version of my M.A. Thesis (Magisterarbeit). See Maurer 2006/2009.

[346]In the context of his ant colony metaphor, the term "subsymbolic" is found for the first time in Hofstadter 1985, where it already stands in the context of connectionism.
The term "subsymbolic approach" can be found in Smolensky 1988b with reference to the fundamental description of the "subsymbolic paradigm" in Smolensky 1988a, as well as in Smolensky 1988c, and

search Group" in the 1980s (Rumelhart and McClelland 1986a, b), is outlined as a connectionist model of cognition in his 1988 position paper "On the Proper Treatment of Connectionism (PTC)"[347] and in subsequent papers. It was then further developed into an "Integrated Connectionist/Symbolic Cognitive Architecture (ICS)" in his main work: "The Harmonic Mind: From Neural Computation to Optimality-Theoretic Grammar" (Smolensky and Legendre 2006a, b)[348].

Against the backdrop of the "Connectionist/Classical Debate"[349] during the 1980s and 1990s, Paul Smolensky, connectionsm's most prominent advocate, advanced his Subsymbolic Paradigm as an alternative theory of cognition. The central problem here is whether, and to what extent, the conception of an internal mental representation (in the sense of the Classical Symbol Theory) can be applied to the connectionist model (Goschke and Koppelberg 1990). While representations are regarded as syntactically structured symbols in "symbol-oriented Classical Artificial Intelligence" (Symbolism), in "subsymbol-oriented 'newer' Artificial Intelligence" (Connectionism) the concept of classical representation is applied to dynamic artificial neural networks in neuroinformatics. An important distinguishing feature between symbolism and connectionism is the respective model-technical realization of information or information processing (Romba 2001). In other words, it is about answering the question: How does intelligent information processing, or neurocognition, work in humans?

Based on the basic assumption in modern cognitive science that neurocognition is computation, the fundamental question for Smolensky is: What kind of computation takes place in the human brain or mind, i.e. which model of a cognitive neuroarchitecture is to be preferred (Smolensky and Legendre 2006a)?

6.1.2 SYMBOLISM VS. CONNECTIONISM DEBATE

The core of the Symbolism vs. Connectionism Debate comprises the dispute between Smolensky's Subsymbolic Paradigm and "Fodor/Pylyshyn Challenge"[350], which has

---

Smolensky 1989a.
For a basic introduction to the subsymbolic paradigm, see Clark 1993.

[347] See Smolensky 1988a.
See also P. Smolensky's reply to the "Open Peer Commentary" in Smolensky 1988c.
A beginner's guide to the PTC version of the subsymbol paradigm can be found, for example, in Dorffner 1991.

[348] In summary, see Smolensky 2012a and Smolensky 2012b.
The "ICS-Architecture" is first published by Smolensky in his article Smolensky 1995.
See also Smolensky et al. 1992, 1994.

[349] For an introduction, see Eliasmith and Bechtel 2003, von Eckardt 2003, Horgan and Tienson 1994a, Dyer 1991, Dinsmore 1992, Vadén 1996, Verdejo 2013, Maurer 2006/2009.

[350] See Fodor and Pylyshyn 1988.
Referring to this Fodor and McLaughlin 1990: "(...) Paul Smolensky reponds to a challenge Jerry Fodor and Zenon Pylyshyn (...) have posed for connectionist theories of cognition: to explain the existence of systematic relations among cognitive capacities without assuming that cognitive processes are causally sensitive to the constituent structure of mental representations. This challenge implies a dilemma: if connectionism can't account for systematicity, it thereby fails to provide an adequate basis for a theory of cognition; but if its account of systematicity requires mental processes that are sensitive to the constituent

formulated the Classical Symbol Theory for a Connectionist Theory of Cognition. In order to be an adequate alternative cognitive theory, Smolensky's Subsymbolic Paradigm would have to explain the existence of systematicity or systematic relations in cognitive performance without the assumption that cognitive processes are causally sensitive to the classical constituent structure of mental representations. In other words, the Subsymbolic Paradigm would have to explain the existence of systematicity without being based on the mere implementation of a classical cognitive architecture. This challenge implies a dilemma: if the Subsymbolic Paradigm could not contribute to systematicity, it would be insufficient as a basis for an alternative theory of cognition. However, if its contribution to systematicity requires mental processes that are sensitive to the classical constituent structure of mental representations, the theory of cognition it offers would at best be an implementation architecture for a classical model of Symbol Theory.

The general structure of Fodor and Pylyshyn's standard argumentation (in which the classical symbol-oriented model is characterized by (1) a "combinatorial syntax and semantics of mental representations"[351] and (2) mental operations as "structure-sensitive processes"[352]) is that, based on this fundamental principle of "(syntactic and semantic) constituent structure of mental representations", the following closely related characteristics of human cognition can be explained: (1) productivity, (2) systematicity, (3) compositionality and (4) inferential coherence (Fodor and Pylyshyn 1988) (see chap. 3.1.4).

---

structure of mental representations, then the theory of cognition it offers will be, at best, an implementation architecture for a 'classical' (language of thought) model."

More descriptions of the "Fodor/Pylyshyn Challenge" can be found in McLaughlin 1993a, b, which points out that besides Smolensky's position, there are also those which reject Fodor's and Pylyshyn's conditions of adequacy for a cognitive theory, especially the condition that an adequate theory of cognition must explain the principle of systematicity.

For an introduction, see also Calvo and Symons 2014, von Eckardt 2003, Matthews 2003, Smolensky and Legendre 2006a, Phillips and Wilson 2016.

[351] According to Fodor and Pylyshyn 1988, one has to postulate a combinatorial syntax and semantics of mental representations, since otherwise certain features of propositional attitudes would not be explainable, and define them as follows:

(1.1) "There is a distinction between structurally atomic and structurally molecular representations."

(1.2) The "structurally molecular representations have syntactic constituents that are themselves structurally molecular or are structurally atomic".

The first two conditions are usually described as the demand for a (syntactic) constituent structure of mental representations.

(1.3) "The semantic content of a (molecular) representation is a function of the semantic contents of its syntactic parts, together with its constituent structure."

The third condition is usually referred to by the authors as the demand for a compositional semantics.

[352] See Fodor and Pylyshyn 1988 which considers (1) and (2) as the requirements for a classical cognitive model definition, i.e. they constrain the physical realizations of symbol structures in the sense of a physical symbol system as defined by A. Newell.

The classical concept of a structure-sensitive process in cognitive science, is, for example, the conclusion, the "logical inference".

See also chap. 3.1.4.

6.1.3 INTEGRATED CONNECTIONIST/SYMBOLIC (ICS) COGNITIVE ARCHITECTURE

The initial, and fundamental, question is which method of computation more accurately represents human cognition: the numerical cognitive neuroarchitecture of connectionism ("brain-as-numerical-computer") which describes the processing of the brain, or the symbolic cognitive architecture of symbolism which describes the processing of the mind ("mind-as-symbolic-computer")? In response to this question, Smolensky takes up a conciliatory position (Smolensky and Legendre 2006a). In an overall view of human cognition, the brain and mind are one and the same complex system. It is a massively parallel, numerical "computer" at a lower formal level of description (in relation to the biophysical level), and at the same time, at a higher level of description (in relation to the mental level), it is a rule-based traditional "computer" of discrete symbol structures. The relationship between these two descriptions can be given with mathematical precision in analogy to the relationship between classical and statistical thermodynamics.

For this reason Smolensky developed his "Integrated Connectionist/Symbolic (ICS) Cognitive Architecture" (hereinafter referred to as "ICS Architecture") (Smolensky and Legendre 2006a, b), first published "Reply: Constituent Structure and Explanation in an Integrated Connectionist/Symbolic Cognitive Architecture" (1994; cited after Smolensky 1995). The decisive characteristic of the ICS architecture is that the representations can be subjected to either a functionally-relevant or a process-relevant analysis method. The symbolically structured representations are decomposed into their constituents only in the context of the functional analysis method, as in symbol theory, so that the productivity of cognition can be explained using the combinatorial syntax and semantics of mental representations and structure-sensitive processes. In the context of the process-related analysis method, however, the representations are not executed in a serial process as in symbol theory, in which constituent by constituent is processed using symbolic algorithms. On the contrary, the moment by moment causal operating dynamic of cognition requires connectionist algorithms. These algorithms do not decompose a representation into its constituents, but into its process-relevant vectorial activation values and neural activation patterns, and numerically weighted connections of synapses. Thus, learning can be interpreted as the determination of the appropriate weights of the connection matrix via a statistical analysis of the experience-based data material.

The basic working hypothesis of the ICS architecture, according to which "cognition is massively parallel numerical computation, some dimensions of which are organized to realize crucial facets of symbolic computation" (Smolensky and Legendre 2006a), is divided into the following four ICS subhypotheses. These also represent the four principles of the ICS theory.

(1) The first ICS principle deals with the integration of symbolic and connectionist forms or formalization of mental representations. This is the central problem of the relation between these two types of representation.

(1.1) The first ICS principle is presented informally as follows[353]:

---

[353] See Smolensky and Legendre 2006a.

P_1. Rep$_{ICS}$: Cognitive Representations in the ICS Architecture

In the ICS architecture, information processing is performed by representing information using widely distributed activation patterns in the form of vectors. In central aspects of higher cognition, these patterns have a global structure which can be described by discrete symbols and symbol structures of symbolic cognition theory. In other words, these vectors realize the symbol structures in terms of a mathematical isomorphism.[354]

(1.2) In the case of more complex connectionist representations, this global structure is formally as follows (Smolensky and Legendre 2006a):
If several symbols are combined into an *unstructured* collection of elements, this constituent combination is based on a pattern superposition using the vector addition operation of activation patterns[355] ("Superposition Principle").

(1.3) However, if several symbols are combined to form a more complex symbol structure (e.g. a symbol sequence or a symbol string), the different syntactic positions or structural roles that a symbol token can occupy in the overall structure must be taken into account (Smolensky and Legendre 2006a). Such a more complex symbol structure s is defined by a set of structural roles $\{r_i\}$ (as variables), which are each bound to individual fillers $\{f_i\}$ (as values) for individual instances of the structure, thus individualizing it. In other words, a string can be considered as having a set of roles $\{r_i, r_2, ...\}$, whereby r_i is the role of the ith element in the string. A single string of length n causes the first n rolls to bind to individual fillers. For example, the string 'aba' will cause the bindings $\{a/r_1, b/r_2, a/r_3\}$, using a notation in which f/r denotes the binding of the instance or filler f to the syntactic position or role r.[356] The symbol structure s thus consists of a set of symbol constituents, each of which corresponds to a filler/role binding $\{f_i/r_i\}$. This filler/role binding f/r is realized by means of a (binding) vector $\boldsymbol{b} = \boldsymbol{f}/\boldsymbol{r}$, consisting of the tensor product[357]

See also, the principle Rep$_{pdp}$ in Smolensky 1995.

[354] For the distinction between "representation" and "realisation" see Smolensky and Legendre 2006a. See also, the detailed criticism by McLaughlin 2014, whose accusation is that Smolensky and Legendre "have a tendency to run together talk of activation vectors with the activation states that they represent."

[355] The activation vectors that realize the atomic symbols are linearly independent. See Smolensky and Legendre 2006a.

[356] See Smolensky 1990.
Both the filler vector and the role vector are usually vectors in the sense of the "fully distributed subsymbolic representation type".
See the remarks in chap. 3.2.2.

[357] For the "tensor product" see e.g. Smolensky and Legendre 2006a with a simple sample calculation. Further examples can be found in Smolensky 1990, in Smolensky 1994, and in Sougné 2003.
For an introduction, see also Plate 1994.
For the definition of a "tensor", see e.g. Lang and Pucker 1998, Nolting 2016a, 2017a.
In Cartesian coordinates, the tensor product can be computed as follows:

$$\boldsymbol{c} = \boldsymbol{a} \otimes \boldsymbol{b} = \begin{pmatrix} a_x \\ a_y \\ a_z \end{pmatrix} \otimes (b_x b_y b_z) = \begin{pmatrix} a_x b_x & a_x b_y & a_x b_z \\ a_y b_x & a_y b_y & a_y b_z \\ a_z b_x & a_z b_y & a_z b_z \end{pmatrix}. \tag{6.1}$$

This means that each vector component of the (filler) vector $\boldsymbol{a}$ is multiplied by each vector component of the (role) vector $\boldsymbol{b}$, where each vector component represents a neuron.

of the (filler) vector $\mathbf{f}$ (which realizes a filler f) and the (role) vector $\mathbf{r}$ (which realizes a role r). Thus $\boldsymbol{b} = \boldsymbol{f}/\boldsymbol{r} = \boldsymbol{f} \otimes \boldsymbol{r}$. This means that the connectionistic realization of a symbol structure s corresponds to an activation vector:

$$s = \sum_i f_i \otimes r_i. \qquad (6.2)$$

This vector consists of the sum of the binding vectors as a vector addition which realizes the filler/role bindings, provided that one identifies the symbol structure s with the conjunction of the bindings which it contains (see Fig. 6.1).

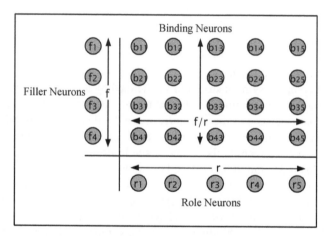

Figure 6.1: The Tensor Product Representation for a filler/role binding consisting of 4 filler neurons, 5 role neurons and therefore $4 \times 5 = 20$ binding neurons (following Smolensky and Legendre 2006a and Smolensky 1990).

This "Tensor Product Representation (TPR)", being a fully distributed subsymbolic representation scheme[358] for variable binding, is already treated as fundamental in Smolensky's article: "Tensor Product Variable Binding and the Representation of Symbolic Structures in Connectionist Systems"[359] (1990) and in various other publications[360].

---

[358] See Smolensky 1990.
For the concept of the "fully" or "fully distributed subsymbolic representation scheme", see the explanations in chap. 3.2.2.

[359] A short introduction can be found in e.g. Huang et al. 2017a, Maurer 2016, 2018, Sougné 2003, Petitot 1994, 2011.
See also, Kralemann 2006.

[360] See Smolensky 1987a, which is almost identical in content to Smolensky 1990, Smolensky 1987b, Dolan and Smolensky 1989a, b, Tesar and Smolensky 1994, Smolensky and Legendre 2006a.
The TPR has been applied in the context of the so-called "Facebook bAbI tasks". See Lee et al. 2015 and Smolensky et al. 2016.

(1.4) It is crucial that each binding vector encodes an exact syntactic position in the activation vector s by means of its role vector, which corresponds to the position of a symbol constituent in a binary parser structure tree (see Box 6.1.3). Smolensky argues that this ensures an independent type of a subsymbolic systematicity (Smolensky 1991). In other words, if r_{x_i} defines the syntactic or positional role in a binary parser structure tree with nodes x_i, the tree s with the atomic filler f_i at node x_i is represented by the tensor product

$$s = \sum_i f_i \otimes r_{x_i}. \tag{6.3}$$

The recursive structure of the binary parser structure tree is constructed (adopting the LISP convention with the functions 'car' and 'cdr') by encoding the position of a node by only two roles. Specifically, the role r_0 encodes a position in the left subtree and the role r_1 encodes a position in the right subtree, so that even fillers that themselves have a more complex structure can be presented.[361]

This is explained by Smolensky (1995) with the following example: Following the LISP convention, the proposition 'Sandy loves Kim' can be illustrated by the following symbolic representation:

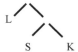

This tree is now represented by the expression $[L, [S, K]]^{362}$, and is abbreviated in the predicate calculus notation by L(S, K). The atomic symbol 'L' denotes the 2-ary relator, which represents the verb 'loves'. The atomic symbols 'S' and 'K' each denote the two individual constants representing the subject 'Sandy' and the object 'Kim' of the sentence.

According to Smolensky, the proposition[363] p = [L, [S, K]] is mirrored exactly in the following connectionist (compositum) vector:

$$p = r_0 \otimes L + r_1 \otimes [r_0 \otimes S + r_1 \otimes K] \tag{6.4}$$

Based on the general technique of TPR, a network architecture, the "Tensor Product Generation Network (TPGN)" is proposed, which that can be interpreted as generating sequences of grammatical categories and retrieving words by their categories from an image. The key ideas of TPGN are an unsupervised learning of role-unbinding vectors of words via a TPR-based deep neural network, and an integration of TPR with typical Deep Learning (DL) architectures. See Huang et al. 2018, Huang et al. 2017.
For an encoder-decoder model based on TPRs for Natural- to Formal-language generation, called TP-N2F, see Chen et al. 2019, Chen et al. 2020.

[361] See Smolensky and Legendre 2006a.
See also, Petitot 1994.
See also, the detailed criticism by McLaughlin 2014.
For an introduction to LISP programming language, see e.g. Mitchell 2003.

[362] The traditional LISP notation for this symbol structure would actually be: (L . (S . K)).

[363] The term "proposition" is used here in the sense of "statement" or "expression".

If they are linearly independent base vectors, the two (role) vectors r_0 and r_1 determine the exact syntactic position of the corresponding (filler) vectors (here L, S and K), in analogy to the position of the symbols 'L', 'S' and 'K' in the tree.[364]

Thus, the vector representing the constituents in the left sub-tree, here the vector L, is bound to the (role) vector r_0 by means of the tensor product when the tree is branched. This vector determines that the resulting constituent vector $r_0 \otimes L$ branches to the left in the tree. In other words, the vector r_0 represents the "left branch role". Accordingly, the more complex (filler) vector, here $[r_0 \otimes S + r_1 \otimes K]$, which represents the right subtree [S, K], is bound to the (role) vector r_1. This vector determines that the resulting (and more complex) constituent vector, here $r_1 \otimes [r_0 \otimes S + r_1 \otimes K]$, branches to the right in the tree. That is, the vector r_1 represents the "right branch role". Both constituent vectors can then be linked to the compositional vector p by means of vector addition[365], as soon as the more complex vector $[r_0 \otimes S + r_1 \otimes K]$ (which represents the right subtree [S, K]) has also been subjected to decomposition.

---

[364] See Smolensky 1995: "The two vectors r_0 and r_1 are the fundamental building blocks in terms of which the representations for all positios in binary trees are recursively defined (...). Obviously, it will not do for r_0 and r_1 to be one and the same vector; we would have no way of distinguishing left from right in that case. Indeed, since we are working in a vector space, what is required is that r_0 and r_1 be *independent* as vectors (...)."

Smolensky (1995) thereby constructs the binary parser structure tree such that each symbol S_k is coded by means of a number k, and each possible syntactic position in the tree is coded by a prime number. The root node is pre-initialized with the binary number '1', which corresponds to the first prime number '2' for the first position in the tree. And then, on the basis of the corresponding (role) vectors r_0 and r_1 (each of which prescribe a branch to the left and right, respectively), the further positions in the structure tree are determined by reading the respective index of the role vectors '0' or '1' as a binary number and appending it to the previous binary number from the right. For example, the binary number '1' in the root node (when branching to the left) results in the binary number '10' whose number value '2' corresponds to the second prime number '3', and which thus precisely determines the second position in the tree structure. In Smolensky's example, this is taken by the symbol 'L'. Correspondingly, the symbols 'S' and 'K' take the positions '110' and '111', respectively. Read as binary numbers, these are the 6th and 7th positions in the tree, to which the prime numbers '13' and '17' correspond, so that with the following assignment of the numbers for the symbols 'L' = 3, 'S' = 2 and 'K' = 5 in the alphabet, the expression $[S_3, [S_2, S_5]] \equiv$ [L, [S, K]] is assigned the Gödel number

$$p_{10}^3 \, p_{110}^2 \, p_{111}^5 = 3^3 \, 13^2 \, 17^5. \tag{6.5}$$

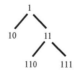

[365] Following Smolensky (1995) it has to be considered that in a recursive tree structure, tensor products with different ranks and thus with a different number of components have to be added depending on the depth of the tree in which they are positioned, which is why, in this case, the direct sum $\oplus$ has to be used. For details, see Smolensky et al. 1992: "The crux of the idea is to add to the fundamental role vectors $\{r_0, r_1\}$ of the stratified representation a third vector v which serves basically as a place holder, like the digit 0 (...) [and] using as many vs as necessary to pad the total tensor product in order to produce a tensor of some rank $D + 1$. Now, atoms at all depths are represented by tensors of the same rank (...).

Trees up to depth D can now be represented with complete accuracy (assuming the three vectors $\{r_0, r_1, v\}$ are linearly independent). The stratified representations (...) can be straightforwardly embedded as a spe-

This (filler) vector itself represents a recursive tensor product representation with the same structure as the compositional vector p: a vector addition of two constituent vectors, here $r_0 \otimes S$ and $r_1 \otimes K$, which represent the left constituent 'S' and the right constituent 'K' respectively, each determined by corresponding (role) vectors r_0 and r_1, which prescribe a branching to the left and to the right respectively. Since both constituents are atomic, no further decomposition takes place.

(2) The second ICS principle, which runs parallel to the first ICS principle P_1. Rep$_{ICS}$, deals with the mental processes to which mental representations are subject.

(2.1) The second ICS principle is as follows[366]:

P$_2$. Pro$_{ICS}$: Cognitive Processing in the ICS Architecture

In the ICS architecture, information is processed by means of widely distributed, weighted connection patterns in the form of matrices. These patterns have, in central aspects of higher cognition, a global structure that can be described by symbolic, recursive functions of symbolic cognition theory. In other words, information processing in PDP networks takes place through the propagation of activations in the form of vectors and weight matrices, based on the tensor calculus (see chap. 6.1.3 [1.3-1.4]). Thus, the connectionistic processes use the central operation of vector space theory, matrix multiplication.[367]

(2.2) The purest formal appearance of the global structure of a process in a connectionist PDP network is in a linear associator (Smolensky and Legendre 2006a). This consists of a set of m input neurons with the activation values $(i_1, i_2, ..., i_a, ..., i_m)$ which form the input vector i, a set of n output neurons with the activation values $(o_1, o_2, ..., o_b, ..., o_n)$, which form the output vector o, and the respective connection weight W_{ba} to the output neuron b from the input neuron a. The sum of all activation values that an output neuron o_b receives from an input neuron i_a can thus be expressed using the equation:

$$o_\beta = \sum_\alpha W_{\beta\alpha} i_\alpha = W_{\beta_1 i_1} + W_{\beta_2 i_2} + ... + W_{\beta\alpha} i_\alpha + ... \qquad (6.7)$$

---

cial case of this new fully distributed representation by mapping $r_0 \rightarrow (r_0, 0)$, $r_1 \rightarrow (r_1, 0)$ and by setting $v \equiv (0, 1)$ where 0 is the zero vector with the same dimensionality as r_0 and r_1."
For the "direct vector sum", see e.g. Smolensky and Legendre 2006a, and McLaughlin 1997 with a simple case study.
See also, the detailed criticism by McLaughlin 2014.

[366] See Smolensky and Legendre 2006a.
See also, the principle Alg$_{pdp}$ in Smolensky 1995.
See also, the criticism by McLaughlin 2014.

[367] The product matrix C from the multiplication of the matrices $A = (a_{ij}) \in \mathbb{R}_{n,m}$ and $B = (b_{jk}) \in \mathbb{R}_{m,r}$ is defined by

$$C = A\,B := \sum_{l=1}^{m} a_{il} \cdot b_{lk} \qquad (6.6)$$

In other words, the output vector o results from the multiplication of the input vector i with the matrix of the connection weights W:

$$o = W \cdot i, \tag{6.8}$$

wherein "$\cdot$" denotes the matrix multiplication.

(2.3) The central aspects of higher cognition, above all language processing with its recursive structure, are thus realized using weight matrices with recursive structure. On the one hand, these are the feed-forward networks (Smolensky and Legendre 2006a), which realize a large class of recursive functions (without the use of closed loops in the activation flow) and have the following form:

$$W = I \otimes \underline{W}. \tag{6.9}$$

An example of this is "PassiveNet", which is able to convert passive sentences into active sentences. On the other hand, these are the recurrent networks (Smolensky and Legendre 2006a) which realize the other large class of recursive functions (with the use of closed loops in the activation flow), and have the following form:

$$W = \underline{W} \otimes R. \tag{6.10}$$

This also includes the important subclass of "harmonic networks" (Smolensky and Legendre 2006a), which realize symbolic functions concerning the optimization of grammatical structures (see chap. 6.1.3 (3)). In both cases, W represents a finite weight matrix that computes the respective recursive cognitive function that can be described using a sequential symbolic program. The recursion matrices I and R are fixed, i.e. these are identical identity matrices for all cognitive functions.

(3) The third ICS principle focuses on whether the widely distributed activation patterns (which take the form of tensor product representations) actually have a combinatorial syntax structure. In other words, can such representations be used in a PDP-connectionist system to generate formal languages in the sense of the Chomsky hierarchy (Smolensky and Legendre 2006a)? The central concept of the ICS theory of language, that of "relative well-formedness" or "harmony", affirms this question. By identifying connectionist well-formedness with linguistic well-formedness, not only can a new approach be formulated in the theory of grammar, but in contrast to the first two principles – a contribution can also be made from connectionist cognitive theory towards symbolic cognitive theory.[368]

(3.1) The third ICS principle is informally represented as follows (Smolensky and Legendre 2006a):
P₃. HMax: Harmony Maximization

---

[368] See Smolensky and Legendre 2006a, which, according to Smolensky, is one of the reasons why the claim of (mere) implementationism has to be rejected.
However, see the detailed criticism by McLaughlin 2014.

(3.1.1) General Harmony Maximization: Information processing in the ICS architecture is done by constructing a net output as the result of the activation flow for which the pair consisting of net input and net output is optimal. In information processing, each activation pattern in the network can be assigned a numerical "harmonic value" that measures the degree to which the "constraints" are satisfied. The activation spread in the network maximizes a connectionistic measure of well-formedness called "harmony" (see chap. 10.2). This means that the goal of the activation propagation is to achieve an output activation pattern with a maximum harmonic value. In other words, the construction of a perceptual interpretation of some stimulus presents itself as the problem of finding an interpretation that simultaneously best satisfies a set of numerically weighted constraints that define the harmonic function, and does so to an optimal degree.

(3.1.2) Harmonic Grammar: Among the cognitive application areas that fall under the principle of harmony maximization are also central aspects of language knowledge, in particular the construction of a grammar. The harmony function, here the "harmonic grammar", is defined as a function which maps a net input (consisting of a sequence of words) to a net output (consisting of a structural analysis of this input), to create the "parser." An example of this would be a parser structure tree that groups words into phrases according to Chomsky's phrase structure grammar (see chap. 3.1.1). The principle of harmony maximization claims that the output, i.e. the correct analysis of the grammatical structure, consists of the parser structure tree, which best satisfies a set of constraints defining the harmony function to a maximum degree. This is why these constraints are the "harmonic grammar".

(3.2) The formal structure of grammar theory in ICS architecture begins with Smolensky's intuitive characterization of the concept of connectionist well-formedness, i.e. harmony (Smolensky and Legendre 2006a). The harmony of an activation vector in a connectionistic network is a numerical measure of the degree to which this vector observes the constraints encoded in the connection matrix. That is, the harmony is a numerical measure of the degree to which the vector is well formed in relation to the connection weights.

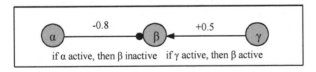

Figure 6.2: Schematic representation of a network example for "Harmony Maximization" of an activation vector. For an explanation see the text (following Smolensky and Legendre 2006a).

Smolensky describes an example (see Fig. 6.2) of a network consisting of three nodes α, β and γ (Smolensky and Legendre 2006a, Smolensky 1995). It has a negative connection weight of -0.8 from the unit α to the unit β, which can thus be interpreted as a constraint such that if the unit α is active, then the unit β should not be active. This means that the unit β is inhibited from being active when α is active. Furthermore, β also has a positive connection weight of +0.5 to another unit γ, which can thus be interpreted as a constraint in the opposite direction: if γ is active, β should also be active. So if both units α and γ were active, β would be exposed to conflicting constraints. And, assuming that the activation values for the two units α and γ are the same, the negative activation that β receives from unit α via the higher connection weight value of -0.8 would "suppress" the positive activation that β receives from γ (via the lower connection weight value +0.5).

An example of an activation pattern that violates the constraint would be, for instance, a pattern a in which both units α and β are active simultaneously, e.g. with the activation value of the unit α of $a_\alpha = +0.7$ and the activation value of the unit β of $a_\beta = +0.4$. Hence the activation pattern a is assigned with a negative harmony:

$$H_{\beta\alpha}(a) = a_\beta W_{\beta\alpha} a_\alpha = (+0.4)(-0.8)(+0.7) = -0.224 \qquad (6.11)$$

Assuming that in the same activation pattern a, the activation value of γ is +0.7, a satisfies the other constraint, according to the positive connection strength of +0.5 from β and γ. Thus, in view of this constraint, the harmony of a would be positive:

$$H_{\beta\gamma}(a) = a_\beta W_{\beta\gamma} a_\alpha = (+0.4)(+0.5)(+0.7) = +0.140 \qquad (6.12)$$

The harmony of the overall network under consideration of both constraints then results from the addition of the single harmony values:

$$H(a) = H_{\beta\alpha}(a) + H_{\beta\gamma}(a) = (-0.224) + (+0.140) = -0.084 \qquad (6.13)$$

Since a satisfies the weaker constraint between β and γ, but violates the stronger constraint between β and α, this leads to an overall negative harmony of the network.

In contrast, consider the activation pattern a', which differs from the previous one only in that the unit β is assigned a negative activation value of $a'_\beta = -0.4$ instead of a positive one. This leads into a situation where the new activation pattern a' violates the weaker boundary condition, according to which, if γ is active then β should also be active. At the same time, it fulfills the stronger constraint under which, if the unit α has a positive activation, this should not be true for β. Since the sign of the activation value a'_β is reversed, all signs of the harmony values in the above equations are also reversed, so that the harmony value $H(a') = +0.084$ is overall positive. This means that the new activation pattern a' is more well-formed than the other, considering the present constraints. In other words, it better matches the set of the two constraints. The combined activation flow in the network of the two units α and γ would now inhibit β, so that the activation flow creates the new activation pattern a'. This means that the activation propagation creates an activation pattern that has maximum harmony. Thus, since this pattern is the one which best satisfies the set of the two constraints simultaneously, it can generally be said that the propagation of activation (according to the harmony function) is a process of parallel soft-constraint satisfaction with different weighting.[369] These constraints are encoded in the connection matrix and applied to the entire set of connections in a network. The total Harmony of a pattern a, in a network with a connection weight matrix W, is therefore simply the sum of the harmony values of a considering all single connections in a network.

One thus obtains the following definition of well-formedness or harmony of a total activation vector a in a PDP network (Wf$_{PDP}$):

$$H(a) = \sum_{\beta\alpha} H_{\beta\alpha} = \sum_{\beta\alpha} a_\beta W_{\beta\alpha} a_\alpha = a^T \cdot W \cdot a. \tag{6.14}$$

Here $\sum_{\beta\alpha}$ means: the sum of all pairs of units β, α. The last term expresses this sum more compactly, using the matrix multiplication operation and the matrix transposition operation (Smolensky and Legendre 2006a).

(3.3) According to Smolensky, the "Harmony Maximization Theorem" is obtained from this harmony maximization process.[370] It means that in "harmonical nets"[371] the harmony of the total activation vector a increases or remains the same at any point of processing time. Furthermore, the total activation of the network – for a very large set of activation rules – "plateaus" to a final vector which maximizes $H(a)$, among all the total activation vectors a that are completions of an input activation vector i. This computation of a complement in the form of a vector a also includes a mapping of the input vector i to the output vector o, which represents the harmonic function f computed by the (harmonical) network.

(3.4) The reconsideration of the formal structure of a grammar theory in Smolensky's ICS architecture has led to the following consequences for the two connectionist principles of harmony maximization and tensor product representation (in relation to the harmony of symbolic structures in the sense of a "harmonic grammar"). These are summarized in the "Harmonic Grammar

---

[369] See Smolensky 1995: The constraints are "soft" in the sense that each of them can be rejected by other constraints and thus violated in the final pattern, but at the costs of a lesser harmony, e.g. by a value depending on the strength of the violated constraints. This means that the violation of a constraint is not impossible, as with "hard" constraints.
See the remarks in chap. 3.2.5.2, 1.1.5.

[370] A formal summary of the third ICS principle P3. HMax of harmony maximization can be found in Smolensky and Legendre 2006a.

[371] Following Smolensky and Legendre 2006a, a "harmonical net" is defined as follows:
A PDP network is harmonious if it has the following characteristics:
(1) Activation function: If the total input flowing into any unit is positive, the activation increases and, if negative, decreases.
(2) Connectivity: The connection pattern is either feed-forward, i.e. without closed loops, or symmetrical feedback: $w_{\beta\alpha} = w_{\alpha\beta}$, i.e. the connection weight from β to α is equal to that from α to β.
(3) Updating: The units change their activation values once at a certain time or by a small value at each time.

Soft Constraint Theorem" (Wf$_{\text{ICS}}$ (HC)) (Smolensky and Legendre 2006a): One considers a tensor product vector $\boldsymbol{a}$ according to the first ICS principle Rep$_{\text{ICS}}$, which realizes a symbolic structure s with the constituents c_j and c_k.

(3.4.1) The harmony of this representation is then computed using the formula

$$H(s) \equiv H(\boldsymbol{a}) = \sum_{j \leq k} H(c_j, c_k). \tag{6.15}$$

Here, $H(c_j, c_k)$, the harmony resulting from the simultaneous occurrence of the constituents c_j and c_k, is constant for all symbol structures s in each case.

(3.4.2) Accordingly, the harmony of s can be computed using the following rules:

R_{jk}: If s contains the constituents c_j and c_k at the same time, then the numerical value $H(c_j, c_k)$ must be added to H.

Each rule R_{jk} is now called a soft rule, and the set of soft rules defines a harmonic grammar. Thus, in order to compute the harmony of a structure s, one must first find all the rules R_{jk} that can be applied to s, and then add up the respective corresponding harmony contributions $H(c_j, c_k)$.

(3.4.3) The soft rules can also be transformed into soft constraints. If the harmony $H(c_j, c_k)$ assumes a positive (negative) value w_{jk} ($-w_{jk}$), then the rule R_{jk} is interpreted as the following positive (negative) constraint, whereby w_{jk} denotes a connection weight:

C_{jk}: The symbol structure s should (not) simultaneously contain the constituents c_j and c_k.

In this case, the harmony of the symbol structure $H(s)$ is computed by adding the connection weights of all positive constraints that satisfy s, and subtracting the weights of all negative constraints that violate s.

(3.4.4) Considering the lower level of a connectionistic network, each harmonic value $H(c_j, c_k)$ is a measure of the degree to which the pair of vectors $\boldsymbol{c_j}$ and $\boldsymbol{c_k}$ (which realize the constituents c_j and c_k) have conformed to the soft constraints encoded in the weight matrix $\boldsymbol{W}$. The value can be computed using the following formula

$$H(c_j, c_k) = H(\boldsymbol{c_j}, \boldsymbol{c_k}) = \sum_{\beta\alpha} [c_j]_\beta \, (W_{\beta\alpha} + W_{\alpha\beta}) \, [c_k]_\alpha. \tag{6.16}$$

Here, $[c_k]_\alpha$ is the activation value of the unit α in the vector $\boldsymbol{c_k}$, which realizes the constituent c_k.

(3.4.5) The harmony value $H(c_j, c_k)$ can be interpreted as the "interaction Harmony" of the pair (c_j, c_k). This is the value of harmony contributed by the constituents c_j and c_k when they occur together, and which exceeds the sum of the harmony values of the two constituents c_j and c_k when they occur independently.

This, therefore, corresponds to a simple case of compositionality – the harmony of a structure as a whole consists of the sum of the harmony values contributed by all its constituents.

To explain the theorem, Smolensky refers to such soft constraints, which correspond to the conventional rules of Chomsky's phrase structure grammar.[372] Under these rules, a sentence (S) consists of a Noun Phrase (NP) and a Verb Phrase (VP):

$$S \rightarrow NP\ VP$$

Two corresponding soft constraints representing instances of the general scheme of the soft rule R_{jk} are therefore informal:

(1) $R_{S, NP}$: If the symbol structure s contains a constituent marked S and its left subconstituent is marked NP, then +2 is added to H.

(2) $R_{S, VP}$: If the symbol structure s contains a constituent, denoted by S, and its right subconstituent is denoted by VP, then +2 is added to H.

Box 6.1.3 Gödel Number Encoding:

Following Smolensky (1991), the TPR scheme can be understood in analogy to the so-called "Gödelization" or "Gödel number encoding", according to which a formal structure, e.g. a grammar or even a symbol structure, is mapped to a Gödel number. This means that it is mapped to a natural number from which the structure can be clearly reconstructed again. A character string, a concatenation of symbols, a "string", e.g. 'ab...x...' a number $s = p_1^a\, p_2^b \dots p_i^x \dots$ is assigned, in which an integer code $a, b, ..., x, ...$ is precisely assigned to each symbol in the alphabet 'a, b, ..., x, ...' . By means of prime number coding, every possible position i in the string corresponds to a certain prime number p_i. Thus the i-th symbol of the string can be effectively reconstructed due to the explicit prime factor decomposition of natural numbers. In the tensor product scheme, this string is represented by a (compositum) vector

$$s = p_1 \otimes a + p_2 \otimes b + \dots p_i \otimes x + \dots . \tag{6.17}$$

Each symbol is encoded by the respective (filler) vector (consisting of activation values instead of a number), and each syntactic position i is encoded by the respective (role) vector p_i (consisting of activation values instead of a prime number). Thus, from the (compositum) vector s, if the (role) vectors $\{p_i\}$ are linearly independent, the (constituent) vectors $\{p_i \otimes x\}$ can be reconstructed in a precise way. In order to get from the Gödel scheme to the tensor product representation scheme, the numbers are replaced by vectors, the exponentiation of which ensures the binding of a symbol to its respective syntactic position, by the tensor product. The tensor product now also serves to precisely bind a filler vector to its respective syntactic position, encoded by the corresponding linearly independent role vector. The multiplication, which makes the connections of the symbol/position-bindings, is replaced by the vector addition, which now links the connections of filler and role vectors with each other.

For the Gödel number coding, see e.g. Aizawa 2003 with a lot of examples, van Gelder 1990a.

For an introduction to Gödel number encoding, see e.g. Hofstadter 2007, Erk and Priese 2000.

---

[372] According to Smolensky and Legendre 2006a, any context-free language can be specified using a harmonic grammar.

By applying the harmony maximization theorem, according to Smolensky[373], the functioning of the harmonic grammar can (in principle) be explained as follows: A PDP network receives the input of any symbolic structure s (coded as an input activation vector i), whose syntactic structure it has to analyze with respect to its harmonic grammar (coded in the connection matrix W). In other words, the network achievement is that this input activation vector i is to be computed towards a total activation vector a, which should have a maximum harmony in order to produce an output activation vector o with a maximum harmonic symbol structure. The higher the harmony value of this symbol structure, the better the generated parser structure tree maximally fulfills a set of constraints (in other words, the conflicting requirements of the constraints are optimally "balanced"). The better the structure tree fulfills these constraints, the more the harmonic grammar will judge the input as well-formed.

(4) The fourth ICS principle – just like harmonic grammar – concerns an optimization-based grammar theory, the so-called "Optimality Theory (OT)". However, it deals with a non-numerical optimization. It represents a comprehensive language theory, which includes phonology, semantics and pragmatics. But it is not yet fully integrated into the computational method of connectionism, which is why it is only briefly discussed here (Smolensky and Legendre 2006a).

P₄. OT: Optimality Theory

At its core, a grammar consists of a set of universal, soft or violable constraints that are applied in parallel to create the optimal well-formedness of a linguistic structure. In contrast to the harmonic grammar, the conflicts between the constraints are solved within the framework of the optimality theory by means of a language-specific "strict domination hierarchy". This means that each constraint that ranks above the other has absolute priority over all others that rank lower in the hierarchy. In other words, what determines the criterion of optimality is no longer the numerically weighted connection strength, but only the rank of a constraint in the hierarchy (Smolensky and Legendre 2006a, b).

6.1.4 IMPLICATIONS OF THE ICS COGNITIVE ARCHITECTURE

According to Smolensky, the ICS theory provides a comprehensive theory of a cognitive neuroarchitecture that solves the dilemma associated with the Fodor/Pylyshyn Challenge (Smolensky and Legendre 2006a). This is done by rejecting the extreme

---

[373]Following Smolensky and Legendre 2006a, it can now be shown that the theorem Wfics(HC) can be derived from the two ICS principles P₁. Repics and P₃. HMax by assigning the following form to the vector a in the formula of the harmony function WfPDP according to Repics:

$$a = \sum_i c_i = \sum f_i \otimes r_i, \tag{6.18}$$

in which the vectors $\{c_i\}$ in the form of the filler/role binding realize the constituents $\{c_i\}$ which are elements of a symbol structure s, which is realized by a total activation vector a.

For an application, see Lalisse and Smolensky 2018.

positions of Eliminativism (Churchland 1989, Ramsey et al. 1990), according to which symbols should not be used in cognitive theory because of their lack of neurobiological plausibility, and Implementationism (McLaughlin 1997), according to which artificial neural networks "merely implement" symbolic structures (see Box 6.1.4). Rather, the ICS theory combines the advantages of both symbolic and connectionistic computation methods. It preserves the former's ability to provide mental explanations, and it retains the latter's attribution of cognition to neurobiologically plausible elementary computations.

Box 6.1.4 Smolensky's Limitivist Position:

Paul Smolensky's subsymbolic theory of (neuro-)cognition stands to classical symbol theory (e.g. from Fodor, Pylyshyn and McLaughlin), in the relationship between micro- and macrotheory, e.g. in analogy to the relationship between classical and statistical thermodynamics in physical chemistry. Smolensky assumes a "limitivist position" with the "Principle of Approximate Explanation". This means that a macro theory only "approximates" a micro theory in the sense that the laws of a macro theory apply only up to a certain degree of approximation. The micro theory limits the applicability of the macro theory, and its relation to the macro theory represents a "refinement".
For detailed information, see Smolensky 1988a.

According to Smolensky (in reference to the American neuroinformatician and mathematician, David Marr), a cognitive theory has to be analyzed on three levels.[374] The functional level[375] describes the combinatorial syntax and semantics of mental representations, as well as the mental structure-sensitive processes. The physical level must describe the neurobiological structure. Finally, the computational level[376] must be described, which is where the ICS theory analysis differs significantly from that of the "Purely Symbolic Architecture (PSA)" (hereinafter referred to as "PSA theory"), in contrast to the other two analysis levels. While the PSA theory does not meet the requirements of the neuronal computation mode of neurobiological systems (because of its symbolically-based method of computation), Smolensky's ICS theory does. This is because ICS bridges the gap between the abstract cognitive functions of symbolism and the neuronally more plausible, elementary connectionist process operations. For this purpose, the computational level of ICS theory has to be divided into two sublevels. At the higher sublevel, representations are activation vectors that can be decomposed into constituent vectors by tensor product representation. This is done in a way that corresponds to the isomorphic decomposition that takes place

---

[374] See Smolensky and Legendre 2006a, b.
See also, the detailed criticism by McLaughlin 2014.
See the remarks in chap. 1.3.

[375] With D. Marr, however, this is referred to as the "computational level"!
For more details, see the explanations in chap. 1.3.

[376] With D. Marr, however, this is referred to as the "algorithmic level"!
For more details, see the explanations in chap. 1.3.

at the functional level by decomposing complex symbolic structures into their constituents. For example, the vector $s = r_0 \otimes A + r_1 \otimes B$ expresses a decomposition of the vector s into its constituent vectors $r_0 \otimes A$ and $r_1 \otimes B$, which is isomorphic to the decomposition of the symbol structure s = [A, B] into its constituents A and B. At the same time, the decomposition on the lower sublevel is completely different, since the representation, an activation pattern, is decomposed into the individual activation values of the network units on the basis of which the pattern is realized. For example, the activation vector s can be divided into a list of number values $(s_1, s_2, ...)$, each of which corresponds to an activation value of an individual connectionistic neuron. While Smolensky argues that this decomposition is isomorphic to the decomposition of a neurobiological activity pattern into a list of numerical activation values of individual neurons, there is no isomorphic relation between the two sublevels of the computational level. This is due to the completely distributed representation format in a connectionistic architecture. For example, a constituent vector $r_0 \otimes A$ to be classified on the higher sublevel corresponds to a multitude of activation values of the individual neurons, which form the activation pattern $r_0 \otimes A$. And vice versa, an activation of a singular neuron k belonging to the lower sublevel corresponds to a multitude of activation patterns in whose generation it is involved, i.e. to a multitude of constituent vectors, e.g. $r_0 \otimes A$ and $r_1 \otimes B$. Smolensky describes this result of the analysis on the computational level by saying that "the decompositions on the higher and the lower levels crosscut one another."

Therefore, according to Smolensky, the ICS theory involves a split-level architecture, whereby only the higher computational sublevel provides a functionally-relevant structure and only the lower computational sublevel provides a process-relevant structure.[377] The decomposition of representations into their constituents, which takes place in both, the PSA theory and the ICS theory on the higher sublevel, is thus decisive for determining the functional significance of the representations, including their compositional semantics. On the other hand, the decomposition into individual neuron activities that takes place on the lower sublevel is decisive for determining the cognitive processes or the process algorithms that actually produce the representations, namely the connectionist algorithms. This internal causal structure (as vectorial activation propagation in a connectionistic network), which models information processing in a neurobiological system more plausibly than the symbolic algorithms, therefore has no equivalent at the higher symbolic level.

Smolensky concludes that the ICS theory operating on subsymbols in the form of vectors is an alternative (micro-)theory of cognition (Smolensky and Legendre 2006a, b). Their constitutive elements do not consist of classical constituents with a classical constituent structure and classical inferential processes, but they can be transformed into connectionistic forms of representation at the higher computational sublevel by means of a homomorphic transformation, so that "symbols are computationally relevant" (Smolensky and Legendre 2006b). In my opinion, however,

---

[377] See Smolensky and Legendre 2006a, b.
Smolensky and Legendre 2006a, in my view, wrongly use the term "physically relevant structure" since they themselves previously used the term "process-relevant decomposition" for that fact.
See also the detailed criticism by McLaughlin 2014.
See the remarks in chap. 6.1.3.

this is merely an unrestricted "implementation connectionism" (in the sense of the American philosopher and cognitive scientist, Brian P. McLaughlin [1997]) if one assumes that an ultralocal representation form is used, since in this case one would have constructed a classical constituent structure architecture in the sense of Fodor and Pylyshyn. In contrast, a fully distributed representational format that would normally be used by Smolensky would possess a sub-symbolic systematicity, compositionality and productivity of one's own type.[378] This is because it is not the symbolic constituent structure based on the process-relevant concatenation principle, but rather the fully distributed representational format of connectionism based on the superposition principle.[379] Furthermore, on the lower computational sublevel, connectionist and non-symbolic algorithms are process relevant. According to Smolensky, the reduction from the higher to the lower computational sublevel is achieved by a formal realization mapping (Smolensky and Legendre 2006b). This "allows a reduction of a symbolic structure to connectionistic neurons", but due to the distributed form of connectionist representation it does not represent an isomorphic reduction, but rather a homomorphic reduction. In other words, the lack of a structure-identical correspondence of the components to each other implies that the symbolic analysis cannot be mapped isomorphically, but only homomorphically, to the process-relevant vectorial analysis.

6.1.5 CRITICISM AND EVALUATION OF THE ICS COGNITIVE ARCHITECTURE

Thus, in my opinion, the ICS architecture has – in analogy to an optical hologram – a "holistic" or "holographic information process structure" which generates a mathematically exact numerical distance metric. For example, it may be based on Euclidean distance, which is why it is able to execute a type of sub-symbolic systematicity, productivity, and strong compositionality of its own on the basis of precise differential equations of Dynamic Systems Theory, and is aligned to the harmony maximization theorem. Following R.J. Mathews' (2003, 2001, 1994) extended concept of a cognitive explanation, the ICS architecture thus also explains the main features of cognition as defined by Fodor, Pylyshyn and McLaughlin. Decisive for the "holographic character" of the ICS architecture, however, is the use of fully distributed representations with their superposition of vectorial information elements, as well as the use of processes of Parallel Soft Constraint Satisfaction Modeling (see

---

[378] Agreeing with respect to a sub-symbolic constituent structure of its own type: Horgan and Tienson 1992a, 1996.
In my opinion, it should also be considered that perhaps the fundamental characteristic of artificial neural networks is that they "extract" the relevant statistical structural relations "derived" from the symbolic structures of human language to be learnt, and that this is precisely where their competence with regard to a sub-symbolic systematicity is to be seen.

[379] Smolensky and Legendre 2006b describe this as "impairment to parts versus wholes", since the damage of process relevant constituents in PSA theory leads to an interruption of the overall processing within the framework of a cognitive function. This is in contrast to ICS theory, in which the superposition principle can result in an error in a partial processing step being eliminated in the course of the overall processing ("resistance to noise").
See also, McClelland et al. 1986.

chap. 3.2.5.2, 6.1.3 3[1.1], [3.4]) as soft rules. In addition, it should be noted that the analytical decomposition of classical symbol theory into discrete symbol representations and processes sensitive to symbol structures can no longer be maintained in connectionist theory. This is because of their use of so-called "fluid" or "fluent architectures"[380] characterized by a constantly flowing transformation of vector and tensor matrices, which cancel the analytical decomposition between the information representation and the information process. In other words, the subsymbol, in the form of the neuronal activity, is both a (micro-)processor and a representational (micro-)engram.

6.2 HOLOGRAPHIC REDUCED REPRESENTATIONS BY T.A. PLATE

Following Smolensky's tensor product representation (see chap. 6.1.3 (1.3)) and G.E. Hinton's reduced descriptions (see chap. 3.2.4.6) (Plate 2003a), the Canadian computer scientist, Toni A. Plate developed a distributed representation form with similarity preservation for recursive, compositional symbolic structures. This representational form is based on the bilinear, associative operation of "circular convolution"[381] and is referred to as "Holographic Reduced Representations (HRRs)"[382] (hereafter abbreviated as "HRRs architecture"). In contrast to Smolensky's tensor product representation, this form is characterized by the fact that the resulting vector of the circular convolution of two vectors of length or dimensionality n (in other words "rank") also has the same length or dimensionality n (Plate 1997a). Thus, the length or dimensionality n of the vector representation remains constant even when applied to recursive structures (see Fig. 6.3) (Seiler 1996).

The circular convolution of an n-dimensional vector $z = x \circledast y$ (also called by its German name, "Faltung") can be understood as a compression or contraction of the

---

[380]For detailed information, see Maurer 2019, 2018, 2016, 2014a.
See also, Chrisley 2000, McClelland et al. 1986.
See also, the remarks on Liquid Computing and the Liquid State Machine (LSM) in chap. 9.1. and chap. 11.1

[381]For the term "circular convolution", see e.g. Plate 1994, 1995, 1997a, 2003b.
For the mathematical properties, see e.g. Plate 1995.
For an introduction to the mathematical operation of circular convolution, see e.g. Plate 2006, 2003a, Smolensky and Legendre 2006a, Kvasnička and Pospíchal 2004, Hölldobler 2004, Seiler 1996.
See also Jaynes 2010.
Since the operation of the circular convolution is used in physical laser technology and optical holography, one speaks therefore also of "holographic models".
See e.g. Willshaw 1981.
For the term "bilinearity", see e.g. Plate 2003b.

[382]First published in Plate 1991.
For details, see Plate 1994, 1995, 1997a, 2003b.
For an introduction, see e.g. Plate 2006, 2003a, Smolensky and Legendre 2006a, Eliasmith 1997, Kvasnička and Pospíchal 2004, Hölldobler 2004, Seiler 1996, Besold and Kühnberger 2013b, Maurer 2016, 2018.
See also, Stewart and Eliasmith 2012 with a calculation example.
For critical information, see e.g. van der Velde and de Kamps 2006b.

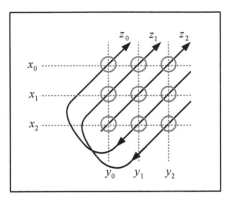

Figure 6.3: Schematic diagram of a circular convolution as a compressed vector product, which is explained using the example (formulas 6.20-6.23). The circles represent the components of the vector product of the vectors x and y. The components of the convolution consist, in each case, of the sum of the components of the vector product along the folded diagonals (following Plate 2006, see also Plate 1994, 2003b).

tensor product or of the outer product of two n-dimensional vectors x and y. The circular convolution is defined as follows (Plate 2003b, 2006):

$$z_i = \sum_{k=0}^{n-1} x_k y_{(i-k) \bmod n}. \tag{6.19}$$

The German computer scientist and logician, Steffen Hölldobler (2004) gives the following simple example: The two vectors $x = (x_0, x_1, x_2)$ and $y = (y_0, y_1, y_2)$ result in the circular convolution

$$z = x \circledast y \quad \text{with} \tag{6.20}$$

$$z_0 = x_0 y_0 + x_1 y_2 + x_2 y_1, \tag{6.21}$$

$$z_1 = x_0 y_1 + x_1 y_0 + x_2 y_2, \tag{6.22}$$

$$z_2 = x_0 y_2 + x_1 y_1 + x_2 y_0. \tag{6.23}$$

For more information, see Fig. 6.3 with a graphical interpretation.

In Plate's HRRs architecture, the circular convolution operation is used to create filler/role bindings in the sense of variable binding[383], like the tensor product operation in Smolensky's ICS architecture. In contrast to the tensor product representation, any filler vector can be recalculated due to the existence of an (approximative) inverse in the circular revolution operation.[384]

---

[383] See e.g. Plate 1994, 1991, 1995.
An example is given in Plate 2003b, 1995, 2003a.

[384] The (approximative) inverse x^T of the n-dimensional vector x is defined as follows:

$$x_i^T = x_{(-i) \bmod n}. \tag{6.24}$$

For details, see Plate 1994, 2003b.
For an introduction, see e.g. Plate 2006, 2003a, Werning 2012, Seiler 1996.
An example of this calculation can be found in e.g. Plate 1994, 2003b, Stewart and Eliasmith 2012.

The model of holographic reduced representations has been combined with El-man's Simple Recurrent Network to form the "Holographic Recurrent Networks (HRNs)" (Plate 1993, 1994). In this model, sequences of symbols are generated along a predetermined trajectory in a continuous vector space using the method of circular convolution ("trajectory associated sequences").

In conclusion, one can say that, in contrast to Smolensky's tensor product representation, the dimension of the resulting vector representation remains constant even when applied to complex, i.e. recursive, compositional vector structures (Plate 1994). Furthermore, any filler vector can be recalculated, at least approximately, by means of "convolution decoding" (Plate 1994, 1995) (see chap. 6.3).

6.3   NEURAL ENGINEERING FRAMEWORK BY C. ELIASMITH AND T.C. STEWART

With their "Neural Engineering Framework (NEF)"[385], the Canadian philosopher and theoretical neuroscientist, Chris Eliasmith and the Canadian computer scientist and cognitive, Terrence C. Stewart have developed a neurobiologically plausible architecture for the non-symbolic, neuronally inspired theory[386] of semantic compositionality within the framework of variable binding (hereinafter referred to as "NEF architecture"). They combine this framework model with Plate's HRRs, based on the mathematical operation of circular convolution. It is based on the book "Neural Engineering: Computation, Representation, and Dynamics in Neurobiological Systems" (2003) by Eliasmith and the American neurobiologist, Charles H. Anderson. The NEF architecture can be described by the three main principles of "neural engineering" in the context of Theoretical Neuroscience, namely[387]:

---

[385]For detailed information, see e.g. Eliasmith 2013, 2003, 2009, 2010, Stewart and Eliasmith 2012, 2008, Stewart et al. 2011. See also Eliasmith 2005, 1995.
For an introduction, see Voelker 2019, Thagard 2012, Maurer 2016, 2018.
The NEF can be also subsumed under the classification of "Spiking Neural Networks (SNN)" (see chap. 9).

[386]See e.g. Stewart and Eliasmith 2012.
See, also, the comments in Werning 2012.

[387]For detailed information, see Eliasmith and Anderson 2003.
For an introductory discussion, see Eliasmith 2003: "The resulting framework is effectively summarized by the following three principles:

1. Neural representations are defined by the combination of nonlinear encoding (exemplified by neuron tuning curves, and neural spiking) and weighted linear decoding (over populations of neurons and over time).

2. Transformations of neural representations are functions of the variables represented by neural populations. Transformations are determined using an alternately weighted linear decoding.

3. Neural dynamics are characterized by considering neural representations as control theoretic state variables. Thus, the dynamics of neurobiological systems can be analyzed using control theory.

In addition to these main principles, we take the following addendum to be important for analyzing neural systems: Neural systems are subject to significant amounts of noise. Therefore, any analysis of such systems must account for the effects of noise."
For more details, see e.g. Eliasmith 2013, 2010, 2009.
For an introduction, see e.g. Eliasmith 2005.

1. A neuronal representation related to the behavior of a population of neurons over a period of time is defined by a combination of nonlinear encoding (see formula 6.25) and optimally weighted linear decoding (see formula 6.26 and 6.27).

2. A transformation of a neuronal representation consists of the function of a variable represented by a neuronal population and is characterized by an alternative weighted linear decoding (see formula 6.28 and 6.29).

3. The neuronal dynamics of a neurobiological system can be characterized in that a neuronal representation is regarded as a control-theoretical state variable in terms of "(Mathematical) Control Theory"[388].

According to Eliasmith and Anderson, one can define these three principles quantitatively by trying to reproduce the biophysical data of a neuronal system as realistically as possible (Eliasmith 2009). This definition is given in terms of information and signal theory, as follows. Within the framework of the first principle the *encoding* process, which is the process that describes the response of a (sensory) neuron to a physical environment variable based on a sequence of neuronal action potentials (so-called "spike train (analysis)"), has to be considered. The *decoding* process, however, also has to be considered. This is the process which, in principle, describes the reconstruction of the originally encoded stimulus, starting from the action potential sequences. Furthermore, two aspects of neuronal representation have to be distinguished, namely the temporal[389] and the distributive[390] aspect. Thus, the quantitative analysis has to assume a population or group of neurons. The neuronal activity $a_i(x)$ of one of the neurons i, i.e. its "tuning curve"[391] (constructed in the context of a "Leaky Integrate-and-Fire (LIF) Model"[392]), which encodes a stimulus vector x(t), is defined as follows (Stewart and Eliasmith 2014, 2012, Eliasmith and Anderson 2003, Eliasmith 2005, Eliasmith 2013):

$$a_i(x(t)) = G_i \left[\alpha_i \tilde{\phi}_i \cdot x(t) + J_i^{bias} \right], \qquad (6.25)$$

For an introduction to "theoretical neuroscience", see e.g. Dayan and Abbott 2001.

[388] See e.g. Eliasmith and Anderson 2003.
For a fundamental discussion, see e.g. Kalman 1960a, b.
For an introduction, see e.g. Sontag 1998, Hinrichsen and Pritchard 2010.

[389] See e.g. Eliasmith 2009, which refers to the basic mathematical concept of the "tuning curve" in the context of temporal encoding and to the two basic methodical concepts of the "rate code view" vs. "timing code view" in the context of temporal decoding.
See the explanations in chap. 4.2, 4.2.4 (1).

[390] See e.g. Eliasmith 2009, which refers to the basic experiments on the "population vector" according to Georgopoulos et al. 1986, 1989.
See the explanations in chap. 4.2.4 (1).

[391] See in detail, e.g. Kandel et al. 2013, Pouget and Latham 2002.
See also, Eliasmith and Anderson 2003, Stewart et al. 2011.

[392] See e.g. Eliasmith and Anderson 2003.
Regarding the question of whether, in the context of the (general) binding problem in the neurosciences and cognitive sciences, a temporal synchronization mechanism in the sense of temporal coding is preferable to (mean) firing rate coding, Eliasmith and Anderson regard this as irrelevant for their approach.
See e.g. Eliasmith and Anderson 2003.

G_i is the nonlinear response function and α_i is the "gain" or "sensitivity factor" of the neuron i, ϕ_i refers to the initialized "encoding vector" (also called "preferred direction vector") allocated to each of the neurons in the population, which is assigned to the neuron that fires the most during the presentation of a particular stimulus:

"(...) the response function $G[\cdot]$, is determined by the intrinsic properties of the neuron. These include the resistances, capacitances, absolute refractory period, etc. that are typically used to model single neuron behavior. Notably, this framework does not depend on the response function being determined by any particular set of intrinsic properties. (...) various neural models, each with their own characterization of $G[\cdot]$, can be used to model single neuron behavior. (...) The vector $\tilde{\phi}_i$ is called the *preferred direction vector* of a cell with this kind of response. This is because, for a given vector magnitude, the cell responds most strongly to inputs whose direction aligns with the preferred direction vector (...). So, the vector is 'preferred' because it causes the highest firing rate for a given magnitude and it is a 'direction' because it has a particular orientation in some (possibly high-dimensional) vector space (Eliasmith and Anderson 2003)."

J_i^{bias} is a "'background' current", which models the neuronal background activity. Thus, a group of neurons can represent a complete vector, but its number of dimensions is different from the number of neurons in the group, and its representation accuracy increases with the number of neurons (see Fig. 6.4).

For a given activity pattern consisting of spike trains $\delta(t - t_{in})$ (in which the index i denotes the neurons in a population, and the index n denotes the spikes that are passed from one population to the next), one can, conversely, determine which previously coded stimulus vector $x(t)$ is currently represented by means of an approximation. This is achieved by means of a "decoding function" $h_i(t)$ within the framework of an "optimal linear decoder" ϕ_i^x (Stewart and Eliasmith 2014, 2012, Eliasmith and Anderson 2003, Eliasmith 2005, Eliasmith 2013):

$$\hat{x}(t) = \sum_i a_i(x(t))\phi_i^x \text{ with } a_i(x(t)) = \sum_n h_i(t) * \delta(t - t_{in}) \text{ and } \phi_i^x = \Gamma^{-1}\Upsilon, \quad (6.26)$$

$$\text{with } \Gamma_{ij} = \int a_i(x)a_j(x)dx \text{ and } \Upsilon_j = \int a_j(x)f(x)dx. \quad (6.27)$$

"It is important to emphasize that analyzing neurons as decoding signals using (optimal) linear or nonlinear filters does not mean that neurons are presumed to *explicitly* use optimal filters. In fact, according to our account, there is no directly observable counterpart to these optimal decoders. Rather, the decoders are 'embedded' in the synaptic weights between neighboring neurons. That is, coupling weights of neighboring neurons indirectly reflect a particular population decoder, but they are not identical to the population decoder, nor can the decoder be unequivocally 'read-off' of the weights. This is because connection weights are determined by both the decoding of incoming signals and the encoding of the outgoing signals (...) (Eliasmith and Anderson 2003)."

In order to obtain a neurobiologically plausible model consisting of compositional representations, the optimal synaptic connection weights between two groups of neu-

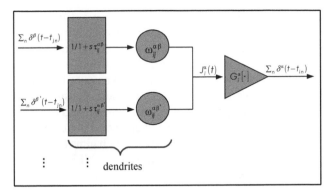

Figure 6.4: Schematic diagram of a "neuronal standard population subsystem" within the framework of the Neural Engineering Framework (NEF) according to Eliasmith and Anderson, which provides a typical neuroscientific description of neuronal function on a basal level. Spike trains $\sum_n \delta^\beta (t - t_{jn})$ from different upstream populations β reach the synaptic cleft and induce a voltage change in the postsynaptic dendrites of the neurons of the population α by releasing neurotransmitters. The resulting Postsynaptic Currents (PSCs) $1/1 + s\tau_{ij}^{\alpha\beta}$ are thus filtered versions of the presynaptic spike trains that can cause gradual effects on the somatic current $J_i^\alpha(t) = \alpha_i \tilde{\phi}_i^\alpha \cdot x^\alpha(t) + J_i^{\alpha bias}$ of the postsynaptic neuron, which can be modelled by synaptic weights $\omega_{ij}^{\alpha\beta}$. After that, a highly nonlinear process in the form of the nonlinear response function $G_i^\alpha [\cdot]$ develops in the soma of the postsynaptic neuron, resulting in a series of spike sequences $\sum_n \delta^\alpha (t - t_{in})$, which migrate to the subsequent neural populations (following Eliasmith and Anderson 2003).

rons have to be determined in such a way that a desired transformation function $f(x)$ is defined. According to Stewart and Eliasmith (2012), the following formula is used:

$$\omega_{ji} = \alpha_j \tilde{\phi}_j \cdot \phi_i. \tag{6.28}$$

This corresponds to a transfer of information from a group A with i neurons to a group B with j neurons. According to Stewart and Eliasmith (2008), one can also use an adaptive transformation function:

$$\Delta\omega_{ij} = -\kappa \left(\sum_i \omega_{ij} a_i - \sum_j \omega_{ij} b_j \right), \tag{6.29}$$

in which (a_i) represents a desired input activation and (b_j) represents the corresponding output activations. In this case, the function of a circular convolution of two input vector variables is defined, so that the activity values from these two neural groups can be bound together to a compositional HRRs structure, appropriate to an "optimal linear function decoder" (Eliasmith and Anderson 2003, Stewart and Eliasmith 2012, Eliasmith 2005, Eliasmith 2013):

$$\hat{f}(x(t)) = \sum_i a_i(x(t))\phi_i^f \text{ with } \phi_i^f - \Gamma^{-1}\Upsilon, \tag{6.30}$$

$$\text{with } \Gamma_{ij} = \int a_i(x)a_j(x)dx \text{ and } \Upsilon_j = \int a_j(x)f(x)dx. \tag{6.31}$$

The NEF architecture has been applied in various ways (Eliasmith 2013, Stewart and Eliasmith 2012), e.g. in a model of the auditory system of the barn owl (Fischer 2005), in the path integration mechanism of the rat (Conklin and Eliasmith 2005), in the swimming and escape mechanism of the zebrafish (Kuo and Eliasmith 2005), in the translational vestibulo-ocular reflex of the macaque (Eliasmith et al. 2002), as well as in a model of working memory (Singh and Eliasmith 2006) and in the implementation of a neuronal production system (Stewart and Eliasmith 2008)).

A further development of the NEF is the "Semantic Pointer Architecture (SPA)" (Eliasmith 2013, Gosmann and Eliasmith 2016), which aims to demonstrate how the functions implemented in the neuronal structures of the NEF architecture can generate higher cognition or complex cognitive behavior (and is based on the "Semantic Pointer Hypothesis"):

"Here is a simple statement of the semantic pointer hypothesis:
Higher-level cognitive functions in biological systems are made possible by semantic pointers. Semantic pointers are neural representations that carry partial semantic content and are composable into the representational structures necessary to support complex cognition (Eliasmith 2013)."

"Semantic pointers can be understood as being elements of a compressed neural vector space. Compression is a natural way to understand much of neural processing. For instance, the number of cells in the visual hierarchy gradually decreases from the primary visual cortex (V1) to the inferior temporal cortex (IT), meaning that the information has been compressed from a higher-dimensional (image-based) space into a lower-dimensional (feature) space. This same kind of operation maps well to the motor hierarchy, where lower dimensional firing patterns are successively decompressed (for example, when a lower-dimensional motor representation in Euclidean space moves down the motor hierarchy to higher dimensional muscle space) (Eliasmith 2013, Eliasmith et al. 2012)."

From this, the "Semantic Pointer Architecture Unified Network (SPAUN)"[393] has also developed. This network is a large-scale cognitive neuroarchitecture with 2.5 million neurons and 60 billion synapses, which aims to consider neuroanatomical and neurophysiological aspects, as well as psychological aspects, of behavior (see Fig. 6.5). Eight different experimental tasks are performed. These include visually presenting randomly selected handwritten characters and reproducing them motorically with a simulated arm (with 94% accuracy, compared to 98% accuracy in human subjects) ("copy drawing"), or solving simple induction problems, such as those present in the "Raven's Progressive Matrices (RPM) test for fluid intelligence" (with 88% accuracy, compared to 89% accuracy in human subjects) ("fluid reasoning") (Eliasmith 2013 with reference to Forbes 1964, Eliasmith et al. 2012).

---

[393]For a fundamental discussion, see e.g. Eliasmith et al. 2012.
For detailed information, see e.g. Eliasmith et al. 2016, Stewart and Eliasmith 2014, Eliasmith 2013, Rasmussen and Eliasmith 2013, Eliasmith and Trujillo 2013.
For the philosophical implications, see e.g. Eliasmith 2015.

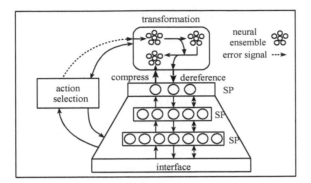

Figure 6.5: Schematic diagram of a standard SPA ("Semantic Pointer Architecture") subsystem or module of the "Semantic Pointer Architecture Unified Network", the details of which depend on the brain area being modelled. High-dimensional information from the system environment or another subsystem reaches the relevant subsystem via the "interface". This information input is then compressed by means of applied functions by creating semantic pointers within a hierarchical structure. So if one moves up or down in the module hierarchy, the representations, which are generated by the semantic pointers, are either compressed or decompressed (or dereferenced). In the course of the module hierarchy, the generated semantic pointers can now be extracted and transformed by other system elements (in the rounded rectangle), e.g. by the action selection system. All these transformations can also be updated using error signals, either generated internally or coming from the action selection system (following Eliasmith 2013).

Furthermore, Eliasmith and Stewart offer an open source software package called Neural ENGineering Objects (NENGO)[394], which provides a graphical interface for the construction of cognitive network models based on NEF and SPAUN.

In summary, it can be said that the combination of NEF with HRRs has resulted in a neurobiologically plausible model of semantic compositionality (Stewart and Eliasmith 2012, Eliasmith 2009). Corresponding to the experimental data from the cognitive neurosciences, it proves to be highly robust against an increasing loss of neuronal resources ("graceful degradation") or increasing "(background) noise". The performance accuracy of the model also increases with increasing neuronal resources, as has already been touched upon, but this accuracy decreases with increasing complexity of the vector structures. The model has been calculated to use the equivalent of 1.4 million neurons, which would correspond to an area of 9 mm^2 of the cortex. This neuronal population is used for complex and implemented algebraic operations between different neuronal groups, i.e. the same neuronal population can be used for each instance of variable coding and decoding. Finally, from the perspective of the philosophy of science, the NEF is an empirically testable theory because it employs a variety of measurable neurophysiological variables, such as "tuning curves", "spike rates", "spike patterns", "somatic currents", etc.

---

[394] See the website https://nengo.ca/ for more information.
For an introduction, see also, Bekolay et al. 2014, Eliasmith 2013, Sharma et al. 2016, Rasmussen 2019.

6.4 DYNAMIC LINK ARCHITECTURE BY C. VON DER MALSBURG

The German physicist and neuroinformatician, Christoph von der Malsburg has further developed his "Correlation Theory of Brain Function" with the "Dynamic Link Architecture (DLA)"[395]. This architecture is an abstract mathematical model type, which, in contrast to the "classical neural networks", tries to solve the binding problem in the form of "feature binding" by generating flexible dynamic neural connections to increase the temporary weight ("Rapid Reversible Synaptic Plasticity [RRP]") due to stochastic convergence processes in short time periods.[396] Therefore, signal intensity (in the sense of the increase of the fire rate) over a certain time interval and the fast increase of the temporal signal correlations (as synchronous neuronal activity) are decisive for feature binding. Thus the corresponding dynamical links reach their maximum connection strength within the framework of convergence-competitive self-organization processes, resulting in a permanent change of the synapse weights ("permanent weight"):

"Under the influence of signal exchange, graphs and their units and links are subject to dynamic change, constituting a game of network self-organization (...). The dynamic links have a resting strength near the value of the permanent weight. (...) Links are subject to divergent and convergent competition: links converging on one unit compete with each other for strength, as do links diverging from one unit. This competition drives graphs to sparsity. Links are also subject to cooperation. Several links carrying correlated signal structure cooperate in imposing that signal structure on a common target unit, helping them all to grow. Because the ultimate cause for all signal structure is random, correlations can only be generated on the basis of common origin of pathways. Thus, cooperation runs between pathways that start at one point and converge to another point. The common origin of converging pathways may, of course, be an event or a pattern in the environment. (...) In classical neural architectures, learning is modeled by *synaptic plasticity*, or the change of permanent synaptic weights under the control of neural signals. This general idea is also part of the dynamic link architecture. However, DLA imposes a further refinement in that a permanent weight grows only when the corresponding dynamic link has converged to its maximum strength, which happens only in the context of an organized graph structure. For a permanent link to grow, it is thus not sufficient for the two connected units to have high intensity in the same brain state; in addition, their signals must be correlated and their link must be active (von der Malsburg 2002a)."

---

[395] For basic information, see e.g. von der Malsburg 1981, 1985, 1986.
For detailed information, see e.g. von der Malsburg and Schneider 1986, von der Malsburg and Bienenstock 1987, Bienenstock and von der Malsburg 1987.
For an introduction, see e.g. von der Malsburg 1995a, 2002a, 1999, 1996.
See the remarks in chap. 4.3 (1).

[396] According to von der Malsburg (2002a) there is no canonical mathematical form yet, which is why a multitude of model variants can be subsumed under it, e.g. Hopfield architectures.
See also, e.g. von der Malsburg 1999.
See the explanations in chap. 4.3.

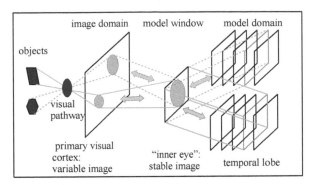

Figure 6.6: Schematic diagram of the "Dynamic Link Matching (DLM)": The image domain consists of the primary visual cortex and the peripheral visual pathway, symbolized by the grey lens through which a sensory stimulus from the environment enters the brain. The model domain corresponds to the areas of the temporal or parietal lobe of the brain and contains a large number of object models. The model window, the "inner eye", mediates between the two domains. Between the domains and the window, ordered point-to-point connections are established by a fast self-organization process, dynamic links, indicated by the double arrows. This happens anew with every eye movement and every shift in attention. The solid and dotted lines represent two different "moments". The links between the image domain and the model window handle all changes in position, orientation, and size of the image created by the eye. The links to the model domain and within it regulate model-dependent changes such as object shape, pose and lighting (following von der Malsburg 2003b).

One application of the Dynamic Link Architecture is the method of "(Extended) Dynamic Link Matching ((E)DLM)"[397] in the context of human face recognition. This consists of a neuronal dynamic for a translation invariant object recognition that is robust against image distortions (see Fig. 6.6) (Lades et al. 1993, Wiskott and von der Malsburg 1996a, b). The already mentioned fast synaptic plasticity (on the basis of the self-organization dynamics of the network, in which a point-to-point matching between the image and model domain is performed on the basis of temporal neuronal signal correlations), is a decisive advantage here. This matching occurs through the establishment of neighborhood connections between neurons and fast dynamic links. Each of the connection weights represents a system variable whose dynamics are controlled by competitive and cooperative parameters (Zhu and von der Malsburg 2002).

The first model level is the image domain, which corresponds to the primary visual cortex. This level contains a two-dimensional rectangular grid of neurons. Since those neurons whose receptive fields are centered at the same position of the retina

---

[397]For basic information, see Lades et al. (1993).
For detailed information, see e.g. Yue et al. 2012, Zhu and von der Malsburg 2002, Wiskott and von der Malsburg 1996a, b.
For an introduction, see e.g. von der Malsburg 2003b, 1999.
On a variant of Dynamic Link Matching, the so-called "Morphological Dynamic Link Architecture (MDLA)", see Kotropoulos et al. 1997.

are combined into a feature package by means of a dynamic binding mechanism, these neurons generate a specific activity signal when a certain "package" of features is detected. In the model, these packages of features consist of so-called "Gabor wavelets"[398] (called "jets" here), i.e. activity vectors encoding the position, orientation and size of a point on the retina (von der Malsburg 2003b, Lades et al. 1993). The entire image of an object is therefore represented by a field of feature packages in the image domain. The second model level is the model domain, which also contains a two-dimensional rectangular grid of neurons and which may be located in the temporal lobe or lateral parietal lobe. This level also consists of feature packages that form a separate field for a large number of already stored classifying object models (von der Malsburg 2003b). The third model level is the model window (also called "inner eye"), which mediates between the two domains. The perceived stable image of the observed object is created from current visual data in the image domain and data stored in the memory of the model domain (von der Malsburg 2003b). The function of the dynamic links is establishing a smooth field of point-to-point connections between the image domain and the model domain in a rapid self-organization process (von der Malsburg 2003b, Lades et al. 1993 with reference to Häussler and von der Malsburg 1983). This means that the connection weights of the fast connections between the corresponding neurons of the image domain and the model domain, which encode similar feature packages, increase rapidly. This is because they tend to be synchronously active with an increased probability by means of positive feedback mechanisms (Lades et al. 1993).

This stabilises certain connectivity structures ("connectivity patterns") which maximise cooperative binding tendencies and minimise competitive binding tendencies (Lades et al. 1993). The total similarity between all feature package-pairs of the associated image and model domain neurons is calculated continuously at a certain point in time, and the best fitting object model is then determined using a "Winner-Take-All (WTA) mechanism"[399]. This means that the object model with the highest similarity to the current image data is detected (von der Malsburg 2003b, Wiskott and von der Malsburg 1996a). This ultimately leads to a situation in which the object model constructed in the model window is optimized for the greatest similarity with the projected image area. Thus the image constructed from the current image data and the stored model data in the model window is given a stable impression of the objects and remains unaffected by eye movements (von der Malsburg 2003b). In other words, in order to recognize a face in a perceived image, the current signal has to be compared with the already known object models in the model level. If cer-

---

[398] For details, see Lades et al. 1993.
A "Gabor wavelet" named after the Hungarian-British electrical engineer and physicist, Dennis Gabor is defined according to Daugman 2013:

$$f(x) = e^{-(x-X_0)^2/a2} e^{-ik_0(x-x_0)} \tag{6.32}$$

For general information on the term "wavelet", see e.g. Burrus et al. 1998, Burke Hubbard 1997, Freeman and Quian Quiroga 2013.
For information on the terms "Gabor function," "Gabor filter" and the relationship to the term "Gabor wavelet," see e.g. Manjunath et al. 2005.

[399] An example for the computation principle of the "Winner-Takes-All (WTA) (computing)" is the Kohonen algorithm or the Grossberg algorithm.
See the explanations in chap. 3.2.4.4 and chap. 3.2.4.5.

tain matches have been found, these object models, e.g. a certain face, are projected onto the model window via these dynamic links. Thus, the adaptations of the connections with respect to the pose, illumination or shape enable the recognition of a face in spite of slight changes in perspective, with predominantly the same reaction accuracy and reaction speed, as in experiments with human test subjects (von der Malsburg 2003b, Wiskott and von der Malsburg 1996a).

The system dynamics of the "DLM Face Recognition System" can be formulated as a set of coupled differential equations (Wiskott and von der Malsburg 1996b, Wiskott and von der Malsburg 1996a):

"Layer Dynamics:

$$
\dot{h}_i^p(t) = -h_i^p + \sum_{i'} \max_{p'} \left(g_{i-i'} \sigma(h_{i'}^{p'}) \right) - \beta_h \sum_{i'} \sigma(h_{i'}^p) - \alpha s_i^p
$$

$$
+ \kappa \max_{qj} \left(W_{ij}^{pq} \sigma(h_j^q) \right) + \kappa_{ha}(\sigma(a_i^p) - \beta_{ac}) - \beta_\theta \Theta(r_\theta - r^p)
$$

(6.33)

Attention Dynamics:

$$
\dot{a}_i^p(t) = -a_i^p + \sum_{i'} g_{i-i'} \sigma(a_{i'}^p) - \beta_a \sum_{i'} \sigma(a_{i'}^p) + \kappa_{ah} \sigma(h_i^p)
$$

(6.34)

Link Dynamics:

$$
W_{ij}^{pq}(t_0) = S_{ij}^{pq} = S(\mathcal{J}_i^p, \mathcal{J}_j^q)
$$

(6.35)

$$
\dot{W}_{ij}^{pq}(t) = \lambda_W W_{ij}^{pq} \sigma(h_i^p) \sigma(h_j^q)
$$

(6.36)

$$
W_{ij}^{pq} \to W_{ij}^{pq} \min_{j'}(S_{ij'}^{pq}/W_{ij'}^{pq}, 1)
$$

(6.37)

Recognition Dynamics:

$$
\dot{r}^p(t) = \lambda_r r^p \left(F^p - \max_{p'}(r^{p'} F^{p'}) \right)
$$

(6.38)

$$
F^p(t) = \sum_i \sigma(h_i^p)
$$

(6.39)

(...) *Variables*: h: internal state (membrane potential) of neurons; s: delayed self-inhibition; a: attention variable; W: synaptic weights between the image and model layers; J: feature jet; r: recognition variable; F: summed activity of each layer. *Indices*: $(p; p'; q; q')$: layer indices, 0 indicates image layer, 1, ..., M indicate model layers; $(p; p'; q; q') = (0;0;1,...,M;1,...,M)$ for image layer dynamics; $(p; p'; q; q') = (1,...,M;1,...,M;0;0)$ for model layer dynamics; $(i; i'; j; j')$: two-dimensional indices for the individual neurons in layers $(p; p'; q; q')$, respectively. *Functions*: $g_{i-i'} = exp(-(i-i')^2/(2\sigma_g^2))$: Gaussian interaction kernel; $\sigma(h) = 0$ for $h \leq 0$, $\sqrt{h/\rho}$ for $0 < h < \rho$, 1 for $h \geq \rho$: nonlinear squashing function; $\Theta(r)$: Heaviside function; $S(\mathcal{J}, \mathcal{J}')$: similarity between jets $\mathcal{J}$ and $\mathcal{J}'$. *Parameters*: β_h: strength of global inhibition; β_a: strength of global inhibition for attention blob; β_{ac}: strength of global inhibition compensating the attention blob; β_θ: global inhibition for model suppression; r_θ: threshold for model suppression; α: strength of self-inhibition; κ: strength of interaction between image and model layers; κ_{ha}: effect of the attention blob on the running blob; κ_{ah}: effect of the running blob on the attention blob; λ_W: time constant for the link dynamics; λ_r: time constant for the recognition dynamics; $\lambda_\pm$: decay constant for delayed self-inhibition $-$ $\lambda_\pm = \lambda_+$: if $h - s > 0$; $\lambda_\pm = \lambda_-$: if $h - s < 0$; ρ: slope radius of squashing function."

In later publications (Zhu and von der Malsburg 2003, 2004), these dynamic links were further developed into higher-order, so-called "maplets", which are defined in terms of the map parameters that specify relative position, orientation and scale referring points in the image and the object model. Thus one obtains a correspondence-based, homeomorphic system for visual object recognition with invariance to position, orientation, scale and deformation, and which is based on a principle of network self-organization (for an overview, see Fernandes and von der Malsburg 2015).

7 Systematic Class of Attractor-Based Architecture Types

The systematic class of attractor-based architectural types contains those connectionist models that attempt to apply the mathematical concept of the attractor to the problem of the analysis and representation of (neuro-)cognitive concepts within the framework of the theory of nonlinear dynamic systems. The models are applied in the representation of percepts in the context of perception ("low-level cognition") (chap. 7.1) and in the representation of sentences in the context of language cognition ("high-level cognition", e.g. the problem of syntactic constituency [chap. 7.2], and especially the problem of the representation of context-sensitive semantic concepts [chap. 7.3]).

7.1 K0-KV SET ATTRACTOR NETWORK MODELS BY W.J. FREEMAN[400]

On the basis of neurophysiological findings (especially in rabbit olfaction (Skarda and Freeman 1987)) the American neurobiologist, Walter J. Freeman, constructed a model of the olfactory system (his "K0-KV (Katchalsky) Set Attractor Network Models"[401]). This model describes the olfactory brain of a rabbit as a nonlinear dynamic system (Yao and Freeman 1990, Skarda and Freeman 1987).

The experimental setup (Freeman 2000a, Huber 2000) involves the placement of up to 64 electrodes over a large area of the rabbit's olfactory bulb so that a common record of the EEG curves of very large assemblies of neurons, in the range of several hundreds of neurons, can be made while the rabbit is perceiving a particular odor. After the presentation of a smell stimulus, a uniform spatiotemporal activity pattern of the entire olfactory bulb is observed, with synchronous oscillations in the frequency range around 40 Hz occurring for a short period of time. The resulting

---

[400]The line of thought in the chapter essentially follows Huber 2000.

[401]For fundamental information, see Yao and Freeman 1990, Freeman 1987.
For detailed information, see Freeman 1995, 2000a, b.
For an introduction, see e.g. Gómez Ramírez 2014, Hardcastle 1998, Jaeger 1996, Huber 2000, Kolo et al. 1999, Rockwell 2005, Schierwagen 1993.
For a brief introduction, see Maurer 2014a.

computer analysis of the data is presented in a 64-dimensional graph (corresponding to the number of electrodes), so that the activity of each electrode corresponds to one dimension of the graph. This analysis shows the statistical frequency profile of the synchronous oscillations in the EEG activity, a common waveform characteristic of a particular scent perception, the "carrier wave," which differs only in the amplitude measured at each electrode. A statistical profile of the carrier wave amplitude modulation is then constructed (in the form of a contour diagram) by plotting the (mean) amplitudes of the EEG curves in the third dimension (with reference to a specific brain section of the olfactory bulb under investigation). Thus a spatial contour line pattern of the carrier wave with "mountains" and "valleys" is obtained.

The analysis of the EEG activity is based on a 3-dimensional profile of the amplitude modulation (AM) of the carrier wave of the brain section under investigation, e.g. the olfactory bulb. Under the model, a 64-dimensional attractor phase space is constructed, which is dominated by a single global chaotic attractor.[402] This attractor consists of a large number of "(attractor) wings" which span an "attractor landscape". The wings represent the behavior of the system under the influence of a certain input stimulus, and are generated by the corresponding neural assemblies. These assemblies have merged into a group during previous (perceptual) experiences (with reference to a certain olfactory stimulus).

If the olfactory system is in its resting state, it has a preferred amplitude modulation profile, which is determined by a specific attractor wing with a corresponding attractor basin. When encountering a new stimulus, the olfactory system suddenly "jumps" or "drifts" from the basin of one attractor wing to another, depending on the initial conditions, which corresponds to a rapid change in system state. This change in system state is brought about by the dynamic construction of a local neuronal topographic representation scheme that encodes a class of certain (new) stimuli received during training:

"To use the language of dynamics (...) there is a single large attractor for the olfactory system, which has multiple wings that form an 'attractor landscape' The system has a preferred basal AM (= amplitude modulation (author's note)) pattern between inhalations, which is governed by one wing of the large attractor. When an inhalation brings in background air, the bulb transits to the basin of another attractor wing that gives the control AM pattern, and it returns to the basal wing after release during exhalation. This attractor landscape contains all the learned states as wings of the olfactory attractor, each of which is accessed when the appropiate stimulus is presented. Each attractor has its own basin of attraction, which was shaped by the class of stimuli the animals received during training. No matter where in each basin a stimulus puts the bulb, the bulb goes to the attractor of that basin, accomplishing generalization to the class (Freeman 2000a)."

The learning of a certain olfactory stimulus thus consists of the stochastic tendency of the system to stabilize under certain conditions. The system's stabilization tendency

---

[402]For detailed information, see e.g. Freeman and Schneider 1982, Freeman 1978, Freeman and Viana di Prisco 1986.
For an introduction, see e.g. Bechtel and Abrahamsen 2002, McGovern and Baars 2007.

is generated by the learning process itself, in a certain attractor wing or in a certain attractor region which is smaller in phase space volume. Thus, different odours associated with "meaning" are encoded by different attractor regions assigned to them (Freeman 2003a, b, Schierwagen 1993, Hardcastle 1998):

"The meaning is not the pattern, nor is it in the pattern. It is the set of relations expressed by the pattern and enacted by the neurons sustaining it, which may include the entire forebrain, if one allows that neurons participate not only by discharging but also by actively remaining silent under inhibition, when that is required of them to form a pattern (Freeman 1995)."

This attractor-based, nonlinear, neurodynamics (which, according to Freeman, provides a new view of neurocognitive functions) is characterized by two factors.[403] Firstly the fact that the olfactory bulb remains involved in the entire perceptual process until recognition and action. This happens by means of a high number of parallel feedback fiber connections between the olfactory cortex and the olfactory bulb. Thus, the incoming olfactory stimuli are already assigned a "meaning" at this early stage of information processing. And secondly, these neurodynamics are characterized by the fact that the temporal synchronization mechanisms of the collective neuronal activity, which bind together the individual excitations caused by the same olfactory stimulus, make it possible for a meaningful perception to stand out against the background of the other neuronal activity[404].

"My view is that nonlinear dynamics despite its difficulties (...) and limitations (...) provides the best available new tools to explore brain function. It enable us to use deterministic equations to create novel patterns that are analogous to the novel patterns created by brains using neurons. Owing to the power of its tools, nonlinear dynamics may play a pivotal role in studies of intentionality by providing a language for making bridges between measurements of brain activity and observations of behavior, including introspection, falling in and out of love, and dealing with hatred as it comes (Freeman 1995)."

Recently, the same types of textured AM patterns and phase modulation (PM) patterns are being measured in scalp EEGs with human subjects and categorized with respect to visual, tactile and auditory conditioned stimuli.[405]

Since the 1970s, Freeman has developed a hierarchy of architectural models of cortical nonlinear neurodynamics that is closely oriented to the neurophysiological

---

[403] See e.g. Freeman 2000b.
For an overview, see Freeman 2013.
See also, Abrahman et al. 1990, Başar and Haken (1999).
See in summary with regard to the interpretation of this new view of functional neurodynamics in the sense of Freeman e.g. Breidbach 1996.

[404] For detailed information, see e.g. Freeman 2003a,b.
For an introduction, see e.g. Huber 2000.
Furthermore, Davis et al. 2013 cite neurophysiological evidence that these neural synchronization mechanisms could represent a potential manifestation of the so-called "aha effect".

[405] For an overview, see Freeman 2015.
For detailed information, see e.g. Pockett et al. 2009, Ruiz et al. 2010, Brockmeier et al. 2012, Zhang et al. 2015, Freeman 2005.

findings (Yao and Freeman 1990 with reference to Freeman 1972, 2000a) of the so-called "K0-KV (Katchalsky) Set Attractor Network Models"[406] These models are based on the "Katchalsky sets" with the components K0, KI, KII, KIII, KIV and KV. These components model the cortical architecture with increasing complexity and functionality:

"The basic K-unit, called K0 set, models a neuron population of about 10^4 neurons. (...) Coupling two or more K0 sets with excitatory connections, we get a KI. The next step in the hierarchy is the KII model. KII is a double layer of excitatory and inhibitory units. In the simplest architecture, there are 4 nodes: two excitatory, denoted e, and two inhibitory, denoted i, nodes. The excitatory and inhibitory nodes in a KII set are arranged in corresponding layers, so KII has a double-layer structure. Given proper initial conditions, this model may produce sustained periodic oscillations, the frequency and magnitude of which are determined by the interconnection weights between units. KIII consists of three double layers of KII sets that are connected with no-delay feed-forward connections and delayed feedback connections. Properly tuned KIII models typically exhibit non-convergent chaotic behavior due to the competition of KII oscillators. KIII is the model of sensory cortices. Finally, several KIII and/or KII sets form the multi-sensory KIV set (...) which is capable of exhibiting intermittent spatiotemporal synchronization, as the result of interacting chaotic KIII and KII oscillatory units (Kozma and Freeman 2009)."

The basic component, K0, describes a cortical microcolumn whose dynamics are determined by a second order ordinary differential equation (Kozma and Freeman 2009 with reference to Freeman 1975):

$$a \cdot b \frac{d^2 P(t)}{d^2 t} + (a+b) \frac{dP(t)}{dt} + P(t) = F(t), \qquad (7.1)$$

wherein a and b are biologically determined time constants, $P(t)$ denotes the activation of a node as a function of time, and $F(t)$ is the summed activation of neighboring nodes and the other weighted input.

Furthermore, the basic component K0 has an asymptotic, sigmoid output function $Q(x)$ with a slope parameter q (Kozma and Freeman 2009 with reference to Freeman 1975):

$$Q(x) = q \cdot \left\{ 1 - \exp\left(\frac{-1}{q(e^x - 1)}\right) \right\}. \qquad (7.2)$$

7.2 MORPHODYNAMIC ATTRACTOR MODEL BY J. PETITOT

The French mathematician and cognitive scientist, Jean Petitot-Cocorda studied the problem of syntactic constituency in linguistics with his "Morphodynamic Attractor

---

[406]For fundamental information, see e.g. Freeman 1975, 1987, Yao and Freeman 1990, Kozma and Freeman 2009.
See also, Freeman 2000a.
An overview can be found e.g. in Kozma and Freeman 2009, Perlovsky and Kozma 2007.
For an introduction, see e.g. Gómez Ramírez 2014.
Named after the Israeli physicochemist, Aharon (Katzir-) Katchalsky. See e.g. Kozma and Freeman 2009.

Model",[407] which combines concepts from R. Thom's "catastrophe theory"[408] and R.W. Langacker's "cognitive grammar".[409] Within the framework of this dynamic model of syntax and semantics, it is assumed that a sentence of a natural language is neuronally instantiated on the basis of dynamic attractor and bifurcation concepts, so-called "(elementary) catastrophes" (Petitot 2011). In other words, the syntactic structure of a sentence is dominated by critical and dramatic phase transitions, which are caused by certain control parameter settings in differential equations. These transitions result in complete qualitative transformations in the dynamic configuration of attractors in phase space. These transformations are the elementary catastrophes mentioned above. The geometric interpretation of these critical parameter values in the structurally stable polynomials of the differential equations of the system then generates complex, archetypal geometric objects (according to the "classification theorems"[410] of R. Thom, E.C. Zeeman and V.I. Arnold), e.g.

(1) the "cusp" according to a fourth degree differential equation (Petitot 2011):

$$f_{u,v}(x) = x^4 + ux^2 + vx, \tag{7.3}$$

wherein the control parameters u, v are referred to as "splitting factor" and "normal factor" according to Zeeman[411],

(2) the "swallowtail" according to a fifth degree differential equation (Petitot 2011):

$$f_{u,v,w}(x) = x^5 + ux^3 + vx^2 + wx, \tag{7.4}$$

(3) the "butterfly" according to a sixth degree differential equation (Petitot 2011) (see Fig. 7.1):

$$f_{t,u,v,w}(x) = x^6 + tx^4 + ux^3 + vx^2 + wx. \tag{7.5}$$

---

[407] For fundamental information, see e.g. Petitot 2011, 1995, 1993.
For a brief introduction, see Maurer 2014a.
On an "Active Morphodynamical Semantics", based on coupled oscillators with (phase gradient) synchronization, see Doursat and Petitot 2005.

[408] For fundamental information, see e.g. Thom 1972/1980, 1975, 1983, 1989.
For an introduction to mathematics, see e.g. Gilmore 1980, Jetschke 1989.
For an introduction to linguistics, see e.g. Wildgen 1985, 1987, Wildgen and Plath 2005.
Catastrophe theory can be seen as a branch of bifurcation theory in the analysis of nonlinear dynamic systems.
See e.g. Haken 2004.
See the remarks in chap. 2.

[409] For basic information, see e.g. Langacker 1987, 1991.
For an introduction, see e.g. Wildgen 2010.

[410] For fundamental information, see e.g. Thom 1972/1980.
For detailed information, see e.g. Petitot 2011.
For an introduction, see e.g. Wildgen and Plath 2005, Wildgen 1985, 1987
The theorem is also called "unfolding theorem".

[411] See e.g. Zeeman 1976.
For an introduction to the approach of catastrophe theory in the sense of E.C. Zeeman, see Jantsch 1979/1980.

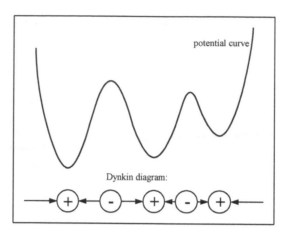

Figure 7.1: Schematic diagram of the potential curve of the "butterfly" (above) with the corresponding Dynkin diagram (below) (following Wildgen and Plath 2005).

Under the assumption that the neuronal system can be described as a gradient system, there are only a small number of transformations from one attractor configuration to another. These transformations are regarded as universal cognitive archetypes of relations between the syntactic functions or actantial roles, such as agent, recipient, etc. This can also be used to address the problem of filler/role-bindings. However, Petitot argues that this is less important than the main problem, which is that the relations of actant interactions are specified by the configurational definition of syntactic functions. This means that the relations of the actant interactions are specified on the basis of a single position within a configuration of different positions, in the terms of attractor topology ("attractor syntax"). In other words, the relations of actant interactions are specified by a sequence of bifurcations of complex attractors within the framework of neuronal algorithmic system dynamics ("dynamical functionalism") (Petitot 2011, Petitot 1991, 1994):

"If the actants A_i of a process are modeled by attractors A_i, a dynamical system, is it possible, within the framework of the mathematical theory of dynamical systems, to elaborate a geometric theory of actantial interactions – i.e. a theory of the verb and its participants?

In many dynamical models, the situation can be greatly simplified if one makes the hypothesis that the dynamics X defining the attractors A_i admits a global Lyapunov function (...) or, even more simply, that $X = -\mathrm{grad} f$. The A_i are then the minima m_i of the potential function f. The main question can thus be simplified: *If the actants A_i of a process are modeled by the minima m_i of a potential function, is it possible, within the framework of the dynamical theory of potential functions, to elaborate a theory of actantial interactions – i.e., a theory of the verb?*

The mathematical challenge is therefore to develop a theory of interactions of attractors, what we call an *attractor syntax*. (...)

Note that we will not be discussing here, what has come to be known as the *binding problem*. The way by which one can bind a role label with a filler term is certainly a fundamental issue. But the main focus of this chapter is that of the configurational definition which can substitute the role labels. We will see that, in such a definition, roles are identified with positions – places – in configurations of positions. Of course, these places have to be filled by terms (particular attractors; see Contents and Complex Attractors, below).

(...)

Contents and Complex Attractors: In brain modeling, we can suppose, owing to the oscillatory nature of the brain, that the attractors come from the coupling of limit cycles. (...) *The (complex) topology of such a strange brain attractor can be identified with the content of the correlated mental state.* In reducing the attractors to points in a quasi-gradient model, *we therefore reduce these mental contents to unanalyzable units.* This reduction is equivalent, in the morphodynamical approach, to the classic reduction of semantic units to formal symbols. The main difference is that the *relations* between these units *are no longer of symbolic nature*: they are dynamically generated by an optimization device (minimizing a Lyapunov function) (Petitot 1995)."

"(...) the main problem is the configurational definition of roles, which can substitute for the classical role labels. (...) in such a configurational definition, roles are identified with positions or 'places' in configurations of positions. Of course, these places have to be filled by fillers, but the key difficulty is to elaborate a CN [connectionist (author's note)] theory of such positional relations without taking for granted any prior CL [classic (author's note)] representation of them.

(...)

(...) the problem is (...) to give a correct, purely CN account of the *relations of actantial interactions* which are involved in syntactic structures. These relations are not binding. They are concerned with the roles independently of their fillers. The PTC [Proper Treatment of Connectionism (author's note)] agenda (...) must also be applied to the configurational definition of the actantial roles.

(...)

Morphodynamics aims at explaining natural morphologies and iconic, schematic, Gestalt-like aspects of structures, whatever their underlying physical substrate may be, using the mathematical theory of dynamical systems. Syntactic structures can be treated as Gestalts and can be morphodynamically modeled.

One must carefully distinguish between the formal description of symbolic structures on the one hand and their dynamical explanation on the other. It is not because the former is correct that one is committed to a symbolic conception of mental states and processes. In morphodynamics, the conceptual contents of mental states are no longer identified with symbols. Their meaning is embodied in the cognitive processing itself. More precisely, it is identified with the topology of the complex attractors of the underlying neural dynamics, and the mental events are identified with sequences of bifurcations of such attractors. Symbolic structures are conceived of as macro-structures emerging from the underlying micro-neurodynamics. Information processing is therefore thought of, not as an implemented symbolic processing, but as a *dynamical process* (Petitot 2011)."

An introductory paraphrase is as follows:

"For classes of very elementary dynamical systems – namely, 'gradient descent' systems, in which the only form of behavior is settling into a point attractor – it is possible to classify the various kinds of interactions of attractors. For each of these 'elementary' catastrophes, there is just a small set of qualitatively different ways in which boundaries can be crossed; or in other words, a small set of transformations from one qualitative arrangement of attractors to another. Now, let us hypothesize that the behavior of the brain can be described, at some suitable high level, in terms of gradient systems. From this it follows that there is a strictly limited set of ways in which the dynamics of the brain transforms from one qualitative arrangement to another.

In Thom and Petitot's theory, these transformations are treated as universal cognitive archetypes for relations between semantic roles. Each basic elementary and nuclear sentence of natural language, as the expression of a possible thought, is syntactically structured by one of these cognitive archetypes. The main verb corresponds to the catastrophe transformation as a whole, while the individual terms correspond to the distinct attractors. Since there is a vast number of distinct sentences, many sentences correspond to each cognitive archetype. Differences in the particular semantic content of a sentence falling under a common archetype (i.e., the difference between 'John gives the book to Mary' and 'Mary sends e-mail to Bob') correspond to differences in the global semantics of the scene (in Fillmore's sense) and in the internal nature of the attractors themselves.

In the limited set of basic catastrophe transformations, there is only a fixed number of positions that attractors can occupy with respect to other attractors (e.g., one being swallowed up by another). A key claim of Petitot's morphodynamical approach to syntax is that these positions correspond to what European linguists call 'actants' or 'actantial roles' and American linguists often refer to as case roles (Agent, Patient, etc.). Thus the morphodynamical approach can account for the fact that all natural languages appear to draw their cases from a limited set of universal types. Further, the approach provides what Petitot calls a 'configurational definition' of case roles. An Agent is an Agent because of the particular place of the corresponding attractor within a specific catastrophe transformation of attractor arrangements or configurations (Petitot 1995)."

According to Thom's catastrophe theory, the attractors (as minima of a potential function) are then regarded as actants of a syntactic position. These are the generated potentials of a potential function or Lyapunov function, which act as a producer for the relations between the actants (Petitot 2011). Furthermore, a vector flow-time path of the potentials is regarded as a transformation process of these relations between the actants, and the interactions of the actants at the bifurcations as verbs:

"For topological models of syntax, Thom's main idea was the following: We start with a general morphodynamical model of gradient type. Let f be a (term of) potential on an internal manifold $\mathcal{M}$. (...) Let (f_w, W, K) be the universal unfolding of f (...). (...) we consider the product $\mathcal{M} \times W$ of the internal space $\mathcal{M}$ (on which the f_w are defined) by the external space W. (...) We have seen (...) that connectionist models have also used this idea, but only for the theory of learning (W is then the space of synaptic weights which vary slowly, adiabatically, along the trajectories of the back-propagation dynamics). Here, it is used for a completely different purpose: to model the *categorial difference between actant and verb*.

We use then the universal unfolding (f_w, W, K) as a geometrical generator for *events of interaction between attractors*. We introduce temporal paths $\gamma = w(t)$ in the external space W and consider that they are driven by slow external dynamics. When γ crosses K, bifurcation events occur. They are events of interaction of quadratic critical points. Thom's idea is then to interpret the minima of the f_w – the attractors of the internal dynamics – as 'actants', the generating potential f_w as a generator of *relations* between them, a temporal path $f_{w(t)}$ as a *process* of transformation of these relations, and the interaction of actants at the crossing of K as a *verbal node* (Petitot 2011)."

"If one interprets the stable local regimes (of the fast internal dynamics) as actants, it becomes possible to give the qualitative appearance of catastrophes a semantic interpretation, expressed in natural language. If (...) one introduces time (i.e. a slow external dynamics), the bifurcations (author's note) are interpreted as verbs.
(...)
Thus, one gets what I think is the universal structural table, which contains all types of elementary sentences (Petitot 2011 with an English translation of a French quotation from Thom 1980)."

Based on Thom's catastrophe theory, the German linguist, Wolfgang Wildgen also developed a dynamic attractor model of cognitive linguistics with his "Archetypal Semantics" (Wildgen 1985, Wildgen 1987, Wildgen and Plath 2005).

7.3 MODULAR NEURODYNAMICAL SYSTEMS BY F. PASEMANN[412]

The German theoretical physicist and cognitive scientist, Frank Pasemann, also characterized a cognitive system based on the mathematical theory of dynamic systems, the "modular neurodynamic system"[413]. This system is given in the form of very small "Modular Neural Networks (MNN)", so-called "neuromodules".[414] These neuromodules can be described by a discrete "(formal) modular neurodynamics"

---

[412]This chapter is a partially revised version of the chapter in Maurer 2006/2009, 2014a.

[413]For fundamental information, see e.g. Pasemann 1995.
For a detailed description of the synchronization dynamics between "chaotic neuromodules", see e.g. Wennekers and Pasemann 1996, Pasemann 1998, 1999, Pasemann and Wennekers 2000.
See also Pasemann and Stollenwerk 1998.
For the synchronization of a robot population using a "coupled oscillator architecture", see e.g. Wischmann et al. 2006, Pasemann et al. 2003, Negrello et al. 2008.
For an introduction, see e.g. Pasemann 1996.

[414]For fundamental information, see e.g. Pasemann 1995, 1998, 2002, Stollenwerk and Pasemann 1996, Wennekers and Pasemann 1996, Pasemann and Stollenwerk 1998, Negrello et al. 2008.
For a detailed description of "coupled neuromodules", see e.g. Pasemann and Wennekers 2000.

(also in the sense of chaos theory), and are characterized by their high degree of "functional flexibility with the constant structure of the system elements"[415]:

"Since, on the one hand, the input signals to cognitive systems change because of the constantly changing environmental situations, and on the other hand, the internal activity of the system influences each subsystem because of the multiple couplings, the dynamics of such a subsystem will usually run close to an attractor and rarely reach it; i.e. neurodynamics is essentially a transient dynamics. We will ascribe 'meaning' to the dynamics of a subsystem if it enables a behavior-relevant performance of the system, and we assume that a transient dynamics that runs in the same basin of the subsystem ultimately produces the same behavior-relevant performance and thus carries the same meaning. 'Signifier' is thus the basin of an attractor, i.e. the set of all states, which is unambiguously (...) characterized by the attractor. The semantic area of a subsystem is then defined by the basin of an attractor whose transients all have the same meaning for the realization of an adequate behavior (Pasemann 1996)."

The neuromodules serve as basic building blocks for larger artificial neural networks whose more complex, continuous neurodynamics they can reflect. The network dynamics are then given by the following:

$$a_i(t+1) = \sum_{j=1}^{N} w_{ij}\sigma_{a_j}a_j(t) + \bar{\theta}_i + I_i, \qquad (7.6)$$

wherein t denotes the discrete time; the set of control parameters ρ consists of the fixed connection weights w_{ij}, a fixed threshold term $\bar{\theta}_i$ and a stationary input I_i, for all neurons $i = 1,...,n$. And with

$$\sigma_{a_j} := \frac{1}{1+e^{-a_j}} \qquad (7.7)$$

the system uses a strictly positive, sigmoidal transfer function.

"In the following we will concentrate on discrete activation dynamics given by a parameterized family of maps $f_\rho : A \to A$, where ρ denotes a set of control parameters.
(...)
For every given set of parameters ρ the dynamics (formula 7.6; author's note) is again dissipative and can be characterized by its attractors. They can be fixed point attractors (stationary states) or periodic attractors (a sequence of p states, p the period), quasi-periodic attractors (fractal sets). The basin of an attractor is the closure of the set of states which approach this attractor with increasing time. If there are coexisting attractors, their corresponding basin structure will be of interest because it reflects the partition of state space into domains of different system behaviour. One

---

[415] See e.g. Pasemann 1995: The modular (chaotic) neurodynamics is determined by a dissipative activation and propagation function.
See also, Pasemann 1996.
See the explanations in chap. 3.2.1, esp. formula 3.3 and 3.7.

has to keep in mind that for nonlinear systems, basin boundaries can have a fractal structure.

If we vary control parameters, the attractors, together with their basin structure, will vary, and we will observe bifurcations at critical parameter values i.e., attractors will suddenly vanish and/or new ones will appear. This corresponds to the change in the qualitative behaviour of the system (sometimes referred to as phase transition). Often, we will observe a whole sequence of bifurcations (...).

In fact, for real neural systems, the actual dynamics will usually run on transients and not on an attractor itself. What we call a *semantic state* of the network will thus be represented by the basin of an attractor (Pasemann 1995)."

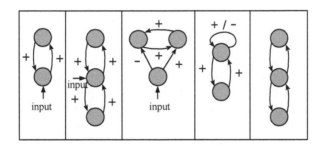

Figure 7.2: Schematic diagrams of different neuromodules (from left to right): (1) an excitatory 2 neuromodule with the classical or simple hysteresis effect which serves as a model of short-term memory, (2) an excitatory 3 neuromodule with the multiple hysteresis effect, (3) a predominantly excitatory 3 neuromodule with general hysteresis, which can be regarded as a dynamic mechanism underlying perspective ambiguity in the sense of the Necker cube or the ambiguity of figure-ground phenomena, (4) an excitatory 2 neuromodule with an inhibitory or excitatory self-feedback connection that generates chaotic neurodynamics; and (5) a 3 neuromodule that generates an even more complex chaotic neurodynamics. These examples of very small artificial neural networks with a very complex behavior suggest that periodic and chaotic neurodynamics play a crucial role in the information processing of higher cognition. These examples also suggest that inhibitory connections in feedback loops are responsible for the generation of this complex behavior (following Pasemann 1995).

To illustrate the neurodynamic effects, the following examples are demonstrated and analyzed in the figure above (Pasemann 1995, 1996, 1998, 2002): classical or simple hysteresis[416] (see Fig. 7.2 (1)), multiple hysteresis (see Fig. 7.2 (2)), general hysteresis (see Fig. 7.2 (3)) and chaotic neurodynamics (see Fig. 7.2 (4) and (5)).

These modular neurodynamic systems are therefore also referred to as "autotropic systems", i.e. the cognitive competences are based on "a self-organizing process of neuromodular structures".

---

[416]The term "hysteresis" is commonly defined as a persistent and variant delaying system behaviour in which a system phenomenon depends, not only on the independently variable parameters influencing it from outside, but also on the previous state of the system. The system can thus – depending on the previous system states – take different possible system values with identical energy supply from outside. For an introduction, see e.g. Krasnosel'skiĭ and Pokrovskiĭ 1989.

"With the term 'autotrop' we want to describe the specific ability of a system to purposefully adapt its self-organization process to the constantly changing boundary conditions with the help of this inner flexibility. Self-organisation in autotropic neuronal systems is therefore, not based on the reaction of the system to a given external boundary condition caused by a clearly defined interaction of the elements, but in particular on the manifold possibilities for influencing 'inner' parameters of its elements, which, in turn, determine the strength of the interactions (synaptic strengths) via their respective dynamic features (Pasemann 1996)."

Thus, according to Pasemann (1996) (and following the German neurobiologist and philosopher, Gerhard Roth [1992, 1994]), the concept of internal representation is best understood in the sense of a "semantic configuration of coherent (synchronous) module dynamics." "The meaning of signal sequences can create a situated system (...) only for itself and out of itself (...). This is the essential contribution that the reflexive, situated self-organization process has to make (...) which is called adaptation (...)." The classical concept of static representation can therefore hardly be maintained, since representation is "rather to be seen as something volatile" and is an "expression of coherence between internal neurodynamic processes and the dynamics of the external environment, reflected in changes in receptor activity." Moreover, one and the same neuromodule can fulfil different functions as a structural element, due to the multifunctionality of neuromodules for different sensory information. And, furthermore, one and the same function can be fulfilled by very different structural elements. "However, representation thus loses the characteristic of being bound to specific static structural elements and having a structural system intrinsic meaning. (...) If a representation appears as semantic configuration in a cognitive process, then it can be assumed that it can never be identified as distinct, always the same partial dynamic. It will fulfil its function as transient dynamics in the form of a dynamic process that is constantly changing."

The neuromodule approach is applied in the context of robotics, in particular in modelling the neural control of the information flow of behavior for complex robots, e.g. the humanoid Myon Robot (Pasemann et al. 2012, Rempis et al. 2013a, b, Toutounji and Pasemann 2014).

Based on this evolutionary robotics techniques, F. Pasemann introduced a concept of a "synchronization core (...) to represent a whole family of parametrized neurodynamical systems." These neurodynamical systems are characterized by a synaptic, recurrent coupling of synchronized dynamics of neuromodules into a composed system (Pasemann 2018). The systems should switch from one "dynamical form" to another, more complex dynamical form of a (global) attractor landscape (Pasemann 2017) "to enlarge the behavioral or cognitive capacities of neural control systems". As an example for these neuromodules which can create the complex dynamics essential for (higher) cognition, F. Pasemann (2018) refers to Freeman's Katchalsky K-sets (see chap. 7.1) and shows that "two neuromodules (...) can be synchronized by appropriate interconnections," such that "the composed system can have a dynamical spectrum which is much broader than that of the original components."

8 Systematic Class of Oscillator-Based Architecture Types

The focus of the following discussion in the systematic class of oscillator-based architecture types is three architectures of oscillatory artificial neural networks which model the binding problem in the form of the problem of "feature binding". These architectures effectively model the binding problem by means of an integrative synchronization mechanism (chap. 8.1, 8.2 and 8.3), as well as developing a "emulative neurosemantics" (chap. 8.14).[417]

The systematic class of oscillator-based architecture types is based on the model of a neural oscillator, which is an instance of the more general "(nonlinear relaxation) oscillator" (Pikovsky et al. 2001, Buzsáki 2006). This represents a large class of nonlinear dynamic systems that occur in a variety of physical and biological systems.[418] Such an oscillator, which shows a "self-sustained oscillation" (Pikovsky et al. 2001), goes back to an investigation of B. van der Pol's triode circuit (van der Pol 1926, Burg et al. 2009, Fitzhugh 1961). It is characterized by two time phases: a slow time phase which is needed to charge the capacitor, and a fast time phase for its sudden discharge. The period of oscillation is proportional to the relaxation time required to charge the capacitor, from which the name of the model derives.[419] The general mathematical form of this oscillator model, which adequately models the

---

[417]There is also a class of oscillatory networks consisting of coupled oscillators, which is summarized under the heading "Visual Image (Scene) Segmentation Analysis" (Wang 2002, Ermentrout 1994). Furthermore, a large number of research groups in computational neuroscience are investigating synchronization phenomena using artificial networks with (coupled) neural oscillators (Ermentrout 1994, 1998, Ermentrout and Terman 2010, Gómez Ramírez 2014), e.g. B. Ermentrout and N. Kopell (Ermentrout and Kopell 1984, Kopell and Ermentrout 1986), D. Somers and N. Kopell (Somers and Kopell 1993, 1995, Kopell 2000) and P. Goel and B. Ermentrout (Goel and Ermentrout 2002).
For a general introduction to the synchronization mechanisms of oscillators, see e.g. Ermentrout and Terman 2010, Pikovsky et al. 2001.
For general information, see e.g. Petitot 2011.

[418]For an introduction to the mathematical analysis of the oscillator, see e.g. Khalil 2002.
A detailed theoretical analysis of the oscillatory dynamics and the associated synchronization mechanisms of neural activity can be found in Sturm and König 2001.

[419]Therefore, the term "accumulate-and-fire oscillator" or "integrate-and-fire oscillator" is also used, which represents an adequate model of an "integrate-and-fire neuron".
See e.g. Pikovsky et al. 2001.

neural activity in the form of a pulsed sequence of action potentials, can be given by the following differential equation system (van der Pol 1926, Fitzhugh 1961, Maye and Engel 2012):

$$\frac{dx}{dt} = f(x,y) + I, \tag{8.1}$$

$$\frac{dy}{dt} = \varepsilon g(x,y), \tag{8.2}$$

wherein I is the input the oscillator receives from the stimulus, ε is a parameter and x,y are two state variables. The first variable x describes the fast time phase, while the latter, y, describes the slow time phase.

The "Wilson-Cowan Network Oscillator Model", developed by H.R. Wilson and J.D. Cowan in 1972, simulates neuronal oscillations of cortical neurons using the following system of coupled differential equations (Wilson and Cowan 1972, Ermentrout and Terman 2010, Wilson 1999) (see formulas 8.3 and 8.4). This system models the action potential activity, in the form of the average fire rate between two subpopulations of excitatory neurons x and inhibitory neurons y. These neurons are interconnected via recurrent feedback connections within a total neural population (Wilson and Cowan 1972, Maye and Engel 2012):

$$\tau_x \frac{dx_i}{dt} = -x_i - g_y(y_i) + J_0 g_x(x_i) + \sum_j J_{ij} g_x(x_j) + h_i + \eta_x, \tag{8.3}$$

$$\tau_y \frac{dy_i}{dt} = -y_i + g_x(x_i) - \sum_j W_{ij} g_y(y_j) + \eta_y, \tag{8.4}$$

wherein the time constant τ can be adapted to match the oscillation frequency to the physiological data values. The transfer functions $g_y(y_i)$ or $g_x(x_i)$ assign an output value to the activation of the respective cell population. J_0 denotes a self-excitation to obtain stable limit-cycle oscillations. The summation terms denote the input that the respective excitatory (inhibitory) population receives from the other excitatory (inhibitory) populations. The term h_i is the input the oscillator receives from the stimulus. The terms η_x or η_y, which describe the noise, model the variability in neuronal activity. Thus, the coupling of oscillators in the subpopulation of excitatory (inhibitory) neurons results in the (de-)synchronization effect of oscillations (Kopell 2000, Buzsáki 2006).

A simplified model for this purpose, described using only the phase variable ϕ, is the "phase-coupled oscillator model" (Pikovsky et al. 2001); it can be given in general mathematical form as follows (Schuster and Wagner 1990, Maye and Engel 2012):

$$x_i = a_i \sin(\phi_i), \tag{8.5}$$

$$\frac{d\phi_i}{dt} = \omega + f(\phi_i, \phi_j), \tag{8.6}$$

wherein a denotes the amplitude of the oscillation, ω denotes the base frequency of the uncoupled oscillator, and the coupling function f models the effect of the phase of a coupled oscillator j on the phase of the oscillator i. The function f is usually defined with

$$f(\phi_i, \phi_j) = -\sin(\phi_i - \phi_j). \tag{8.7}$$

8.1 OSCILLATORY NETWORKS BY M. WERNING AND A. MAYE

8.1.1 PROBLEM OF SEMANTIC COMPOSITIONALITY

Following Frege (see chap. 8.1.4), the problem of (semantic) compositionality can be briefly described as follows (Werning 2002, 2005b, 2004): The semantic values of complex syntactic terms are determined by, and thus depend on, the semantic values of the elementary terms in the form of a syntax-dependent function. The German philosopher of science and cognitive scientist, Markus Werning, states that this problem is not convincingly solved either by the classical symbolic models, e.g. by Fodor and Pylyshyn, or by the connectionist models, e.g. by Smolensky.[420] Smolensky's strategy to generate syntactic compositionality in his ICS Architecture (by homomorphically mapping the syntax of a systematic language to an algebra of vectors and tensor operations) is not sufficient to achieve systematicity, but requires a form of semantic compositionality (Werning 2001).

According to Werning, the vast majority of semantic theories explain the semantic properties of internal representations in either the sense of covariance, inferential relations, or association (Werning 2001). The question of how the semantic values of elementary representations determine the semantic values of complex representations can thus be traced back to the question of how the causal properties can be passed on. This leads to the development of the concept of "particle constituents", in the sense of physics and chemistry.

This requires that the causal properties of a composite state B are determined and dependent, necessarily and generally, on the causal properties of the simple states $A_1, ..., A_n$ and on their relations to each other. This, in turn, ensures that the states $A_1, ..., A_n$ are understood as the constituents of the state B.

With regards to the problem of compositionality, the connectionist models therefore fail in that the homomorphism between the systematic language to be mapped and the structure of the network in question cannot preserve these required causal constituent relations.

8.1.2 ARCHITECTURE OF THE OSCILLATORY NETWORKS

The reference to diachronic causal relations (in the context of an activation flow in an artificial neuronal network) is therefore not sufficient to constitute constituent relations. Instead, a synchronous relation is required, namely the synchronization relation between the phases of neuronal activity. This synchronization relation can

---

[420] See Werning 2001. See also, Werning 2003a.
See e.g. Fodor and Pylyshyn 1988, Smolensky and Legendre 2006a, b, Smolensky 1991.
See the remarks on sybolism vs. connectionism debate in chap. 6.1.1. and 6.1.3.
For the systematicity and compositionality problem, see e.g. Maurer 2006/2009.

be defined using an "oscillatory network", the architecture of which is now briefly described.[421] An elementary oscillator, which is a model of a neuronal assembly, is realized by coupling an excitatory unit with an inhibitory unit via delay connections (see chap. 8.1.4). This is pre-connected by an additional unit, through which the stimulus can be entered (see Figure 8.1.1).

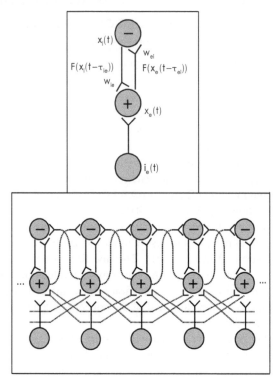

Figure 8.1: Figure 8.1.1 (above): Schematic diagram of an elementary oscillator consisting of a coupled pair of an excitatory (+) and an inhibitory unit (-) together with an input unit: t, time; $x(t)$, activity unit; $F(x)$, sigmoidal output function; w, coupling weight; τ, delay time; $i_e(t)$, stimulus input. Indices: e, excitatory unit; i, inhibitory unit (following Werning 2001). Figure 8.1.2 (below): Schematic diagram of a coupled oscillator: Oscillatory elements coupled by short-range synchronizing connections (dashed) and long-range desynchronizing connections (dotted), without mutual interference at the crossings (following Werning 2001).

The entire network consists of elementary oscillators connected side by side, coupled via short-range synchronizing connections as well as long-range desynchronizing connections (see Figure 8.1.2). An oscillatory network stimulated with sensory

---

[421] For an introduction to the architecture of an oscillatory network, see Werning 2001.
For details, see e.g. Werning 2005c, Maye and Werning 2007.
See also the explanations on the "Self-Organizing Neuronal Oscillator Model" by König and Schillen in chap. 8.2, to which Werning (2001) refers.

information can, therefore, be regarded as a feature module whose oscillators synchronize to represent, for example, one or more features of the same object in the respective receptive field of neurons (Werning 2001). In contrast, those oscillators that represent, for example, a feature of a different object, *desynchronize* their activity. This is because a certain phase of the activity propagates in the network for each represented object, and this phase of activity is reserved only for those oscillators that represent the feature (or features) of the object in question (see the example in Fig. 8.3).

8.1.3   ALGEBRAIC DEFINITION OF THE OSCILLATORY NETWORKS

Werning specifies an abstract algebraic definition of an oscillatory network, called Algebra $\mathcal{N}$, which uses one fundamental operation (Werning 2001, 2003a, Maurer 2016, 2018). This is the operation "being synchronous with" with the corresponding operation symbol "$\approx^N$", which correlates the phases of neuronal activity. Here, the elementary entities of algebra $\approx^N$ consist of

(1) just these phases of neuronal activity, represented by the symbols $\varphi_1^N, ..., \varphi_m^N$, and
(2) the sets of phases of the neuronal assembly, represented by the symbols $F_1^N, ..., F_n^N$, which index or encode a certain feature:

"Oscillatory networks that implement the two hypotheses[422] can be given an abstract algebraic description:

$$\mathcal{N} = \langle N_i, N_p, N_s; \varphi_1, ..., \varphi_m; F_1, ..., F_n; \approx, \not\approx, \varepsilon, \wedge \rangle" \tag{8.8}$$

(Werning 2001, 2003a).

According to Werning, this notation of algebra $\mathcal{N}$ is isomorphic to a compositional and systematic language, referred to as algebra L.[423] Algebra L also uses a fundamental operation, namely "being the same as", with the corresponding operation symbol "$\approx^L$". This operation correlates the indexical expressions (such as "this" and "that"), whereby the elementary entities of algebra L consist of:

(1) just these indexicals, represented by the symbols $\varphi_1^L, ..., \varphi_m^L$, and
(2) the sets of features, represented by the symbols $F_1^L, ..., F_n^L$ that correspond to the predicates:

---

[422] See Werning 2001: "Assuming that elementary oscillators are models of neurons and that oscillatory networks are models of part of the visual cortex, the results of these studies support two hypotheses:
Indicativity - As part of the visual cortex, there are collections of neurons whose function it is to show activity only when an object in the perceptual field instantiates a certain property.
Synchrony - Neurons that belong to two collections indicative for the properties π_1 and π_2, respectively, have the function to show activity synchronous with each other only if the properties π_1 and π_2 are instantiated by the same object in the perceptual field.
The hypotheses are supported by neurobiological evidence."

[423] To prove this, four conditions have to be fulfilled. See Werning 2001. See also Werning 2003a.

"Since languages can be treated as algebras, we may define:

$$\mathcal{L} = \langle L_i, L_p, L_s; \varphi_1, ..., \varphi_m; F_1, ..., F_n; \approx, \neq, \varepsilon, \wedge \rangle"$$ (8.9)

(Werning 2001, 2003a).

In summary, the neuronal representation of an elementary predication $F(a)$ can be described as follows in accordance with Werning (2001): Given an assembly of sensory neurons which show the same facts in the space of perception (i.e. in the respective receptive field, e.g. the same feature of an object), one can say that if a neuron which shows the same synchronous phase activity φ_i^N as the neurons of this assembly isomorphic is an element of the (phase) set F_j^N of the neurons of this assembly. Thus, this neuronal state is represented by the definition of the relation of "pertaining", ε^N, as follows:

$$[\varphi_i \, \varepsilon \, F_j]^N \text{ is the (neuronal) state } [(\exists x)(x \approx \varphi_i \; \& \; x \in F_j)]^N.$$ (8.10)

This is isomorphic to the fact if one combines an indexical expression φ_i^L via the definition of the copula ε^L (English: "is") with a predicate F_j^L into a fact, e.g. the same feature of an object, according to the form: This perceived item is a certain feature at a certain point in time and at a certain place in the space of perception. This means that this synchronicity of the phase activity of neurons guarantees the attribution of a feature to a certain spatiotemporal fact in the space of perception, e.g. an object:

$$[\varphi_i \, \varepsilon \, F_j]^L \text{ is the (linguistic) clause } [(\exists x)(x \approx \varphi_i \; \& \; x \in F_j)]^L.$$ (8.11)

Figure 8.2 presents an example which illustrates the neuronal representation of a complex predication.

According to Werning (2001), this predication process can only be performed if both the individual phase activities and the assembly of neurons to which a set consisting of a certain synchronous phase activity is assigned, occur in the cortex as an actual individual state (a so-called "token"). Thus, the required causal constituent structure of a language is preserved, and oscillatory networks ensure not only syntactic but also semantic compositionality.

Furthermore, according to Werning (2001, 2003a), one can describe the neural representation of a 2-ary relation $R(a,b)$ as follows:

"The representation of relations poses a binding problem of second order. (...) The constituency preserving isomorphism between L and $\mathcal{N}$ straightforwardly generates a prediction of how to realize relational representation by oscillatory networks: After L has been extended by the tools for representing relations known from logic, $\mathcal{N}$ has to be extended in a way that perpetuates the isomorphism and the congruence with respect to constituency structure. The tools needed in the extensions of L and $\mathcal{N}$ are the operation of pairing a higher-order copula and relation constants, or, respectively, their neuronal counterparts. Following Kuratowski (1967), ordered *pairs* are, by common standards, defined as asymmetric sets of second order:

$$[\langle \varphi_i, \varphi_j \rangle]^{L/N} =_{\text{def}} [\{\{\varphi_i, \varphi_j\}, \{\varphi_j\}\}]^{L/N}.$$ (8.12)

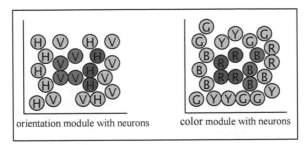

orientation module with neurons   color module with neurons

Figure 8.2: Scheme of a typical neuronal reaction caused by a blue vertical and a red horizontal object: The circles with letters represent neurons with the properties those letters indicate: vertical (V), horizontal (H), red (R), green (G), blue (B) and yellow (Y). Similar hues express synchronous activities: The phases of some blue neurons are synchronized with the phases of some vertical neurons (tinted blue), and some horizontal neurons are in synchronicity with the phases of some red neurons (tinted red).

The figure thus expresses the cortical state: $[\varphi_1 \, \varepsilon \, V \wedge \varphi_1 \, \varepsilon \, B \wedge \varphi_2 \, \varepsilon \, H \wedge \varphi_2 \, \varepsilon \, R]^N$, which corresponds to the sentence: "This is a blue vertical and a red horizontal object," which can be paraphrased: $[\varphi_1 \, \varepsilon \, V \wedge \varphi_1 \, \varepsilon \, B \wedge \varphi_2 \, \varepsilon \, H \wedge \varphi_2 \, \varepsilon \, R]^L$ (following Werning 2001).

With the relations $R_1^L, ..., R_k^L$ being sets of pairs, the higher-order copula links pairs to relations in the manner of set membership. On the neuronal level, the $R_1^N, ..., R_k^N$ can be interpreted as relational modules:

$$[\langle \varphi_i, \varphi_j \rangle \, \varepsilon' R_L]^{L/N} =_{\text{def}} [\langle \varphi_i, \varphi_j \rangle \in R_L]^{L/N} \qquad (8.13)$$

(...) To achieve a distribution of phases this complex, some neurons are required to show a superposition of two phases (Werning 2001, 2003a)."

In summary, a neuronal representation of a relation is ensured, in that the higher-order copula of the relation (in the sense of algebra L) is understood as a set of pairs which connects ordered pairs of indexical expressions on the basis of the set membership to relations. This can be implemented neuronally (in the sense of algebra $\mathcal{N}$) with a relational function module which connects ordered pairs of phase activities by means of the superposition of these two phase activities to relations.

8.1.4 EMULATIVE (NEURO-)SEMANTICS

The model of the "Oscillatory Networks" has been further developed by Markus Werning, in collaboration with the German neuroinformatician, Alexander Maye, into a so-called "emulative (neuro-)semantics".[424] This means that a neurobiolog-

---

[424] For fundamental information, see e.g. Werning 2001, 2003a.
For a detailed description of the model, see Werning 2005c, 2012.
See also Werning 2005a, Maye and Werning 2004, 2007.
For an introduction, see Maurer 2016, 2018.

ically realistic[425], emulative and compositional, model-theoretical semantics for a first-order predicate language is generated. This emulative semantics is non-symbolic in the sense that it adheres to the modern principle of "Compositionality of Meaning" (see Box 8.1.4.1), but not to the "Principle of Semantic Constituency" (see Box 8.1.4.2). The model also shows how its neuronal structure elements (in the form of oscillation functions) covary as internal ("mental") representations with external contents. Thus it becomes clear how these neuronal structure elements can mediate between the expressions of predicate language and the objects of the world referenced by them, the "denotations" (Werning 2012).

Box 8.1.4.1 Principle of Compositionality of Meaning:

See Werning 2012: "Principle 1 (Compositionality of meaning) *The meaning of a complex term is a syntax-dependent function of the meanings of its syntactic parts.*" See also Werning 2005c.

Contrary to the classical formulation of compositionality in Frege (1923/1976), which postulates a correspondence relation between the part-whole relationship in the syntactic realm and that in the semantic realm, one can assume that the modern principle of compositionality of meaning is a homomorphism between two algebraic structures, namely the syntactic structure of terms and the semantic structure of meanings.

The formal definition (Werning 2012) is as follows: "Definition 1 (Formal Compositionality) *Given a language with the syntax* $\langle T, \Sigma_T \rangle$, *a meaning function* $\mu : T \to M$ *is called compositional just in case, for every n-ary syntactic operation* $\sigma \in \Sigma_T$ *and any sequence of terms* $t_1, ..., t_n$ *in the domain of* σ, *there is a partial function* m_σ *defined on* M^n *such that*

$$\mu(\sigma(t_1, ..., t_n)) = m_\sigma(\mu(t_1), ..., \mu(t_n)). \tag{8.14}$$

A semantics induced by a compositional meaning function will be called a compositional semantics of the language."
See also Janssen 2011.

Based on precisely this principle of semantic constituency (as a cornerstone of symbolic theories of meaning), a "Symbolic Semantics" (in the sense of Fodor's "Language of Thought") is defined (see Box 8.1.4.3). Their part/whole-relations can partly be reproduced by means of "Vector Symbolic Architectures", in the sense of Smolensky, Plate, or Stewart and Eliasmith. These architectures use the concept of circular convolution as a binding mechanism, so that an algorithm of unbinding restores the filler vector.

---

[425] See e.g. Werning 2005c, 2012: The architecture of Oscillatory Networks is based on empirical findings from neurobiology, neurophysiology and perceptual psychology, which concern the existence of topographically structured, cortical (feature) maps, the neurophysiological binding mechanism of an object-related synchronization of neuronal activity and the Gestalt principles of perception in the sense of "Gestalt psychology", according to M. Wertheimer, W. Köhler and K. Koffka.
For more details, see the explanations in chap. 4.4.

Box 8.1.4.2 Principle of Semantic Constituency:

Following the classical formulation of compositionality (Frege 1923/1976), one can assume – in contrast to the modern principle of compositionality of meaning – that a correspondence relation exists between the part-whole relationship in the syntactic realm and in the semantic realm, such that this can be described as the Principle of Semantic Constituency.

See e.g. Werning 2012: "Principle 2 (Semantic constituency) *There is a semantic part-whole relation on the set of meanings such that for every two terms, if the one is a syntactic part of the other, then the meaning of the former is a semantic part of the meaning of the latter.*"

The formal definition of a broad concept of a part-whole relationship is (Werning 2012): "Definition 2 (Part-whole Relation) *A relation $\sqsubseteq$ defined on a set X is called a part-whole relation on X just in case, for all $x, y, z \in X$ the following holds*: (...)

$$(i) \quad x \sqsubseteq x \ (reflexivity). \tag{8.15}$$

$$(ii) \quad x \sqsubseteq y \wedge y \sqsubseteq x \ \rightarrow \ x = y \ (anti\text{-}symmetry). \tag{8.16}$$

$$(iii) \quad x \sqsubseteq y \wedge y \sqsubseteq z \ \rightarrow \ x \sqsubseteq z \ (transitivity)." \tag{8.17}$$

See also Werning 2005c.
However, see Werning 2004.

The neuronal structure of oscillatory networks, on the other hand, offers compositional, *non*-symbolic semantics for a first-order predicate language. That means that the elements of the neuronal structure represent internal mental representations, which reliably covary with the external contents which are identical (in the sense of an "isomorphism" [see chap. 1.1.6]) with the standard model theoretical denotations of this language (Werning 2003a).[426] In other words, each denotation of an expression in the language has a possible corresponding neuronal state which covaries with the denotation, so that one can speak of "emulative semantics":[427]

"We will demonstrate that the neural structure provides a compositional semantics of the language. Compositionality of meaning will hence be achieved. It will become obvious that this semantics is non-symbolic in the sense defined above. The principle of semantic constituency is negated. We will also show that the elements of the neural structure are internal representations that reliably co-vary with external contents. These external contents are identical with the standard model-theoretical denotations for the language. The covariation with content is achieved. It will finally become clear that the covariation is one-to-one, such that the neural structure can be regarded as isomorphic to the external denotational structure. These results justify our calling the neural structure an emulative semantics. This is to say that each de-

---

[426] According to Werning 2012, with reference to Fodor 1990, there exists a relation between an internal mental representation and its content in the form of a causal-informational covariation.

[427] For a counterexample from standard model theoretical semantics for a compositional but non-symbolic semantics, see Werning 2012.

notation of an expression in our language has a potential counterpart neural state that co-varies with the denotation (Werning 2012)."

Box 8.1.4.3 Symbolic Semantics:

See Werning 2012: "Definition 3 (Symbolic Semantics) *Given a language with the syntax* $\langle T, \Sigma_T \rangle$, *a thereon defined syntactic part-whole relation* $\sqsubseteq_T$, *and a meaning function* $\mu : T \rightarrow M$, *then its semantics* $\langle M, \Sigma_M \rangle$ *is symbolic if and only if there is a part-whole relation* $\sqsubseteq_M$ *defined on M such that for all terms* $s, t \in T$ *the following holds*:

$$s \sqsubseteq_T t \; \rightarrow \; \mu(s) \sqsubseteq_M \mu(t)." \tag{8.18}$$

The architecture of an oscillatory network, which had already been briefly described (see chap. 8.1.2) as a recurrent neural network, has been further developed in such a way that it can be regarded as a plausible model of information processing in the visual cortex.[428] The dynamics of a single oscillator as an elementary functional unit, whose excitatory and inhibitory technical neuron respectively represent the average activity of a cluster of about 80-200 biological cortical neurons, can now be described in the "Mean-Field Model" using the following differential equations[429]:

"(...) the dynamics of each oscillator can be described by two variables x and y (...) according to the following differential equations:

$$\frac{dx}{dt} = -\tau_x x - g_y(y) + L_0^{xx} g_x(x) + I_x + N_x, \tag{8.21}$$

$$\frac{dy}{dt} = -\tau_y y - g_x(x) - I_y + N_y. \tag{8.22}$$

Here, τ_ξ ($\xi \in \{x, y\}$) are constants that can be chosen to match refractory times of biological cells. The g_ξ are transfer functions that tell how much of the activity of

---

[428]For an introduction, see e.g. Werning 2005c, 2012, 2005a, Maye and Werning 2004. For detailed information, see e.g. Maye and Werning 2007, Maye 2002.

[429]See e.g. Maye and Werning 2007. In the "Model with Phase-Coupled Oscillators", however, the state of an oscillator is given by the phase $\phi(t)$ and the amplitude $a(t)$, (according to Maye and Werning 2007), so that its dynamics are described by the following differential equations:

"(...) the dynamics of an oscillator is given by:

$$\dot{\phi}_i = \omega - \sum_j s_{ij} a_j \sin(\phi_i - \phi_j) + \eta_i \tag{8.19}$$

$$\dot{a}_i = -a_i + h_i. \tag{8.20}$$

Weights s_{ij} comprise couplings within a feature module as well as between feature modules. Synchronizing connections have $s_{ij} > 0$, whereas desynchronizing connections are given by $s_{ij} < 0$. The same connection scheme, as for the mean-field model, is applied. Again, η is a noise term and h_i describes external input from the feature detectors."

a neuron is transferred to other neurons. The constant L_0^{xx} describes self-excitation of the excitatory cell population. I_ξ are static external inputs and N_ξ variable white noise, which models fluctuation within the cell populations (Werning 2005c, Maye and Werning 2007, Maye 2003)."

A feature module, which represents a feature dimension, e.g. a certain color or orientation, consists of a three-dimensional topological grid structure of oscillators. A module layer, constructed as a two-dimensional retinotopic structure, encodes in each case, one feature, e.g. 'red' or 'horizontal.' Thus each oscillator is characterized by its position in the receptive field, whose x,y-coordinates are given in relation to the two-dimensional layer plane. At the same time, each oscillator is also characterized by its feature selectivity, depending on the z-coordinate that determines the respective layer or feature. The implementation of the "Gestalt Principles" therefore takes place in such a way that those oscillators, which are selective for stimulus elements with similar features, tend to form synchronous oscillations if they are stimulated simultaneously. Thus, these oscillations can be regarded as one object (concept).

According to Werning (2005c, 2012, 2005a), the dynamics of an oscillatory network can be described in the context of a "Hilbert Space Analysis"[430] by means of the oscillations or the oscillation functions of the oscillators, and the degree of their synchronous activity. Oscillation functions are regarded as vectors in the Hilbert space, and the Hilbert space $L_2(\Omega)$ of the square-integratable functions (in the sense of the "Lebesgue Integral"[431]) is taken as the basis:

"The oscillation spreading through the network can be characterized mathematically: An oscillation function, or more generally the activity function $x(t)$ of an oscillator, is the activity of its excitatory neuron as a function of time during a time window $\left[-\frac{T}{2}, +\frac{T}{2}\right]$. Mathematically speaking, activity functions are vectors in the Hilbert space $L_2\left[-\frac{T}{2}, +\frac{T}{2}\right]$ of the interval $\left[-\frac{T}{2}, +\frac{T}{2}\right]$ square-integrable functions. This space has the inner product

$$\langle x(t) | x'(t) \rangle = \int_{-T/2}^{+T/2} x(t) x'(t)\, dt. \tag{8.23}$$

The degree of synchrony between two oscillations lies between -1 and +1 and is defined as their normalized inner product

$$\Delta(x, x') = \frac{\langle x | x' \rangle}{\sqrt{\langle x | x \rangle \langle x' | x' \rangle}}. \tag{8.24}$$

---

[430]For an introduction to the mathematical concept of "Hilbert Spaces" in functional analysis, see e.g. Hansen 2016, Werner 2005, Heine 2009, Fischer and Kaul 2008, Wachter and Hoeber 1998.
For a beginner's guide, see e.g. Prigogine and Stengers 1993.
Named after the German mathematician, David Hilbert.

[431]For an introduction to the mathematical concept of the "Lebesgue-Integrals", see e.g. Hansen 2016, Fischer and Kaul 2008.
Named after the French mathematician, Henri Lebesgue.

The degree of synchrony, so defined, corresponds to the cosine of the angle between the Hilbert vectors x and x'. The most important cases are:

$$\Delta(x,x') = 1 \leftrightarrow x \text{ and } x' \text{ are parallel (totally synchronous),}$$
$$\Delta(x,x') = 0 \leftrightarrow x \text{ and } x' \text{ are orthogonal (totally uncorrelated),} \qquad (8.25)$$
$$\Delta(x,x') = -1 \leftrightarrow x \text{ and } x' \text{ are anti-parallel (totally anti-synchronous)}$$

(Werning 2005c)."

In the context of "Synergetics" (Haken 1983, 2004, Maurer 2014a), the dynamics of a complex system are determined (according to the German theoretical physicist, Hermann Haken) on the basis of a few dominant states, the so-called "eigenmode", ordered according to their "eigenvalues" λ.[432] A specific network state can be considered by means of the superposition of the respective eigenvector v_i, which contains the excitatory activities of all the corresponding oscillators as components, weighted with the respective characteristic function $c_i(t)$ (Werning 2005c, 2012, 2005a, Maye and Werning 2004, 2007). The so-called "eigenmode analysis" separates the spatial from the temporal variation in the overall network dynamics, given as a Cartesian vector $x(t)$, consisting of all the oscillation functions of the active oscillators (Werning 2005c). While the eigenvectors are constant over time, but responsible for the changing behavior of the network's spatially distributed oscillators, the characteristic functions are the same for all oscillators, but responsible for the temporal dynamics of the network as a whole[433]:

"The vector $x(t)$ comprises the activities of the excitatory neurons of all k oscillators of the network after a transient phase and is determined by a solution of the system of differential equations[434] (...).
For each eigenmode, the eigenvalue λ and its corresponding eigenvector v are solutions of the eigen-equation for the auto-co-variance matrix $C \in \mathbb{R}^{k \times k}$:

$$Cv = C\lambda, \qquad (8.26)$$

where the components C_{ij} of C are determined by the network dynamics $x(t)$ as:

$$C_{ij} = \langle x_i | x_j \rangle. \qquad (8.27)$$

(...) To assess the temporal evolution of the eigenmodes, the notion of a characteristic function $c_i(t)$ is introduced. The network state at any instant can be considered as a

---

[432]For the concept of the so-called "eigenmode analysis", see e.g. Haken 1983, 2000.
See also, Maye and Engel 2012.
See also, the remarks in Maurer 2014a, 2016.

[433]See Werning 2005c.
A major advantage of eigenmode analysis is that an object representation is no longer identified with the concrete oscillatory behavior of neurons, but with that of the eigenmode-relative, characteristic functions. See Werning 2012.

[434]See the formulas 8.18 and 8.19.

superposition of the eigenvectors v^i weighted by the corresponding characteristic functions $c_i(t)$ (...):

$$x(t) = \sum_i c_i(t) v_i. \tag{8.28}$$

(Werning 2005c)."

According to Werning, the dynamics of an oscillatory network can furthermore be subject to a semantic interpretation (Werning 2005c, 2012, 2005a, Maye and Werning 2004), since it realizes a structure of internal representations which can be expressed by means of a monadic, first order predicate language with identity $PL^=$.[435] The Hilbert space analysis allows oscillation functions to assign individual terms to a predicate language $PL^=$ because they covary with individual objects. Thus a sentence of the predicate language, e.g. $a = b$, expresses a representational state of the system, e.g. the identity of two objects, by means of two individual constants a, b, according to the degree to which two oscillation functions $\alpha(a)$ and $\alpha(b)$ of the system are synchronous:

"Because of Hyp. 5[436] we are allowed to regard oscillation functions as internal representations of individual objects. They may thus be assigned some of the individual terms of the language $PL^=$. Let

$$Ind = \{a_1, ..., a_m, z_1, ..., z_n\} \tag{8.29}$$

be the set of individual terms of $PL^=$, then the partial function

$$\alpha : Ind \rightarrow L_2 \left[-\frac{T}{2}, +\frac{T}{2} \right] \tag{8.30}$$

be a constant individual assignment of the language. By convention, I will assume that, for the domain of α, unless indicated otherwise

$$dom(\alpha) = \{a_1, ..., a_m\} \tag{8.31}$$

so that the $a_1, ..., a_m$ are individual constants and the $z_1, ..., z_n$ are individual variables. (...)
In case of identity sentences, for every eigenmode i and any individual constants a, b, we have:

$$d(a = b, i) = \Delta(\alpha(a), \alpha(b)) \tag{8.32}$$

(Werning 2005c)."

---

[435] See Werning 2005c: "Oscillatory networks (...) realize a structure of internal representations expressible by a monadic first order predicate language with identity $PL^=$."

[436] See Werning 2005c: "Hypothesis 5 (Synchrony). *Neurons of different feature clusters have the function to show synchronous activation only if the properties indicated by each feature cluster are instantiated by the same object in their receptive field.*"

In order to determine to what extent a certain oscillation function $\alpha(a)$, assigned to an individual constant a, belongs to a feature layer which is assigned to a predicate F (in other words, is in the "neuronal extension" of a predicate F), one has to compute the extent to which it is maximally synchronous with one of the existing oscillation functions in the respective feature layer (in other words, in the respective neuronal extension) (Werning 2005c, 2012, 2005a, Maye and Werning 2004).

A (monadic) predicate F denotes a feature of the respective feature layer, and is represented by a neuronal feature cluster in the sense of the diagonal matrix $\beta(F)$, e.g. the red layer within the color module of the network, which thus represents the "neuronal intention" of a predicate:

"Following Hyp. 4^{437}, clusters of feature selective neurons function as representations of properties. They can be expressed by monadic predicates. I will assume that our language $PL^=$ has a set of monadic predicates

$$Pred = \{F_1, ..., F_p\} \tag{8.33}$$

such that each predicate denotes a property represented by some feature cluster. To every predicate $F \in Pred$, I now assign a diagonal matrix $\beta(F) \in \{0,1\}^{k \times k}$ that, by multiplication with any eigenmode vector $\mathbf{v^i}$, renders the sub-vector of those components that belong to the feature cluster expressed by F:

$$\beta : Pred \to \{0,1\}^{k \times k}. \tag{8.34}$$

(...)

Since $\beta(F)$ is a hardware feature of the network and varies, neither from stimulus to stimulus, nor from eigenmode to eigenmode (and is, modeltheoretically speaking, hence constant in all models), it is sensible to call it the *neuronal intension* of F.

The neuronal intension of a predicate, for every eigenmode, determines what I call its neuronal extension, i.e., the set of those oscillations that the neurons on the feature layer contribute to the activity the eigenmode adds to the overall networks dynamics. Unlike the neuronal intension, the neuronal extension varies from stimulus to stimulus and from eigenmode to eigenmode (just as extensions vary from possible world to possible world). Hence, for every predicate F, its *neuronal extension* in the eigenmode i comes to:

$$\left\{ f_j | \mathbf{f} = c_i(t)\beta(F)\mathbf{v^i} \right\}. \tag{8.35}$$

Here, the f_j are the components of the vector $\mathbf{f}$.
(...)

To determine to which degree an oscillation function assigned to an individual constant a is in the neuronal extension of a predicate F, we have to compute how synchronous it maximally is with one of the oscillation functions in the neuronal extension. We are, in other words, justified in evaluating the degree to which a predicative

---

[437] See Werning 2005c: "Hypothesis 4 (Feature maps). *There are many cortical areas that function as topologically structured feature maps. They comprise clusters of neurons whose function it is to show activity only when an object in their receptive field instantiates a certain property of the respective feature dimension.*"

sentence Fa expresses a representational state of our system, with respect to the eigenmode i, in the following way:

$$d(Fa, i) = max\left\{\Delta(\alpha(a), f_j) \mid \boldsymbol{f} = c_i(t)\,\beta\,(F)\,\boldsymbol{v^i}\right\} \tag{8.36}$$

(Werning 2005c)."

Finally, an explicit formal description of the neuronal semantics of an oscillatory network is made. This includes a semantic evaluation of the truth-functional junctors and the predicate logical quantifiers, related to a first order, monadic, predicate language ($PL^=$) with identity, predication, conjunction, disjunction, implication, negation, existential and universal quantifier. Since this requires an infinite, multi-valued semantics in the context of "fuzzy logic"[438], according to Werning (2005c, 2012, 2005a), the intuitionist "Min-Max System"[439] of the German logician, Kurt Gödel, is used for this purpose (see Fig. 8.3):

"(...) the system that fits my purpose best is Gödels (...) min-max-logics.
Here the conjunction is evaluated by the minimum of the values of the conjuncts (...).
Let ϕ, ψ be sentences of $PL^=$, then, for any eigenmode i, we have:

$$d(\phi \wedge \psi, i) = min\{d(\phi, i),\, d(\psi, i)\}. \tag{8.37}$$

The evaluations (...) allow us to regard the first eigenmode of the network dynamics, which results from stimulation with one red vertical object and one green horizontal object (...), as a representation expressed by the sentence

This is a red vertical object and that is a green horizontal object.

We only have to assign the individual terms this ($= a$) and that ($= b$) to the oscillatory functions $-c_1(t)$ and $+c_1(t)$, respectively, and the predicates red ($= R$), green ($= G$), vertical ($= V$) and horizontal ($= H$) to the redness, greenness, verticality and horizontality layers as their neuronal intensions. Simple computation then reveals:

$$d(Ra \wedge Va \wedge Gb \wedge Hb \wedge \neg a = b, 1) - 1.^{440} \tag{8.38}$$

(Werning 2005c)."

"Besides the individual terms of *Ind* and the monadic predicates of *Pred*, the alphabet of $PL^=$ contains the logical constants $\wedge \vee \rightarrow \neg \exists \forall$ and the binary predicate

---

[438]For an introduction, see Gottwald 2001.
See also, chap. 3.2.4.5.

[439]For Gödel's Min-Max System G^∞, see Gödel 1932/1986.
For an introduction, see e.g. Gottwald 2001.

[440]An example is given by presenting a red vertical bar and a green horizontal bar as stimulus to the oscillatory network (see Fig. 8.3).
See e.g. Werning 2005c.

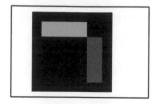

Figure 8.3: Schematic representation of the stimulus, consisting of a red vertical bar and a green horizontal bar (following Werning 2005c).

=. Provided we have the constant individual and predicate assignments α and β of $(8.27)^{441}$ and $(8.31)^{441}$, the union

$$\gamma = \alpha \cup \beta \tag{8.39}$$

is a comprehensive constant assignment of $PL^=$. The individual terms in the domain of α are individual constants, those not in the domain of α are individual variables. The syntactic operations of the language $PL^=$ and the set SF of sentential formulae as their recursive closure can be defined as follows, for arbitrary $a, b, z \in Ind$, $F \in Pred$, and $\phi, \psi \in SF$:

$$(\ldots)\sigma_{pred} : (a, F) \mapsto Fa; \ (\ldots)\sigma_\wedge : (\phi, \psi) \mapsto \phi \wedge \psi; \ (\ldots).^{442} \tag{8.40}$$

The set of terms of $PL^=$ is the union of the sets of individual terms, predicates and sentential formulae of the language. A sentential formula in SF is called a *sentence* with respect to some constant assignment γ if and only if, under assignment γ, all and only individual terms bound by a quantifier are variables. Any term of $PL^=$ is called γ-*grammatical* if and only if, under assignment γ, it is a predicate, an individual constant, or a sentence. Taking the idea at face value that eigenmodes can be treated like possible worlds (or more neutrally speaking, like models), the relation 'i neurally models ϕ to degree d by constant assignment γ' in symbols

$$i \models_\gamma^d \phi, \tag{8.41}$$

for any sentence ϕ and any real number $d \in [-1, +1]$, is then recursively given as follows:

(...)

Predication: Given any individual constant $a \in Ind \cap dom(\gamma)$, and any predicate $F \times Pred$, then

$$i \models_\gamma^d \phi Fa \text{ iff } d = max\left\{\Delta(\gamma(a), f_j) \mid f = \gamma(F) \, \boldsymbol{v^i} \, c_i(t)\right\}. \tag{8.42}$$

Conjunction: Provided that ϕ, ψ are sentences, then

$$i \models_\gamma^d \phi \wedge \psi \text{ iff } d = min\left\{d', d'' \mid i \models_\gamma^{d'} \phi \text{ and } i \models_\gamma^{d''} \psi\right\}. \tag{8.43}$$

(Werning 2005c)."

---

[441] The numbers of the formulas have been adapted to the counting in this chapter.

[442] Only the case of predication and conjunction are shown here.

Emulative neurosemantics has been applied in various ways (Werning 2012), e.g. by extending it from an ontology of objects (localized in the ventral visual pathway) to an ontology of events (localized in the dorsal visual pathway) (Werning 2003b). Another application is the "Theory of (Neuro-)Frames"[443], which shows how a neuronally realized substance concept can be analyzed as a typed "frame" in the form of synchronized neuronal clusters in attributive subconcepts. Finally, applications have been developed to address ambiguous representations and representations based on a sensory illusion (Werning and Maye 2006), or, as already described (see chap. 8.1.3), involving the neuronal representation of a 2-ary relation.

Recently, A. Maye has developed a neurobiological "Oscillator Ensemble Model" (Maye et al. 2019), composed of an ensemble of neural oscillators whose learning rule attunes them to the various rhythms that are generated by a given sequence of number codes like '99392'. In this computational model a mechanism is employed which dynamically adjusts oscillation frequencies and phases: "The main idea is that the phase of the input relative to the ongoing oscillation determines how the synchronization patterns between the neural populations change. (...) The simultaneous tuning of phase and frequency is aptly modeled by a phase-locked loop (PLL). (...) In PLL-based computational models of neural processing, memorized patterns are (...) synchronized oscillatory states with a certain phase relation (...) (Pina et al. 2018)."

8.1.5 CRITICISM AND EVALUATION OF THE OSCILLATORY NETWORKS

In my opinion the model of oscillatory networks follows closely the empirical data from neurobiology and neurophysiology and describes how – in time – an internal compositional representation is generated by neuronal cortical structural elements (Werning 2012). The model refers to a certain fact of visual perception, so that the reference of a linguistic expression (in the context of a first order, monadic, predicate language with identity) is guaranteed to a fact in the world, given on the basis of information in the respective receptive field. Consequently, this model can describe how a certain neuronal, temporal, synchronization process can be assigned a meaning. For example, in the case of visual perception, this semantic content assigns a perceived predication fact to a linguistic expression. This predication fact is what Werning refers to as a neuronal extension. This implies an isomorphic transformation of discrete symbolic structures–and their denotations–of this first order predicate language into continuous oscillations of the network's neurons, because these neuronal structural elements covary (in the sense of an isomorphism) with the external information contents of the perceptive "stimulus" (Werning 2005a). These information contents, in turn, are identical with the standard model theoretical structure of the denotations of the expressions of this predicate language. This means that an oscillatory network, with its neuronal oscillation structure or its eigenmode structure, thus generates a non-symbolic "algebraic emulation" of what it represents within its perception, based on the concept of the receptive field:

"The meaning of a sentence is a set of eigenmodes. We can regard it as an internal propositional representation. Since the meanings of constants and predicates

---

[443] See Werning 2008 in connection with Petersen and Werning 2007, with reference to Barsalou 1992 and Pulvermüller 1999.

are internal representations and co-vary with what they denote, the sets of eigen-modes can be mapped one-to-one to sets of models or possible worlds built from the denoted objects and properties. If one takes propositions to be sets of models or possible worlds, as is commonly done, and if one assumes that propositions are the denotations of sentences, we have a one-to-one mapping between the internal propositional representations of the network and the denotations of the sentences that express them. We may hence infer that the principle of content co-variation is fulfilled for the triples <constant term, internal object representation = oscillation, denoted object>, <predicate, internal object representation = feature layer, denoted property>, <sentence, internal propositional representation = set of eigenmodes, de-noted proposition>.

The co-variation between the internal representations generated by the network and expressed by the terms of the language, on the one side, and the denotations of the expressions, on the other side, are one-to-one. Moreover, the semantic operations used to construct our neuronal semantics are also completely analogous to those used in the denotational semantics of standard model theory. It can thus be immediately shown that the neuronal structure $\mathcal{N}$, which provides a semantics of internal repre-sentations of our language, is strictly isomorphic to the denotational semantics one would get in the standard model-theoretical approach. This isomorphism justifies the claim that the neuronal structure is an emulative semantics of a first-order language. It is non-symbolic because it is isomorphic to a denotational semantics as provided by standard model theory and thus violates the principle of semantic constituency. Each element of a denotational semantics for the perceptual expressions used in our language has a counterpart in the neuronal structure: its emulation (Werning 2012)."

The (simulation) model thus represents a dynamic snapshot of a single visual scene with the constitution of at least two different objects, e.g. a vertical red bar and a horizontal green bar (see Fig. 8.3) (Werning 2005a).

8.2 SELF-ORGANIZING NEURONAL OSCILLATOR MODEL BY P. KÖNIG AND T.B. SCHILLEN

Based on the "Wilson-Cowan Network Oscillator Model", the German physicist and neurophysiologist Peter König and the German physicist and psychiatrist Thomas B. Schillen have developed the "Self-organization Neuronal Oscillator Model".[444] This model simulates the experimental situation of temporal coding of object features by the synchronization of the oscillatory neuronal activity of cortical assemblies in neurophysiology. To solve the binding problem, the model consists of one or more feature modules with coupled nonlinear oscillators in visual scene analysis. The sys-tem dynamics are determined by the following differential equations (Schillen and König 1994, 1991a, König and Schillen 1991):

$$\tau_0 \dot{x}_e(t) = -\alpha_e x_e(t) - w_{ie} F\left[x_i(t - \tau_{ie})\right] + i_e(t) + \eta_e(t) \tag{8.44}$$

$$\tau_0 \dot{x}_i(t) = -\alpha_i x_i(t) + w_{ei} F\left[x_e(t - \tau_{ei})\right] + \eta_i(t), \tag{8.45}$$

[444]For fundamental information, see e.g. Schillen and König 1994, 1993, 1991a, b, König and Schillen 1991.
See also König et al. 1993, König and Schillen 1990, Schillen and König 1990a, b.

where α_e or α_i is a damping constant, w_{ie} and w_{ei} is the coupling strength, τ the delay time, $i_e(t)$ the external stimulus input, F is a non-linear Fermi output function with a slope σ and a treshold Θ[445]:

$$F[x(t)] = \frac{1}{e^{\sigma(\Theta - x(t))} + 1}. \tag{8.46}$$

The architecture of the model serves as a precursor for Werning's and Maye's emulative neurosemantics (see chap. 8.1.2, 8.1.4) (see also Salari and Maye 2008).

8.3 COUPLED PHASE OSCILLATOR MODEL BY H. FINGER AND P. KÖNIG

The German cognitive scientist, Holger Finger and the German physicist and neurophysiologist, Peter König have developed a binding mechanism, the "Coupled Phase Oscillator Model".[446] This model binds a set of neurons by means of the synchronized phase variable within the framework of scene segmentation with an unsupervised learning method (see Fig. 8.4) (Finger and König 2014). The analysis of the network dynamics shows that this increasing phase synchronization establishes a coding of the relational structure of the natural image input data:

"In this study we investigate whether the concept of binding by synchrony, as has been investigated using abstract stimuli, is viable for natural stimuli. The most important novelty of our approach is the combination of these different concepts described above into one single simulation model to allow the investigation of their interplay: Specifically, we combine normative model approaches of unsupervised learning from natural stimuli with the concept of binding by synchrony in a network of coupled phase oscillators. Importantly, the data driven approach, that utilizes general principles, minimizes the number of heuristics and free parameters. We present large-scale simulations of neural networks encoding real-world image scenes. In the first stage of our algorithm, forward projections generate activation levels of neurons corresponding to the primary visual cortex. In the second stage, these activation levels are used in a simulation of tangential coupled phase oscillators. We present results with forward projections based on designed Gabor filters that are a good approximation of receptive fields in the primary visual cortex. To allow later canonical generalization in higher network layers, we also present results with forward projections, learned in a normative model approach with a sparse autoencoder, using natural image statistics. In addition to these learned forward weights, the structural connectivity of the phase simulations is also learned, unsupervised, using the correlated activity induced by natural stimuli. Performance of the network is tested using

---

[445]This (distribution) function, named after the Italian physicist, Enrico Fermi, stems originally from quantum statistics.
See e.g. Scherz 1999, Cohen-Tannoudji et al. 2010.

[446]For fundamental information, see Finger and König 2014, which is based on the model of Sompolinsky et al. 1990.

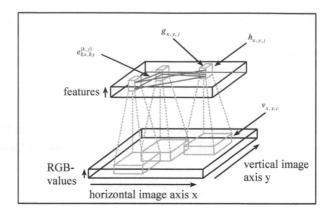

Figure 8.4: Schematic diagram of the network structure of the "Coupled Phase Oscillator Model": Feedforward convolutional filter mechanisms (grey dashed lines) are applied to each RGB color channel of the input image $v_{x,y,c}$ (lower black cuboid) to generate the neuron activations $h_{x,y,j}$ of the feature columns (small grey cuboids) in the subordinated layer (upper black cuboid) representing the primary visual cortex. These activations are then transformed into the oscillator activations $g_{x,y,j}$. The sparse connections $e_{\delta x,\delta y}^{k,j}$ (grey lines in the upper black cuboid) simulate the coupled neural phase oscillators, which bind the corresponding image features by means of the respective phase synchronization (following Finger and König 2014).

images taken from the LabelMe database. Thereby, we can investigate how synchronization phenomena might be utilized in sensory cortical areas to bind different attributes of the same stimulus, and how it might be exploited for scene segmentation (Finger and König 2014)."

The probability of a neuron's fire activity $P_{x,y,k}(t)$ is modelled by an isochronous oscillator (Goldstein et al. 2001), with reference to (1) a particular image position (x,y) and (2) the encoding of an (object) feature type k at a particular time t. The system state of a neuronal oscillator is determined by (1) the activation variables $g_{x,y,k}$ and (2) the phase variables $\Phi_{x,y,k}$, which together define the neurobiological interpretation of the fire probability according to the equation:

$$P_{x,y,k}(t) = g_{x,y,k}\left(1 + \lambda \cdot \cos\left(\Phi_{x,y,k}(t)\right)\right), \tag{8.47}$$

where the parameter $0 < \lambda < 1$ controls the relative strength of the temporal oscillation in relation to the fire probability of a neuron as a whole, and the phase progression is a periodic function according to the equation:

$$\Phi_{x,y,k}(t) = \Phi_{x,y,k}(t + 2\pi). \tag{8.48}$$

9 Systematic Class of System Dynamics-Based and Synapse-Based Architecture Types

The systematic class of system dynamics-based and synapse-based architecture types includes those connectionistic models, that can be subsumed under the classification of "Spiking Neural Networks (SNN)" or "Spiking Neural Models" (chap. 9.1).[447] These neuroarchitectures are characterised by the fact that the dynamic time aspect is implemented as realistically as possible in neuronal network modelling, and thus the exact time of a spike's occurrence is of importance (see chap. 4.1). Furthermore, these neuroarchitectures are characterized by the fact that algorithms which can be subject to "synaptic modulation" in different time scales are used, so that rapid changes in connection weights are possible (see chap. 6.4). Thus, stable synchronization processes can be analyzed within the temporal dynamics of stochastic synapses (chap. 9.2). Furthermore, special recurrent neuroarchitectures that have an internal, recurrent layer of neurons, the "reservoir" (in the context of "Reservoir Computing") are discussed (chap. 9.3 and 9.4). In addition, a dynamic binding mechanism is described by means of synfire waves to construct compositional representations (chap. 9.5). Finally, in contrast to the BBS and CTC hypothesis (chap. 4.4), a novel mechanism based on resonance frequencies is presented (chap. 9.6).

---

[447]For a fundamental discussion, see e.g. Maass 1995, 1996.
For a detailed discussion, see e.g. Maass 2003, 1999, 1997, Gerstner 1999, Gerstner and Kistler 2002.
For an introduction, see e.g. Maass 2002, 2015.
According to Maass 1997, the so-called "Spiking Neural Networks (SNN)" represent the 3rd generation of neural network modeling, in contrast to the "McCulloch-Pitts neurons" (1st generation) and the "feedforward and recurrent sigmoidal neural nets" (2nd generation).

9.1 STOCHASTIC SYNAPTIC MODEL AND LIQUID COMPUTING BY W. MAASS AND A.M. ZADOR

The "Synaptic Stochastic Model (SSM)"[448] has been developed by German mathematician, Wolfgang Maass and American biologist, Anthony M. Zador. In the course of this development, the concept of a nonlinear stochastic (dynamic) synapse (Liaw and Berger 1996) has been added to neuronal information processing (within the framework of SNN) as the third generation of neuronal network modelling (see the intro of chap. 9). The temporal dynamics of a single stochastic synapse is modelled according to the following three formulas (Maass and Zador 1999, 1998):

"The central equation in this model gives the probability $p_S(t_i)$ that the ith spike in a presynaptic spike train $\underline{t} = (t_1, ..., t_k)$ triggers the release of a vesicle at time t_i at synapse S,

$$p_S(t_i) = 1 - e^{-C(t_i) \cdot V(t_j)}. \tag{9.1}$$

The release probability is assumed to be nonzero only for $t \in \underline{t}$, so that releases occur only when a spike invades the presynaptic terminal (*i.e.* the spontaneous release probability is assumed to be zero). The functions $C(t) \geq 0$ and $V(t) \geq 0$ describe, respectively, the states of facilitation and depletion at the synapse at time t (Maass and Zador 1998)."

"The dynamics of facilitation are given by

$$C(t) = C_0 + \sum_{t_i < t} c(t - t_i), \tag{9.2}$$

where C_0 is some parameter ≥ 0 that can, for example, be related to the resting concentration of calcium in the synapse. The exponential response function $c(s)$ models the response $C(t)$ to a presynaptic spike that had reached the synapse at time $t - s : c(s) = \alpha \cdot e^{-s/\tau_C}$, where the positive parameters τ_C and α give the decay constant and magnitude, respectively, of the response. The function C models in an abstract way, internal synaptic processes underlying presynaptic facilitation, such as the concentration of calcium in the presynaptic terminal. The particular exponential form used for $c(s)$ could arise, for example, if presynaptic calcium dynamics were governed by a simple first order process (Maass and Zador 1998)."

"The dynamics of depletion are given by

$$V(t) = \max \left(0, V_0 - \sum_{t_i : t_i < t \text{ and } t_i \in S(\underline{t})} v(t - t_i) \right), \tag{9.3}$$

for some parameter $V_0 > 0$. $V(t)$ depends on the subset of those $t_i \in \underline{t}$ with $t_i < t$ on which vesicles were actually released by the synapse, i.e. $t_i \in S(\underline{t})$. The function

---

[448]For fundamental information, see e.g. Maass and Zador 1999, 1998.
For an introduction, see e.g. Maass 2003.
For a brief introduction, see Maurer 2014a.

$v(s)$ models the response of $V(t)$ to a preceding release of the same synapse at time $t - s \leq t$. As for $c(s)$, one may analogously choose for $v(s)$, a function with exponential decay where $\tau_V > 0$ is the decay constant. The function V models in an abstract way, internal synaptic processes that support presynaptic depression, such as depletion of the pool of readily releasable vesicles. In a more specic synapse model, one could interpret V_0 as the maximal number of vesicles that can be stored in the readily releasable pool, and $V(t)$ as the expected number of vesicles in the readily releasable pool at time t.

In summary, the model of synaptic dynamics presented here is described by five parameters: C_0, V_0, τ_C, τ_V and α (Maass and Zador 1998)."

In order to adequately model the typical computation method for "online computation" and "real-time computing" of a biological organism's neurocognitive system, Wolfgang Maass, Thomas Natschläger and Henry Markram have constructed a "Liquid State Machine (LSM)"[449] (see Fig. 9.1) (in contrast to a traditional Turing-Machine (TM), chap. 1.1.5):

"Like the Turing machine (...), the model of a liquid state machine (LSM) is based on a rigorous mathematical framework that guarantees, under ideal conditions, universal computational power. Turing machines, however, have universal computational power for off-line computation on (static) discrete inputs, while LSMs have, in a very specific sense, universal computational power for real-time computing with fading memory on analog functions in continuous time. The input function $u(\cdot)$ can be a continuous sequence of disturbances, and the target output can be some chosen function $y(\cdot)$ of time that provides a real-time analysis of this sequence. In order for a machine M to map input functions of time $u(\cdot)$ to output functions $y(\cdot)$ of time, we assume that it generates, at every time t, an internal 'liquid state' $x^M(t)$ which constitutes its current response to preceding perturbations, that is, to preceding inputs $u(s)$ for $s \leq t$ (...). In contrast to the finite state of a finite state machine (or finite automaton), this liquid state consists of analog values that may change continuously over time (Maass et al. 2002)."

"The computation of a Turing machine always begins in a designated initial state q_0, with the input x (...) written on some designated tape. The computation runs until a halt-state is entered (the inscription y of some designated tape segment is then interpreted as the result of the computation). This is a typical example for an *offline computation*, where the complete input x is available at the beginning of the computation, and no trace of this computation, or of its result y, is left when the same Turing machine subsequently carries out another computation for another input $\tilde{x}$ (starting again in the state q_0). In contrast, the result of a typical computation in the neuronal system of a biological organism, say the decision about the location y on the ground where the left foot is going to be placed at the next step (...), depends on several pieces of information. (...) In general these diverse pieces of information arrive at

---

[449]For a basic discussion, see e.g. Maass et al. 2002.
For a detailed discussion, see e.g. Maass 2007.
For an introduction, see e.g. Maass 2016, Lukoševičius and Jaeger 2009, Jaeger 2002/2008.
Probst et al. 2012 describes an application case in neurorobotics.

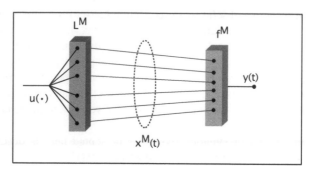

Figure 9.1: Schematic diagram of the architecture of a "Liquid State Machine (LSM)": A function $u(\cdot)$ is fed into the "liquid filter" L^M, which generates a "liquid state" $x^M(t)$ at any time t. This liquid state is transformed into an output $y(t)$ at any given time t by means of a "memoryless readout map" f^M, which has been trained for a specific task (following Maass et al. 2002).

different points in time, and the computation of y has start before the last one has come in. Furthermore, new information (...) arrives continuously, and it is left up to the computational system how much of it can be integrated into the computation of the position y of the next placement of the left foot (...). Once the computation of y is completed, the computation of the location y' where the right foot is subsequently placed is not a separate computation that starts again in some neutral initial state q_0. Rather, it is likely to build on pieces of inputs and results of subcomputations that had already been used for the preceding computation of y.

The previously sketched computational task is a typical example for an online computation (where input pieces arrive all the time, not in one batch). Furthermore it is an example for a realtime computation, where one has a strict deadline by which the computation of the output y has to be completed (...) (Maass 2007)."

The Liquid State Machine can perform continuous computing processes in real time, according to the formula (Maass, Natschläger and Markram 2002):

$$x^M(t) = (L^M u)(t). \tag{9.4}$$

The model shows that a "liquid state" $x^M(t)$ results from the current output of an operator or a time-invariant "liquid filter" L^M, which maps an input function $u(\cdot)$ onto the continuous function $x^M(t)$. This liquid system state consists of all information about the current internal state of a dynamic system, in the form of analog values that can change continuously over time.

The current, liquid, system state $x^M(t)$ is then transformed at any time t into an output $y(t)$ (in a task-specific manner, and by means of a "memoryless[450] readout

---

[450]See Maass et al. 2002: "The term *memoryless* refers to the fact that the readout map f^M is not required to retain any memory of previous states $x^M(s)$, $s < t$, of the liquid. However, in a biological context, the readout map will, in general, be subject to plasticity and may also contribute to the memory

map" f^M), according to the formula (Maass et al. 2002):

$$y(t) = f^M\left(x^M(t)\right). \tag{9.5}$$

C. Fernando and S. Sojakka (2003) have constructed a water tank as a "liquid brain", and have shown that the waves generated on the water's surface can be used as a medium for solving the XOR problem for a liquid state machine. Furthermore, it could be shown that the dynamic properties of the fluid could be used to produce a transient synchrony mechanism that performs a speech recognition task "following the example of the Hopfield and Brody experiments (...) to distinguish a speaker saying the word 'one' from the same speaker saying 'zero'" (Hopfield and Brody 2000).

Recently, Maass has developed a model for variable binding, based on empirical findings, that rapidly recruits assemblies of neurons in subregions of the temporal cortex (Legenstein et al. 2016; see also Müller et al. 2020). These assemblies can act as "pointers" in a neural space, thereby binding a variable that represents a thematic role to a semantic concept ("pointer-based binding"). These assembly pointers provide a model for a neural mechanism that replaces the "copy process" which processes information in a digital computer. The binding process is controlled by the neurophysiological mechanism of top-down disinhibition, and is not based on precise synchronization of spikes in different neural spaces. However, "the synaptic coupling between these spaces together with lateral inhibition leads to some synchronized oscillations of interacting neural spaces in [their] (author's note) simulations. This is consistent with recent experimental data (Friederici and Singer 2015) which suggests that common rhythms in two brain areas support the flow of excitation between these two areas, and also the potentiation of synapses between activated neurons in both areas."

9.2 MODIFIED STOCHASTIC SYNAPTIC MODEL BY K. EL-LAITHY AND M. BOGDAN

The Egyptian technical neuroinformatician, Karim El-Laithy and the German technical neuroinformatician, Martin Bogdan have constructed the "Modified Synaptic Stochastic Model (MSSM)"[451], which is a modified version of Maass and Zador's "Synaptic Stochastic Model (SSM)." They investigated whether and to what extent the concept of temporal synchronicity can be generated by a recurrent artificial neural network using nonlinear stochastic and dynamic synapses. The model consists of two network structures of respectively three and eight neurons[452], where the maximum

---

capability of the system. We do not explore this issue here because the differentiation into a memoryless readout map and a liquid that serves as a memory device is made for conceptual clarification and is not essential to the model."

[451]For a fundamental discussion, see e.g. El-Laithy and Bogdan 2009.
For a detailed discussion, see e.g. El-Laithy and Bogdan 2011a, b, 2010a.
For a brief introduction, see Maurer 2014a.

[452]The assumptions regarding the neurobiologically plausible size of an (artificial) neuronal network in which temporal synchronicity activity of the neurons concerned can be expected to vary between two

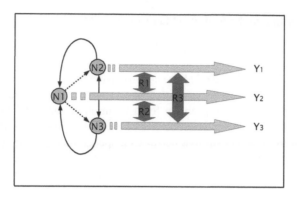

Figure 9.2: Schematic diagram of the "Modified Synaptic Stochastic Model (MSSM)" with a network structure consisting of three neurons. The dashed arrows represent the synapses to be trained between neuron N_1 and neurons N_2 and N_3. The double arrow represents a reciprocal connection between the neurons N_2 and N_3. The horizontal light grey double arrows represent the output signals Y_1, Y_2 and Y_3 of the respective neurons, and the vertical dark grey double arrows represent the corresponding cross correlation coefficients R_1, R_2 and R_3 (following El-Laithy and Bogdan 2009).

of the cross correlation coefficients between the filtered signals is used to indicate the degree of synchronicity (see Fig. 9.2).

The "(Leaky-)Integrate-And-Fire ((L)IAF) Neuron Model"[453] is integrated into the "Synaptic Stochastic Model (SSM)"[454] to produce the "Modified Synaptic Stochastic Model (MSSM)"[451]. The (L)IAF Neuron Model describes the dynamics of the observable excitatory postsynaptic potential E_{psp} by means of the concentration of the neurotransmitter molecules C_{Nt}:

"Each neuron is described by its voltage membrane potential V, that followed the following dynamics:

$$\tau_V \frac{dV}{dt} = -V + E_{psp},$$ (9.6)

---

and about one hundred neurons.

See, for example, the "small network argument" in the sense of Herzog et al. 2007.

See also, Singer and Gray 1995.

[453] See e.g. El-Laithy and Bogdan 2009.

The (L)IAF Neuron Model is one of the most important classes of mathematical neuron models within the Spiking Neural Networks (SNN).

See e.g. Kandel et al. 2013.

See also, Haken 2008.

See the explanations in chap. 9.

In later publications, e.g. El-Laithy and Bogdan 2010b, 2011c, the "Markram-Tsodyks (synaptic) Model" is also used. See Markram et al. 1998.

[454] See e.g. El-Laithy and Bogdan 2009.

See the remarks in chap. 9.1.

For an alteration in the $P(t_i)$ representation in the revisited MSSM, see El-Laithy and Bogdan 2017.

where τ_V is the membrane time constant, and E_{psp} is the total observed excitatory postsynaptic potential from all presynaptic terminals.
(...)
E_{psp} can be expressed as follows (...):

$$\tau_{epsp}\frac{dE_{psp}}{dt} = -E_{psp} + C_{Nt},\tag{9.7}$$

where τ_{epsp} is a decay time-constant. C_{Nt} is the concentration of the Nt in the synaptic cleft (El-Laithy and Bogdan 2009)."

The SSM estimates the transmission probability of an incoming action potential from a presynaptic neuron via a synapse to a postsynaptic neuron, regulated by two compensating mechanisms of "facilitation" $C_C(t)$ (based on Ca^{2+} concentration) and "depression" $C_V(t)$ (based on vesicle concentration) (El-Laithy and Bogdan 2009):

"The probability that the ith spike in the spike train triggers the release of a vesicle at time t_i at a given synapse is given by:

$$P(t_i) = 1 - e^{(-C_C(t_i) \cdot C_V(t_i))},\tag{9.8}$$

where $C_C(t_i)$ and $C_V(t_i)$ represent the facilitation and depression mechanisms respectively at t_i (El-Laithy and Bogdan 2009)."

"$C_C(t_i)$ and $C_V(t_i)$ are expressed mathematically as follows (...):

$$C_C(t) = C_{C_0} + \sum_{t_i} \alpha e^{-(t-t_i/\tau_{C_C})}\tag{9.9}$$

$$C_V(t) = \max\left(C_{V_0} - \sum_{t_i} e^{-(t-t_i/\tau_C)}\right)\tag{9.10}$$

(...) τ_{C_C} and α represent the decay constant and the magnitude of the response respectively. C_{C_0} represents the initial concentration of Ca^{2+} in the pre-synaptic terminal. (...) $C_V(t)$ is the expected number of vesicles of neurotransmitter molecules (Nt) in the ready-for-release pool at time t. C_{V_0} is the max. number of vesicles that can be stored in the pool. τ_{V_C} is the time constant for refilling the vesicles (El-Laithy and Bogdan 2009)."

A Hebb-based learning rule is also introduced, showing how the time parameters and constants of electrochemical mechanisms can be readjusted based on the activity of pre- and postsynaptic neurons. In addition to the learning rate r, a "feedback parameter" K is introduced as modulator. It represents improvements to the extent to which a more frequent, stable, synchronicity is generated between the output signals of the neurons concerned, i.e. a higher mean value R_m of the maximum cross correlation coefficients:

"The update of the contribution values could be mathematically formed as follows: $m_{new} = (1 \pm r) m_{current}$, where r is the learning rate. (...)
We introduce a feedback parameter, K, that represents the advance in the direction of getting both, more and stable synchrony, between the responses (i.e. a higher

cross-correlation coefficient). Thus, it is the difference in the observed synchrony R_m between the current run and the previous one, mathematically expressed as follows:

$$K = R_{m_{current}} - R_{m_{previous}}. \tag{9.11}$$

K is used as a modulator to the learning rate. Thus, the learning rule can be rewritten as follows:

$$m_{i_{new}} = (1 \pm r \cdot K) \, m_{i_{current}}. \tag{9.12}$$

K can reverse the direction of the updating process of the parameters since it is a signed value, and can either accelerate or decelerate the learning process (El-Laithy and Bogdan 2009)."

Based on the LSM by Maass, Natschläger and Markram, El-Laithy and Bogdan (2011d) use a recurrent artificial network as an implementation of an LSM. This network takes the form of a column whose activity is read and transformed by a number of task-specific "side networks", also called "readout maps". These readout maps receive their input from the same overall assembly of internal neuronal activity in the form of spikes, but from a different configuration of neurons of the "core machine", i.e. a subassembly with a collective-synchronous, neuronal activity. This neuronal activity can be defined as a system state, so that a mapping of a finite physical system state space into an infinite informational system state space is possible (El-Laithy and Bogdan 2011d). The synaptic representation of the MSSM proves to be efficient because it is able to generate (at least) two different transient, stable system states in the context of a synchronous activity. Thus, one basic condition of a neuronal dynamic system, the capacity to compute, i.e. the ability to represent sensory information by a specific number of different sets of synchronicity states (El-Laithy and Bogdan 2011d), is fulfilled.

Finally, Friston's "Free Energy Principle" (see chap. 10.3) is used to describe the energetic dynamics of a (stochastic) synapse in the sense of the Binding-By-Synchrony Hypothesis according to Singer et al. One considers a synapse as an open physical dynamic system, which can be described by the system equations of the MSSM explained above. This synaptic system tends to minimize its "Free Synaptic Energy (FSE)" (i.e. the transfer of the excitatory postsynaptic potential [EPSP]) (El-Laithy and Bogdan 2014), or the neuroelectrical energy transfer optimally settles down into local minima in the context of the respective energy functions (Bullmore and Sporns 2012):

"The electrical energy held by (and transferred via) EPSP, consequently represents, in an abstract way, what is termed here the 'free synaptic energy' (FSE) and defined as:

Proposition 1. *As an open thermodynamic system, a synapse has a total free energy that is a function of two parameters: The output state parameter corresponding to the presynaptic input, and the 'recognition density that is encoded by its internal states' (...). When the EPSP(t) is the synaptic response and output state parameter, S(t) is the synaptic dynamic strength (recognition density), and $\tau > 0$ is a presynaptic-dependent constant, the free synaptic energy (FSE) is dened as*

$$\text{FSE} \equiv E_{syn}(t) \approx S(t) \times \text{EPSP}(t) \times e^{\frac{-\Delta_{isi}}{\tau}}, \tag{9.13}$$

where Δ_{isi} is the inter spike interval.
(...)
In other words, the energy represented in EPSP is the bounded function that the biological system (here the synapse) tries to *minimize* and to *stabilize* by optimizing its internal states. These states (in the synapse) are the activity-dependent concentrations of the chemical constitutes holding (and responsible for) the synaptic transmission. E_{Syn} does not represent the thermodynamic free energy of the synapse. The notation 'free' is adopted since the synapse, as a biological system, tries to minimize this exchange energy in a fashion similar to that known from the second law of thermodynamics. This is performed through the minimization of the free energy of a system parallel to the maximization of its entropy (El-Laithy and Bogdan 2014)."

This leads, in a self-organized way, to the inevitable generation of stable synchronous neural activities in the entire network (El-Laithy and Bogdan 2014):

"How can the synaptic energy profile affect the collective network behaviour? In order to answer this question we present the next proposition that represents a theoretical bridge between the internal dynamics from a synaptic level to the top network level.
Proposition 2. *For a given network with n neurons, if s synapses operate at any of the local energy minima and sustain stable synaptic energy E_{Syn} to l neurons, then the rest of the network $((n-l)$ neurons) is forced to follow gradually the stable activity of the l neurons, provided that the temporal features of input signal are maintained. If the coherent activity of these neurons is observed over a time window W, after a suitable time T, where $T \gg W$, a general new state of synchronous discharge from all n neurons should be observed. This defines a network synchrony state* (El-Laithy and Bogdan 2014)."

9.3 ECHO STATE NETWORK AND RESERVOIR COMPUTING BY H. JAEGER

The "Echo State Network (ESN)"[455] has been developed by the German mathematician and neuroinformatician, Herbert Jaeger as an alternative model of the LSM in the context of "Reservoir Computing"[456]. It is a special type of recurrent neural network in the sense of Elman (see chap. 3.2.4.2). This time-discrete model consists of K input neurons, N internal reservoir neurons and L output neurons. The activations of the input neurons at time n are denoted with $\mathbf{u}(n) = (u_1(n), ..., u_K(n))$, the activations of the internal neurons of the dynamic reservoir with $\mathbf{x}(n) = (x_1(n), ..., x_N(n))$,

---

[455] For basic information, see e.g. Jaeger 2001/2010, 2002/2008.
For detailed information, see e.g. Jaeger et al. 2007b, Pascanu and Jaeger 2011.
See also, Jaeger et al. 2007a.
For an introduction, see e.g. Lukoševičius et al. 2012, with additional literature, Lukoševičius and Jaeger 2009, Appeltant 2012, Holzmann 2008.

[456] For an introduction to the concept of "Reservoir Computing", see e.g. Lukoševičius et al. 2012, Lukoševičius and Jaeger 2009, Appeltant 2012, Schrauwen et al. 2007.
For the connection between the concept of "Reservoir Computing" and the "Binding-By-Synchrony (BBS) Hypothesis", see e.g. Singer 2013.

and the activations of the output neurons with $\mathbf{y}(n) = (y_1(n), ..., y_L(n))$. Furthermore, the connection weights of the input neurons to the internal neurons are recorded in an $N \times K$ weight matrix $\mathbf{W}^{in} = (w_{ij}^{in})$, the connection weights of the reservoir neurons in an $N \times N$ weight matrix $\mathbf{W} = (w_{ij})$, the connection weights of the internal neurons to the output neurons in an $L \times (K \times N \times L)$ weight matrix $\mathbf{W}^{out} = (w_{ij}^{out})$. The feedback connection weights of the output neurons back to the internal neurons are recorded in a $(N \times L)$ weight matrix $\mathbf{W}^{back} = (w_{ij}^{back})$. In addition, direct connections from the input neurons to the output neurons and connections between the output neurons are allowed (see Fig. 9.3). It should be noted that the topological structure of the reservoir is not subject to any further conditions. This means that the sparse[457] connection weights between the reservoir neurons are randomly chosen and, contrary to the functioning of traditional recurrent neural networks, these weights are not trained. At most, it is generally intended that the network dynamics generate recurrent pathways between the internal neurons, so that the input signal is projected into a high-dimensional system state space as part of non-linear, transient transformation processes. The advantage of the ESN is that only the connection weights between the internal neurons and the output neurons are adjusted in a supervised learning procedure, so that the training algorithm is a classification by means of a simple "linear regression" (Jaeger 2001/2010, 2002/2008). Finally, it should be mentioned that all input signals, connection weights and activation values are real-valued.

The activation of the internal reservoir neurons is computed as:

$$\mathbf{x}(n+1) = \mathbf{f}\left(\mathbf{W}^{in}\mathbf{u}(n+1) + \mathbf{W}\,\mathbf{x}(n) + \mathbf{W}^{back}\mathbf{y}(n)\right), \tag{9.14}$$

where $\mathbf{f} = (f_1, ..., f_N)$ is the nonlinear activation function[458] of the internal neurons, usually a sigmoid function, such as $f(x) = \tanh(x)$.

The reservoir output is computed as:

$$\mathbf{y}(n+1) = \mathbf{f}^{out}\left(\mathbf{W}^{out}\left(\mathbf{u}(n+1), \mathbf{x}(n+1), \mathbf{y}(n)\right)\right), \tag{9.15}$$

where $\mathbf{f}^{out} = (f_1^{out}, ..., f_L^{out})$ is the linear output function of the output neurons with $f^{out}(x) = 1$, and $(\mathbf{u}(n+1), \mathbf{x}(n+1), \mathbf{y}(n))$ is the serial concatenation of the input vectors, the internal vectors and the preceding output activation vectors.

Application examples in the cognitive neurosciences are the "Temporal Recurrent Network" (Pascanu and Jaeger 2011), a neurodynamic and neurolinguistic model of working memory and grammar construction, by P.F. Dominey (Dominey et al. 2003, 2006, Dominey 1995, Lukoševičius and Jaeger 2009) and the "Predictive Echo State Network Classifier" (Skowronski and Harris 2007) for automatic speech recognition.

---

[457]This means that only about 5-20% of the connections are given.
See e.g. Jaeger 2001/2010, 2002/2008.
See also, chap. 4.2.5.

[458]Sometimes, it is also referred to as the "transfer function" or the "output function".
See e.g. Jaeger 2002/2008.

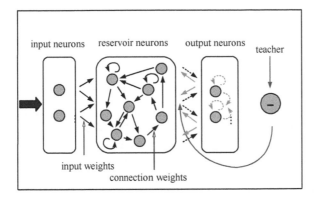

Figure 9.3: Schematic diagram of the basic network architecture of the "Echo State Network": The input is processed via randomly selected connections from the neurons of the input layer to those of the internal neurons of the reservoir. The sparse connections between the reservoir neurons are also chosen randomly and are not trained. The transient, dynamic computation process of the reservoir is then read from an output layer, based on the linearly weighted sum of the respective reservoir system states. This state can finally be compared with a desired output, which is indicated by the grey (curved) arrows. The solid arrows indicate that it is a random, fixed connection, whereas the dashed arrows indicate that it is a connection to be trained (following Jaeger 2001/2010 and Jaeger 2002/2008).

9.4   (REWARD-MODULATED) SELF-ORGANIZING RECURRENT NEURAL NETWORK BY G. PIPA

Based on the architecture of the ESN by Jaeger as part of "Reservoir Computing", the German neuroinformatician, Gordon Pipa, has developed the "Reward-Modulated Self-Organizing Recurrent Neural Network (RM-SORN)" (Aswolinskiy and Pipa 2015) (see Fig. 9.4). It is a further development of the "Self-Organizing Recurrent Network (SORN)"[459]. This model, which uses an unsupervised learning procedure, consists of a recurrent layer (the "reservoir" (Lazar et al. 2009)) which contains neurons with a binary threshold value.

"At each time step the activity of the network is determined both, by the inputs, and the propagation of the previously emitted spikes through the network. This recurrent drive received by unit i is given by:

$$R_i(t+1) = \sum_{j=1}^{N^E} w_{ij}^{EE}(t)x_j(t) - \sum_{k=1}^{N^I} w_{ik}^{EI}y_k(t) - T_i^E(t). \qquad (9.16)$$

---

[459]For fundamental information, see Lazar et al. 2009.
For detailed information, see e.g. Lazar et al. 2007, 2011, Schumacher et al. 2015, Toutounji et al. 2015.
See also, Toutounji and Pipa 2014, Schumacher et al. 2013, Pipa 2006, 2010a, 2010b, Cao 2010.

Based on this, we define a 'pseudo state' x(t) that only depends on the recurrent drive:

$$x'_i(t) = \Theta\left(R_i(t)\right);\tag{9.17}$$

(...) Most of our analysis focuses on the pseudo states $x(t)$ as the network's internal representation of previous inputs (Lazar et al. 2009)."

The model is also designed with three plasticity mechanisms ("Intrinsic Plasticity (IP)", "Synaptic Normalization (SN)" and "Spike-Timing-Dependent Plasticity (STDP)"), and with an output layer (the "readout layer"), which is trained with a supervised learning procedure.[459] The network is trained in two phases. In the first phase, the recurrent layer processes the input signals with permanent plasticity. In the second phase, the permanent plasticity is switched off while the input signals are processed again, but the neuron activations serve to train the output layer. However, while the output signal in SORN is trained with a simple linear regression (see chap. 9.3), in RM-SORN, the plastic connection weights from the recurrent layer to the output layer are adjusted by the plasticity mechanism of the "reward-modulated Spike-Timing-Dependent Plasticity (rm-STDP)". The model also allows this rm-STDP mechanism to be applied to the weight adaptation in the recurrent layer, consisting of N^E excitatory and N^I inhibitory neurons, e.g. in the ratio 5:1. The excitatory and inhibitory neurons are fully connected, in contrast to the number of connections of the excitatory neurons to each other, whose connectivity is sparse (5-10%).[457] From the output layer, whose neurons are not interconnected, a feedback connection to the recurrent layer may be necessary for certain tasks, e.g. if a sequence, such as '1234', is to be generated. A random subset of excitatory neurons of the recurrent layer receives the input (sequence).

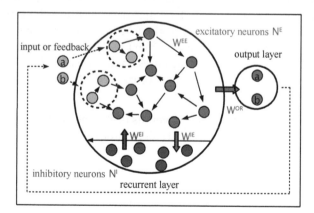

Figure 9.4: Schematic diagram of the basic network architecture of the "(Reward-Modulated) Self-Organizing Recurrent Neural Network (RM-)SORN": Excitatory neurons are shown in blue, inhibitory neurons in red. The black arrows symbolize direct connections with variable connection weights between the neurons. Only the excitatory neurons project to the output neurons. The few excitatory neurons that receive external input signals are displayed in light blue. The dotted arrow indicates the feedback connection to the recurrent layer required for certain tasks (following Aswolinskiy and Pipa 2015).

The activation of the neurons of the recurrent layer is defined according to

$$x_i(t+1) = \Theta \left(\sum_j^{NE} w_{ij}^{EE} x_j(t) - \sum_k^{NI} w_{ik}^{EI} y_k(t) + u_i(t) - T_i^E(t) \right) \qquad (9.18)$$

$$y_i(t+1) = \Theta \left(\sum_j^{NE} w_{ij}^{IE} x_j(t) - T_i^I \right), \qquad (9.19)$$

while the neuron activity of the output layer is computed according to

$$o_i(t+1) = a \left(\sum_j^{NE} w_{ij}^{OE} x_j(t) - T_i^O(t) \right), \qquad (9.20)$$

where x and y represent the activities of the excitatory and inhibitory neurons in the recurrent layer, o represents the activity of the output neurons, u represents the input signals, and T represents the threshold of the respective neurons. The activation function for the excitatory and inhibitory neurons is the threshold or "Heaviside step function" Θ[460]. The activation function for the output neurons is the function a, which is either a Winner-Takes-All (WTA) function[461] (when multiple neurons are used), or the Heaviside step function (when only one neuron is present). At the beginning of the training, the weights are subject to a normal distribution, after which they are changed by three plasticity mechanisms or plasticity rules: Intrinsic Plasticity (IP), Synaptic Normalization (SN) and reward-modulated Spike-Timing-Dependent Plasticity (rm-STDP) (Aswolinskiy and Pipa 2015):

"IP adapts the thresholds so that, on average, each neuron has the firing rate μ_{IP}:

$$\Delta T_i^E(t) = \eta_{IP}(x_i(t) - \mu_{IP}). \qquad (9.22)$$

The threshold is increased when the unit is active and decreased when the unit is inactive, leading to an asymptotic fix point of the average firing rate μ_{IP}. Thereby, IP activates neurons, which would otherwise be inactive, and regulates down neurons which fire too often, enforcing the given average firing rate. During the experiments, μ_{IP} was set to values between 0.05 and 0.25 in the recurrent layer, depending on which value performed best. In the output layer, μ_{IP} was set per neuron to correspond to the expected occurrence probability of the symbol represented by the neuron. η_{IP} is the learning rate for IP.

---

[460]The Heaviside function, also called theta, unit step or threshold function, named after the British mathematician and physicist, Oliver Heaviside, is defined with:

$$H(x) = \begin{cases} 0 & x < 0 \\ 1/2 & x = 0 \\ 1 & x > 0 \end{cases} \qquad (9.21)$$

See e.g. Abramowitz and Stegun 1972, Bracewell 2000.

[461]An example for the computation principle of the "Winner-Takes-All (WTA) (computing)" is the Kohonen algorithm or the Grossberg algorithm.
See the explanations in chap. 3.2.4.4 and chap. 3.2.4.5.

STDP strengthens the connection from x_j to x_i when x_j was active before x_i (x_j causes x_i) and weakens it, when x_j was active after x_i. The main difference to SORN is the remodeling of the output layer as another plastic neuron layer and the reward-modulation of STDP with the modulation m:

$$\Delta w_{ij}^{EE} = m_r * \eta_{STDP}(x_j(t-1)x_i(t) - x_j(t)x_i(t1)) \tag{9.23}$$

$$\Delta w_{ij}^{OE} = m_o * \eta_{STDP}(x_j(t-1)o_i(t)) \tag{9.24}$$

η_{STDP} is the learning rate for STDP. m_r and m_o are the modulation factors for the recurrent and the output layer, respectively. During the simulations, m_r was either set to one (no modulation) or to the same value as m_o. m_o is determined according to a rewarding strategy, which is a function of the reward r. Both modulation and reward can be positive, negative or zero. Depending on the task, different modulation strategies can be chosen for m_o.

After application of STDP the incoming weights to a neuron are scaled to sum up to 1:

$$w_{ij}(t) = \frac{w_{ij}(t)}{\sum_j w_{ij}(t)} \quad \rightarrow \quad \sum_j w_{ij}(t) = 1 \tag{9.25}$$

The relative strength of the synapses remains the same (Aswolinskiy and Pipa 2015)."

A further important field of research consists of being able to adequately describe and model self-organized synchronization processes in neuronal populations (Pipa 2006, 2010a) (in the sense of the Binding-By-Synchrony Hypothesis by Singer, Engel and König et al. [Uhlhaas et al. 2011, 2009, Vicente et al. 2009, Balaban et al. 2010, Korndörfer et al. 2017 with reference to Vinck and Bosman 2016]) with this concept of Reservoir Computing (Pipa 2010b).

9.5   SYNFIRE CHAINS AND CORTICONICS BY M. ABELES

Since a selective sensitivity of cortical neurons towards a more synchronous activity over a high number of interneuron layers had been experimentally demonstrated[462], the Israeli neurophysiologist and technical biomedical scientist Moshe Abeles developed an architectural model, the "Synfire Chain (SFC) Model"[463]. This model

---

[462] See e.g. Abeles et al. 1993, Abeles 1994 with more literature: Koch et al. 1990, Nelken 1988, Reyes and Fetz 1993.
See also Shmiel et al. 2005, 2006.

[463] For fundamental information, see e.g. Abeles 1982b, 1982a, 1991, Abeles et al. 1993.
For detailed information, see e.g. Herrmann et al. 1995, Hertz and Prügel-Bennett 1996, Diesmann et al. 1996, 1999, Hertz 1998, Aviel et al. 2002, 2004, Reyes 2003, Morrison et al. 2005.
For an introduction, see e.g. Abeles 2009, 2003, 1994 with an illustration of the structure of the synfire chains.
For a brief introduction, see Maurer 2014a.
See also, the approach of the "Synfire Braids" in Bienenstock 1995 and the approach of the "Polychro-

is based on studies on the frontal cortex of monkeys.[464] The model consists of a feedforward network with a high number of layers, i.e. a "chain" of "pools" of neurons connected by diverging and converging excitatory synapses. Thus, the dominant neural functional principle is that a single neuron will no longer become active if it "integrates" the incoming, super-threshold excitatory discharges of a large number of preceding neurons over a certain period of time. Such a neuron will be referred to as a "coincidence detector" (Abeles 1982a, 1994, Trappenberg 2010). This means that the neuron becomes active when the synchronous activity of a few excitatory discharges exceeds the threshold value. If a "synfire chain" is now in synchronization mode, then each assembly of neurons will release an approximately synchronized volley within one millisecond, which will activate another assembly synchronously, and so on (Abeles 2003). Thus a depolarizing wave, a "synfire wave," is induced in the next neuron layer (Abeles 2003). At any one time, the same neuron may belong to a multitude of different pools, depending on which assembly its neural activity is currently correlated with (see Fig. 9.5):

"The stability of propagation of activity along a synfire chain was analyzed (...) using a transfer-function $N_{out}(N_{in})$ (The number of active neurons in the post-synaptic pool as a function of the number of active neurons in the pre-synaptic pool). This transfer function is defined solely by the synfire chain architecture. The fixed points of the synfire chain dynamics can be found through this method. This function is only deterministic when there is no noise in the system and activity (if it exists) in each pool is exactly synchronous. When noise is present, responses become probabilistic and activity may be described by the pulse packet model (...). Using this model the transfer function may be replaced by a transfer matrix P_{ij}, where P_{ij} is the probability that j neurons will fire in the next pool within the following τ milliseconds, given that i neurons fired in the pre-synaptic pool at the last τ milliseconds. (...) [It can be shown] that the transfer function is the first moment of the transfer matrix

$$j(i) = \sum_{k=1}^{N} kP_{ik} \tag{9.26}$$

Here, we use i and j instead of N_{in} and N_{out} respectively, and N is the number of neurons in a pool.

To calculate P_{ij}, the pulse packet model (Aertsen et al. 1996) was used. A stable isolated pulse packet was created. Then the post-synaptic firing time distribution was calculated when only i of the W neurons of the pool were active. The total activity within the first 5 milliseconds after the mean firing time of the presynaptic pool

nization" in Izhikevich 2006, Izhikevich et al. 2004, Eguchi 2018 and in Isbister 2018.

For the term "synfire attractor", see e.g. Kumar et al. 2008.

For an application on the compositional structure of hand movements by a monkey, see Abeles et al. 2013.

For the network delay loops mechanism, see Brama et al. 2015.

For a beginner's guide, see e.g. Breidbach 1996, Ziemke and Cardoso de Oliveira 1996, Maye and Engel 2012.

[464] See e.g. Prut et al. 1998, Abeles and Prut 1996, Aertsen et al. 1991.

See also Ikegaya et al. 2004, which presents experimental evidence of synfire chains in the primary visual cortex of mice and cats.

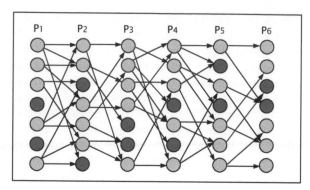

Figure 9.5: Schematic diagram of a "Synfire Chain" (simplified), consisting of inhibitory neurons (dark grey) and excitatory neurons (light grey). Contrary to the classical model of a neuron as an "integrator" according to which a neuron becomes active when its threshold value is exceeded by the incoming excitatory discharges of a high number of preconnected neurons, Abeles' "Synfire Chain (SFC) Model" considers the neuron as a "coincidence detector". Since even a small number of incoming discharges leads to an above-threshold synchronous coactivity of an ensemble of neurons, a transient oscillation of a large neuron population occurs under certain conditions. This happens in such a way that it can lead to further dynamic activity cascades of adjacent neuron populations which are already almost above-threshold. Thus, these clocked, large-scale spatio-temporal wave patterns can generate stable synchronized activity patterns over a large number of interneuron layers (following Abeles et al. 2004).

yielded the mean activity level of the postsynaptic pool (μ_i). Then, using a binomial distribution, we calculated P_{ij}:

$$P_{ij} = \left(\frac{\mu_i}{W}\right)^j \left(1 - \frac{\mu_i}{W}\right)^{w-j} \frac{W!}{j!(W-j)!} \tag{9.27}$$

Using discrete time, a recursive formula may be used to calculate the probability $P(m, t = k+1)$ (the probability that m neurons of the $k + 1$ pool are active):

$$P(m, t = k+1) = \sum_{i=1}^{W} P_{mi} P(i, t = k) \tag{9.28}$$

This method was used to study the effect of a wave in one chain on the velocity of a wave in another one, to study the effect of inhibition on waves, and the spontaneous generation of a wave in one chain by a wave propagating in another chain (Abeles et al. 2004 with reference to Abeles 1991 and Diesmann et al. 1996)."

According to E. Bienenstock (Bienenstock 1995, 1996, Bienenstock et al. 1997) and M. Abeles et al. (Abeles et al. 2004, Maye and Engel 2012), the main application of this model is in the generation of a synfire wave by means of a synchronization of neural activity waves. Because the synfire wave interacts with other waves, the problem of compositionality can be modelled convincingly. There is a "concatenation" in the form of a superposition of several neural assemblies in a synfire chain (see Fig. 9.5) (a "synfire-superposition hypothesis"), based on Hebb's principle of synaptic plasticity (Bienenstock 1995).

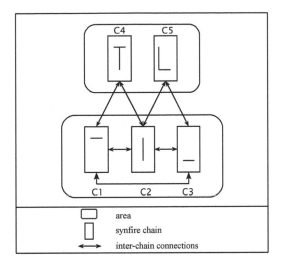

Figure 9.6: Schematic diagram of the network architecture of the "Part Binding Problem": The Synfire chains C1, C2, C3 represent lines, while the Synfire chains C4 and C5 represent symbols. Within an area, all synfire chains are subjected to the same inhibitory activity. Between the first three Synfire chains C1, C2, C3, there is only a weak reciprocal connection, indicated by the arrows. The Synfire chain C4 is reciprocally connected to the Synfire chains C1 and C2 in the lower area, and the Synfire chain C5 is reciprocally connected to the Synfire chains C2 and C3 in the lower area. All these synfire chains contain excitatory and inhibitory neurons (following Hayon et al. 2005 and Abeles et al. 2004).

The basic idea behind the accompanying wave model is that excitatory activity accelerates a wave, which increases its stability (Hayon et al. 2005). Conversely, inhibitory activity decelerates a wave and decreases its stability. A schematic equation of the speed of the ith wave $\dot{w}_i^{\mu}(t)$ in the synfire chain μ can be defined as follows (compare Hayon et al. 2005):

$$\dot{w}_i^{\mu}(t) = \min\{v_{\max}, V_0 + S_i + R_i - Inh\}, \tag{9.29}$$

in which V_0 is the velocity of a single wave, S_i is the acceleration due to waves in other chains, R_i describes the effect of refractoriness due to other waves in the same chain, Inh is the term representing deceleration due to global inhibition in the network, and $v_{\max}$ describes the upper limit of the wave velocity.

Thus, the dynamic binding of elementary components is transformed into a meaningful and compositional mental representation.[465] A simple example is the so-called "Part Binding Problem", according to which activity waves are initiated at the lower level in the three synfire chains that represent three different lines (Hayon et al. 2005, Abeles et al. 2004) (see Fig. 9.6). Due to the synchronization between two of the

---

[465] See e.g. Bienenstock 1995, 1996, Abeles et al. 2004.
For an introduction, see e.g. Abeles 2003.
For the term "compositionality" used here in the LEGO metaphor, see e.g. Bienenstock 1996.

waves, an activity wave is then initiated with a certain probability in one of the synfire chains on the upper level, which represent either the symbol 'T' or the symbol 'L'.

By adding a recurrent graph structure ("reverberating-synfire dynamics"), based on the concept of the attractor, one finally obtains a classical associative memory model:

"(...) one may envisage connectivity graphs intermediate between feedforward synfire chains and random graphs with feedback. Such graphs would contain multiple, irregularly arranged, feedback loops, leading to a reverberating-synfire dynamics (...). A network including a superposition of such graphs would qualify as a classical associative-memory model, with attractors defined in terms of firing rates, and would also retain important features of the synfire model (Bienenstock 1995)."

9.6 MULTI-LAYERED FEED-FORWARD NETWORKS WITH FREQUENCY RESONANCE MECHANISM BY A. KUMAR

The Indian engineer and computational neuroscientist, Arvind Kumar studied the propagation of synchronous spiking activity across diluted feedforward networks (FFNs) with sparse and weak connections between subsequent layers.[466] Each layer consists of two recurrently connected homogeneous neuronal populations; an excitatory (E) and an inhibitory (I) neuronal population, the connectivity within each layer is sparse and random. The connections between layers, which modeled long-range projections between different cortical networks, are also sparse, strictly feedforward and excitatory. These interlayer projections were restricted to a sub-population of randomly-chosen excitatory neurons which are refered to as projecting (P) neurons. The neuron model and synapse model are described as follows (Hahn et al. 2014):

"Neurons were modeled as leaky integrate-and-fire neurons, with the following membrane potential sub-threshold dynamics:

$$C_m V_m = -G_{leak} [V_m(t) - V_{reset}] + I_{syn}(t), \qquad (9.30)$$

where V_m is the neurons membrane potential, I_{syn} is the total synaptic input current, C_m and G_{leak} are the membrane capacitance and leak conductance respectively. When the V_m reached a fixed threshold (...), a spike was emitted and the membrane potential was reset to V_{reset} (...).
(...)
Synaptic inputs consisted of transient conductance changes:

$$I_{syn}(t) = G_{syn}(t) [V_m(t) - E_{syn}], \qquad (9.31)$$

where E_{syn} is the synapse reversal potential (Hahn et al. 2014)."

---

[466]The Synfire Chain Model (chap. 9.5) postulates the existence of dense and/or strong convergent-divergent connections between subsequent layers of feedforward networks, which allow the generation and faithful transmission of synchronous spike volleys. In contrast to this, the cortical connectivity is characterized by a large number of sparsely and weakly connected (diluted) FFNs, so "they would fail to generate enough synchronization to ensure propagation of spiking activity".
See Hahn et al. 2014, 2013.

In contrast to the BBS Hypothesis and the CTC Hypothesis (chap. 4.4.3) which proposes that synchronization and communication between different brain areas is achieved by maintaining a consistent phase relationship (coherence) between population oscillations, Kumar proposed a novel mechanism by which oscillatory stimuli ("pulse packets") exploit the presence of resonance frequencies in diluted FFNs, to locally generate and amplify a weak, slowly propagating synchronous oscillation ("Communication Through Resonance (CTR) Hypothesis") (Hahn et al. 2014, 2019). These network resonance frequencies naturally occurs in oscillating networks due to the interactions between excitatory and inhibitory neurons in each FFN layer. Once the oscillations in the FFNs are strong enough, the pulse packets are transmitted:

"The role of such network resonance is to amplify weak signals that would otherwise fail to propagate. According to our model, coherent oscillations emerge in the network during slow propagation of synchrony, while at the same time, synchrony needs these oscillations to be propagated. Thus, spreading synchrony both generates oscillations and renders them coherent across different processing stages. This abolishes the requirement for separate mechanisms providing the local generation of oscillations and establishing their long-range coherence. Moreover, coherence between oscillations may be viewed as a consequence of propagation instead of being instrumental to establish communication through synchrony. Our results also suggest that the emergence of coherent oscillations is influenced by the dynamical state of the ongoing activity. We propose that changes in the ongoing activity state can have an influence on cortical processing by altering the communication between different brain areas.

(...)

Our results show that oscillations arise in the network as a consequence of the stimulus propagation, and at the same time, the stimulus exploits these oscillations to propagate. Due to this propagation, oscillations in each layer are driven by the previous layer and are hence naturally coherent with a phase that is determined by the conduction delay between the layers (...). From this perspective, coherence becomes a side effect of the propagation dynamics. Thus, a separation of distinct mechanisms that create oscillations and provide coherence is not necessary, as both arise naturally as a consequence of CTR (Hahn et al. 2014)."

10 Systematic Class of Information Based Architecture Types

The systematic class of information-based architecture types contains those connectionist models which strive for a solution to the binding problem by means of a coherent and integrated process organization of the neural information (within the framework of quantitative, information- and probability-theoretical analyses). In this context, there are three possible measures that can be defined. First (chap. 10.1), an information-theoretical measure can be defined on the basis of a reentrant process organization, i.e. the synchronization of neurophysiological activity between groups of neuronal populations. A second possible measure (chap. 10.2) is an "optimally harmonic" information structure. Thirdly (chap. 10.3), the measure of the minimization of "free energy" (on the basis of statistical methods) can be defined.

10.1 FUNCTIONAL CLUSTERING MODEL AND INFORMATION INTEGRATION THEORY BY G.M. EDELMAN, G. TONONI AND O. SPORNS

With a computer simulation model[467] of the cortical reentrant[468] integration in the visual system (by Edelman and Tononi) (see Fig. 10.1), and a much more detailed

---

[467] See Tononi et al. 1992: The model contains about 10.000 neurons in all that are connected to each other by about 1.000.000 links. The activities of the neurons, which respond to different features of the same object, e.g. movement, position, color and shape, are synchronized in the millisecond range. After training, the computer model is able to identify the red cross with 95% probability, approximately 100-250 milliseconds after an optical presentation consisting, for example, of a red cross, a red square and a green cross.
For an introduction, see Edelman and Tononi 2000.
For a brief introduction, see Maurer 2014a.

[468] On the concept of a "reentrant function" in computer science, see e.g. Jha 2005: "A *reentrant* function is one that can be used by more than one task concurrently without fear of data corruption. Conversely, a *non-reentrant* function is one that cannot be shared by more than one task unless mutual exclusion to the function is ensured, either by using a semaphore or by disabling interrupts during critical sections of code. A reentrant function can be interrupted at any time and resumed at a later time without loss of data. Reentrant functions either use local variables or protect their data when global variables are used."
See also, e.g. Edelman and Tononi 2000.
A "reentrant" process organization ("Re-entry") is a spatiotemporal synchronization and coordination of the functions of spatially separated brain maps. These synchronizations and coordinations are based on a

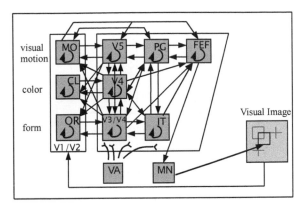

Figure 10.1: Schematic diagram of the (computer simulation) model of the cortical reentrant integration in the visual system: The functionally specialized visual areas are shown here as boxes, the pathways between them, consisting of several thousands of individual fiber connections, as arrows. The model comprises three parallel information processing paths which comprise the analysis of visual motion (upper row), color (middle row), and form (lower row). The visual image, which is scanned by a color camera, is represented by the large box at the bottom right (following Tononi et al. 1992).

computer simulation model[469] on the dynamics of reentrant interactions between cortical areas of the thalamocortical system (by Lumer, Edelman and Tononi) (Walter 2006, Walter and Müller 2012, Edelman and Tononi 2000), the American physician and neurobiologist Gerald M. Edelman and the Italian psychiatrist and neuroscientist Giulio Tononi proposed a solution to the binding problem of the neuronal activities of different and functionally separated cortical areas. The neuronal dynamics of a "reentrant"[468] process organization ("Re-entry"), i.e. the temporal synchronization of activity between groups of neuronal (sub-)populations in the same cortical area or between different cortical areas, are decisive.[470] This is mediated by the existence of interacting or reciprocal, voltage-dependent, (fiber) connections[471] as well as by the rapid change in the strength of these connections. Thus, this coherent process is to be regarded as the fundamental mechanism of neural integration, as the result

---

permanent, simultaneous and parallel selection process of information, processing between the neuronal groups in the networks of these brain maps using a variety of parallel, reciprocal and recurrent fiber connections.
See e.g. Edelman 1987, Edelman and Tononi 2000 with the "String Quartet" metaphor, Sporns 1994.

[469] See Lumer et al. 1997a, b: The model contains about 65.000 neurons in all, which are interconnected by about 5.000.000 links.
For an introduction, see Edelman and Tononi 2000.
For a brief introduction, see Maurer 2014a.

[470] See e.g. Edelman 1987, Tononi et al. 1992, 1998, Edelman and Tononi 2000, Sporns 1994.
See also, fn. 468.
See also, the remarks in chap. 5.4.

[471] See Tononi et al. 1992.
See also, Edelman and Tononi 2000: In the human brain, these connections correspond to the "NMDA(N-methyl-D-aspartate) receptors" for the neurotransmitter glutamate.

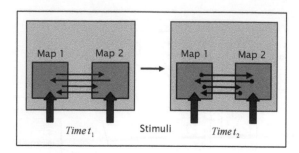

Figure 10.2: Schematic diagram of the concept of "Re-Entry" or "Reentrant Mapping": The maps coordinate themselves spatially and temporally via reciprocal fibre connections by means of a continuous flow of information, where the black dots illustrate the synapses that are thereby amplified (following Edelman and Tononi 2000).

of reentrant interactions between several neuronal (sub-)populations in different (in some cases spatially) and widely separated cortical areas (see Fig. 10.2).

10.1.1 FUNCTIONAL CLUSTERING MODEL BY G.M. EDELMAN AND G. TONONI

In order to define a quantitative criterion for the existence of this coherent, integrated neural process, Edelman and Tononi assume that a (sub-)class of system elements is to be understood as an integrated subsystem if, over a certain period of time, these elements interact very strongly with each other and weakly with the rest of the system (Tononi et al. 1998, Edelman and Tononi 2000). This means that the deviation from the (statistical) independence (in the sense of multivariate statistics [see chap. 3.2.5.1 and chap. 5]) has to be determined simultaneously and generally for all system elements. Thus, such a subpopulation of strongly interacting neurons is called a "functional cluster", i.e. the system elements that have separated themselves from the rest of the system in their function (Tononi et al. 1998). The statistical method in question is also referred to as "functional clustering" (Tononi et al. 1998a, b, Edelman and Tononi 2000) (see Fig. 10.3).

If one considers an isolated neural system X, consisting of n neural system elements $\{x_i\}$ (the neurons), and if one assumes that the activity of these elements is described by stationary, multidimensional stochastic processes, then the probability density function, which describes such a multivariate process, can be understood in terms of the information entropy H, according to C.E. Shannon and W. Weaver.[472] This probability density function is a logarithmic function which calculates the number of discrete system states possible in this system – here, the neural activity patterns – weighted according to the probability of their occurrence.

---

[472]Based on Gauss functions.
For general information, see e.g. Cover and Thomas 2006, Papoulis 1991.
See also, the remarks in chap. 3.2.4.4 and chap. 5.2.

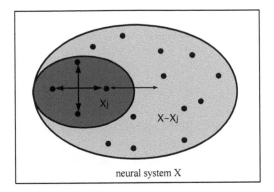

Figure 10.3: Diagram of "Functional Clustering": The small ellipse represents a functional cluster, i.e. a subset of brain regions, represented as points that interact strongly with each other, illustrated by the crossed arrows, and interact only weakly with the rest of the brain, illustrated by the weaker arrow (following Edelman and Tononi 2000).

Under the assumption that in a neural system X, consisting of n neural system elements $\{x_i\}$, whose components are independent of each other, i.e. that each statistically possible system state occurs with equal probability, the number of possible system states N which the system can assume is 2^n. This corresponds to a system entropy

$$H(X) = \operatorname{ld} N = \log_2 2^n = n \qquad (10.1)$$

bits of information, where in this case the entropy of the system $H(X)$ is the sum of the entropies of its individual components $H(x_i)$. The difference between the sum of the entropies of all single, independently considered components $\{x_i\}$ and the entropy of the system as a whole $H(X)$, results in a value for the integration $I(X)$ of the neural system X (Tononi et al. 1998a, b):

$$I(X) = \sum_{i=1}^{n} H(x_i) - H(X). \qquad (10.2)$$

An increasing integration of a partition of the neural system X by an increased interaction (in the sense of an increasing statistical correlation of the individual elements with each other) thus reduces the number of possible states that the system as a whole can take. This is because at least some of the states would thus become more or less probable than if all elements were independent of each other. This also leads to a loss of entropy of the overall system $H(X)$ in comparison to the sum of the entropies $H(x_i)$ of all individual components $\{x_i\}$ considered independently of each other, so that the value for integration $I(X)$ increases.

If one considers a bipartition of the isolated neural system X, i.e. a subsystem or any subset j of k system elements, the integration value $I(X_j^k)$ can be used to calculate the statistical dependency as a whole within the subset and the dependency between the subset X_j^k and the rest of the system, the complement $(X - X_j^k)$. This provides a measure of the mutual exchange of information ("Mutual Information (MI)")[473] between any subpopulation of elements and the rest of the system (Tononi et al. 1998a, b).

It is given by

$$MI(X_j^k; X - X_j^k) = H(X_j^k) + H(X - X_j^k) - H(X), \qquad (10.3)$$

whereby a measure is provided to the extent that the entropy of (X_j^k) is determined by the entropy of its complement $(X - X_j^k)$.

From this, a functional "Cluster Index" (CI) can be defined for any arbitrary subset j (Tononi et al. 1998a, b):

$$CI(X_j^k) = \frac{I(X_j^k)}{MI(X_j^k; X - X_j^k)}, \qquad (10.4)$$

where the two terms $I(X_j^k)$ and $MI(X_j^k; X - X_j^k)$ are to be normalized accordingly in order to take into account the effects of the different sizes of the respective subsets. Accordingly, a functional cluster is identified if its cluster index is statistically significantly above the value one would expect for a homogeneous system, since in this case there is a subpopulation of elements which interact strongly with each other and only weakly with the rest of the system, and which, in turn, contains no smaller subset with a high cluster index.

After the integration of a neural subpopulation with the cluster index can be determined, i.e. a neural process is integrated, Edelman and Tononi define the extent to which the process is integrated (Tononi et al. 1994, Edelman and Tononi 2000). It is calculated on the basis of the total measure of the degree of differentiation of a neural total system, which is calculated by averaging the mutual information $MI(X_j^k; X - X_j^k)$ for each subpopulation of the neural system and the rest of the system for all possible cases of splitting of the total system. Again, a bipartition of an isolated neural system X is considered, i.e. a subpopulation j of k elements of this system (X_j^k) and their complement $(X - X_j^k)$. The mutual information thus expresses to what extent the states of the subpopulation (X_j^k) contribute to the differentiation of the states of the rest of the system, or vice versa.

This total measure of the degree of differentiation of an overall neural system, which Edelman and Tononi refer to as "neural complexity" C_N, can be defined by (Tononi et al. 1994, Tononi et al. 1998b):

$$C_N(X) = \sum_{k=1}^{n/2} \left\langle MI(X_j^k; X - X_j^k) \right\rangle, \qquad (10.5)$$

where the average mutual information between the subpopulations X_k (consisting of k of n elements of the system) and their respective complements, is written as

---

[473] An application of the theoretical measure of mutual information with reference to the so-called "connectome" concept of the human brain according to Sporns can be found in Kolchinsky et al. 2014.

$\langle MI(X_j^k; X - X_j^k) \rangle$, and the index j indicates that the average is determined over all combinations of k elements. Accordingly, the value for the complexity of a neural system will be high if, firstly, both subpopulations, (X_j^k) and $(X - X_j^k)$, can assume as many different states as possible. This means that their entropies must be high, i.e. the subpopulations are specialized. Secondly, the states of (X_j^k) and $(X - X_j^k)$ must be statistically interdependent, i.e., the entropy of (X_j^k) must be determined to a large extent by the interactions with $(X - X_j^k)$, and vice versa, which means that the respective subpopulation is integrated. This leads to the conclusion that a high level of complexity corresponds to an optimal synthesis of functional specialization and functional integration of neuronal processes within a system. A change of the neural degree of complexity as an optimal balance between segregation and integration of functions can be achieved, not only by means of neuroanatomical connectivity, i.e. the respective connection pattern, but also solely by dynamic modulation of neurophysiological activity, i.e. the respective excitation or discharge patterns. In other words, a high level of complexity results from a high number of possible discharge patterns in a subsystem with a different interaction on the whole system:

"Thus, we reach the important conclusion that high values of complexity correspond to an optimal synthesis of functional specialization and functional integration within a system (Edelman and Tononi 2000)."

10.1.2 INFORMATION INTEGRATION THEORY BY G. TONONI AND O. SPORNS

Following up on this, the Italian psychiatrist and neuroscientist, Giulio Tononi and the German neuroscientist and cognitive scientist, Olaf Sporns have developed the "Information Integration Theory (ITT) (of Consciousness)"[474]. In this context the phenomenon "consciousness" is understood as a measurable, intrinsic capacity of a discrete, dynamical, biophysical system: the amount of "integrated information" within the framework of an information process that can be generated, starting from a repertoire of possible states $\{x_i\}$, by moving from one certain (conscious) state to the next.

If one considers a neural system X in the form of a directed graph, consisting of n abstract neural system elements with a finite repertoire of outputs, e.g. '0' and

---

[474]For fundamental information, see e.g. Tononi and Sporns 2003, Tononi 2004a.
For detailed information, see e.g. Balduzzi and Tononi 2008.
For an introduction, see e.g. Tononi 2004b.
For a brief introduction, see Maurer 2014a.
For a beginner's guide, see e.g. Massimini and Tononi 2018.
A further development of this approach to a so-called "Integrated Information Theory (IIT) of Consciousness 3.0" can be found in Oizumi et al. 2014: It is based on phenomenological axioms that are formalized into information theoretic postulates. These postulates then describe how a simple system of biophysical mechanisms, such as neuronal processes or logical gates, must be structured in order to generate (experiential) consciousness.
Albantakis and Tononi 2015 apply this to the analysis of the causal and dynamical properties of a dynamical system, such as adaptive networks consisting of logic gates, so-called "animats."

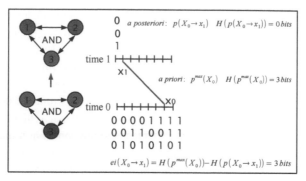

Figure 10.4: Illustration of the generation of "effective information" *ei* using a system of three connected state transitions in the form of AND gates, from state $x_0 = 110$ at time '0' to state $x_1 = 001$ at time '1'. The a priori repertoire consists of the $2^3 = 8$ possible (output) configurations of the system elements, which can occur with the same probability distribution. The system architecture with a causal mechanism (dark red) then specifies that the state '110' is the unique cause of the state x_1, so that the a posteriori repertoire assigns the state '110' the probability '1', and '0' probability to the other states. In other words, by determining one of eight possible configurations as a cause of the current state by the system mechanism and excluding the other seven configurations as a cause, (effective) information is generated by reducing the uncertainty (following Balduzzi and Tononi 2008).

'1', and if one assumes that the elements are equipped with causal mechanisms in the form of AND or XOR activation rules, then the generated information consists of the extent to which the uncertainty of the repertoire is reduced (in the sense of a probability distribution of the set of output states of the system) if the system has passed from a state x_0 to the subsequent x_1 (Balduzzi and Tononi 2008). This reduction is based on measured, causal, element interactions, and is referred to as "effective information" e_i, which is defined as "relative entropy",[475] This is the difference between the potential (a priori) repertoire $p^{max}(X_0)$ and the actual (a posteriori) repertoire $p(X_0 \to x_1)$ (see Fig. 10.4) (Balduzzi and Tononi 2008):

$$ei(X_0 \to x_1) = H\left[p(X_0 \to x_1) \,\|\, p^{max}(X_0)\right].^{476} \qquad (10.6)$$

"The a priori repertoire is the probability distribution on the set of possible outputs of the elements considered independently, with each output equally likely. (...) The a priori repertoire coincides with the maximum entropy (maxent) distribution on the states of the system (...) (Balduzzi and Tononi 2008)."

---

[475]For the definition of "relative entropy", also known as "Kullback-Leibler (KL) divergence (distance)", see e.g. Cover and Thomas 2006, Dayan and Abbott 2001.

[476]According to Balduzzi and Tononi 2008, "effective information" can also be written more simply than a difference of entropies:

$$ei(X_0 \to x_1) = H(p^{max}(X_0)) - H(p(X_0 \to x_1)).$$

"The a posteriori repertoire (...) is the repertoire of states that could have led to x_1 through causal interactions. (...) The a posteriori repertoire is formally captured by Bayes' rule (...) (Balduzzi and Tononi 2008)."

In addition to the effective information, which only indicates how much information has been generated, the extent to which this generated information has been integrated must also be determined. Hence, one has to calculate how much information the system generates as a whole, compared to the information that is generated independently of the combined, individual partitions of the system. This so-called "integrated information" ϕ is defined as the entropy of the a posteriori repertoire of the system as a whole, relative to the combined a posteriori repertoire of the partitions (Balduzzi and Tononi 2008):

$$\phi(x_1) = H \left[p(X_0 \to x_1) \,\|\, \prod_{M_k \in P^{MIP}} p(M_0^k \to \mu_1^k) \right], \tag{10.7}$$

where M and μ are arbitrary partitions and P^{MIP} is the minimum information partition.

"Integrated information (...) represents the natural decomposition of the system into parts. (...) for any system, we need to find the informational 'weakest link', i.e. the decomposition into those parts that are the most independent (least integrated). This weakest link is given by the minimum information partition P^{MIP} (...) (Balduzzi and Tononi 2008)."

Using this, one can identify those subsets S of a system X, which have the capacity to integrate information, namely the "(main) complex" (Balduzzi and Tononi 2008):

$$S \subset X \text{ is a complex iff } \left\{ \begin{array}{c} \phi(s_1) > 0 \\ \phi(t_1) \leq \phi(s_1) \text{ for all } T \supset S \end{array} \right\} \tag{10.8}$$

$$S \subset X \text{ is a main complex iff } \left\{ \begin{array}{c} S \text{ is a complex} \\ \phi(r_1) < \phi(s_1) \text{ for all } R \subset S \end{array} \right\} \tag{10.9}$$

where r_1, s_1 and t_1 denote states:

"At each instant in time, any system of elements can be decomposed into its constituent complexes, which form its fundamental units. Indeed, only a complex can be properly considered to form a single entity. For a complex, and only for a complex, it is meaningful to say that, when it enters a particular state out of its repertoire, it generates an amount of integrated information corresponding to its ϕ value (Balduzzi and Tononi 2008)."

In summary, in IIT, the quantity of consciousness results from computing the quantity of integrated information generated by a complex of elements. More recently, Tononi has described the (causal) structure or quality of the integrated information: the quality of experience and consciousness is specified by the informational relationships which are generated by a complex of informational mechanisms.[477] In other words, according to IIT, generating a large amount of integrated information entails having a highly structured set of causal mechanisms. These mechanisms together generate integrated information by specifying a set of informational relationships that completely and univocally determine the quality of experience. The notion of a quale is introduced "as a shape that embodies the entire set of informational relationships generated by interactions in the system (Balduzzi and Tononi 2009)". Then the mathematical concept of a Qualia Space (Q) is defined as a space with an axis for each possible state of the complex "where each point is a probability distribution on the possible states of the system. The informational relationships can then be thought of as arrows between points in Q generated by causal mechanisms". It is then argued that "each experience or quale corresponds to a particular set of arrows linking points in Q, that is, an experience is a shape in Q-space (Balduzzi and Tononi 2009)".

10.1.3   DYNAMIC CORE HYPOTHESIS BY G.M. EDELMAN AND G. TONONI

The "Dynamic Core Hyphotesis (DCH)", according to Edelman and Tononi, states that the neuronal dynamics of a "reentrant"[468] process organization ("Reentry") of the thalamocortical system (i.e. the synchronization of neurophysiological activity between groups of neuronal (sub-)populations in different (sub-)cortical areas) should be regarded as the fundamental mechanism of neural integration and differentiation (or segregation).[478] This synchronous activity of (only) one of the neuronal groups involved can then contribute directly to the emergence and preservation of conscious experience if it is part of a widely organized "functional cluster", and is in exchange over a period of several hundred milliseconds with a number of other neuronal groups via strong mutual interactions. This presupposes that such a functional cluster (conceived as a neural process, described by Edelman and Tononi as a "dynamic core"), is both highly differentiated (which is expressed in its high level of complexity), and – in spite of its constantly changing composition – highly integrated, and for the most part generated in the thalamocortical system.[479]

---

[477]For detailed information, see Balduzzi and Tononi 2009, Tononi 2010, 2012, Tononi et al. 2016. See also, Tononi 2009.

For PyPhi, a Python software package that implements the framework of ITT, see Mayner et al. 2018.

[478]For detailed information, see e.g. Tononi and Edelman 1998a.

For an introduction, see e.g. Edelman and Tononi 2000.

See e.g. Tononi and Edelman 1998b. See the remarks in chap. 10.1.1.

[479]For detailed information, see e.g. Tononi and Edelman 1998b.

For an introduction, see e.g. Edelman and Tononi 2000.

For an overview of the most recent empirical evidence on the interaction between integration and segregation of neural information against the background of his so-called "Connectome" concept of the human brain, see Sporns 2013. See also, Deco et al. 2015.

10.2   HARMONY THEORY BY P. SMOLENSKY[480]

In his paper "Information Processing in Dynamical Systems: Foundations of Harmony Theory" (1986a) and in various other publications, the American cognitive scientist, Paul Smolensky introduces his "Harmony Theory".[481] It is based on the Theory of Dynamical Systems, Information Theory and Probability Theory. It is a mathematical theory which is able to express various cognitive phenomena in Smolensky's "Subsymbolic Paradigm" and contains the fundamental principles of this paradigm (see chap. 6.1.1).

The mathematical structure of harmony theory is based on the "schema theory" or "script theory" in cognitive psychology and cognitive science[482], whereby a categorial or conceptual knowledge structure can be mapped onto a class of objects, facts or events. This grants a cognitive system a certain degree of flexibility; Smolensky (1986a) assumes that the knowledge base of the system (in the sense of the idea of "memory traces"), at the micro level, consists of a set of so-called "knowledge atoms"[483], or better, of a set of "vectorial information atoms". At the macro level, within the framework of a dynamic construction of scripts (in the sense of R.C. Schank and R.P. Abelson[484]), these cognitive atoms actively and dynamically configure themselves into scripts tailored to the context in question. In other words, by activating stored elementary (schema) constituents in the form of vectorial information atoms, microinference processes are carried out within the framework of perceptual processes. This leads to these cognitive atoms actively and dynamically combining to form coherent and context-sensitive schemata in the sense of J.A. Feldman (1989), M. Minsky (1975) and D.E. Rumelhart (1980).[485] According to Smolensky (1986a), this results in the "Harmony Principle": "The cognitive system is an engine for activating coherent assemblies (see chap. 4.2.4, 4.4.3) of atoms and drawing inferences." The "subassemblies of activated atoms that tend to recur exactly or approximately are the schemata" (Smolensky 1986a) that encode the statistical structure relations of

---

[480]This chapter is a largely adapted and partly revised version of the chapter in Maurer 2006/2009.

[481]See Smolensky 1986a.
See also, e.g. Smolensky 1984a, b, 1995, Prince and Smolensky 1991, Smolensky and Legendre 2006a. The harmony theory is closely related to Smolensky's ICS Cognitive Architecture.
See also, the explanations in chap. 6.1.
For an introduction, see e.g. Bechtel and Abrahamsen 2002.

[482]See e.g. Smolensky 1986a.
For an introduction to the term "schema" or "script" in cognitive and developmental psychology as well as cognitive science, e.g. by Bartlett, Anderson, Piaget, Brewer, Rosch, Bower or Abelson, see e.g. Anderson 2015, Trautner 1991, Miller 2016.

[483]In my opinion, the term "vectorial information atoms" is preferable to the term "knowledge atoms" used by Smolensky 1986a, since the term "knowledge" sounds too anthropomorphic in connection with the theory of artificial neural networks.

[484]According to Schank and Abelson (1977), "scripts" are a conceptual scheme with which prototypical events can be represented, e.g. a visit to a restaurant or cinema

[485]According to Feldman (1989), a "schema" is a form of representation originating from computer science which represents categorial or conceptual knowledge in the form of a structure of slots by assigning attribute values to attributes of the term. For example, the following schema representation results from the term "house": generic term: building/parts: rooms/material: wood, stone, etc.

sensory information. According to Smolensky, this principle thus directs attention to the concept of "coherence" or "consistency".[486] In other words, preference is given to the information structure which is "optimally harmonic", i.e. which violates the fewest constraints, and which is based on the already-generated "knowledge" of the network. An informational atom, e.g. a so-called "digraph"[487], is represented by the vector of a neuron that encodes a "(micro-)feature" which constitutes a very small fragment of the perceptual or task area that the cognitive system deals with.

From the abstraction of typical features of a category, i.e. either an object representation or an episode representation (in the sense of a schema or a script by means of the assignment of attributes to their attribute values), Smolensky (1986a) proposes the probabilistic formulation of schema theory:

"Each schema encodes the statistical relations among a few representational features. During inference, the probabilistic information in many active schemata are dynamically folded together to find the most probable state of the environment (Smolensky 1986a)."

In order to approach the degree of cognitive flexibility present in human action and behavior, it is therefore necessary to return to the description of those knowledge atoms at the micro level, that represent the elements of cognitive computation, and not the schemata and scripts. Thus, the problem of modeling schemata and scripts is subsumed under the problem of modeling vectorial information atoms, whereby this is solved by developing the harmony function as the measure of self-consistency of an (artificial) neural network. According to Smolensky (1986a), a central cognitive process consists of establishing a cognitive state which is "maximally self-consistent", whereby "the self-consistency of a possible state of a cognitive system can be assigned the value of a 'harmony function' H". A state of the system is defined by two layers of neurons (see Fig. 10.5). The second layer consists of a set of knowledge atoms that the system uses to interpret its environment, and a corresponding "activation vector" that indicates whether the information atom is activated or deactivated. The harmony of such a state is the sum of the active knowledge atoms, weighted by the "strength" of the connection of the respective knowledge atom to the input nodes in the first layer, which encode the features to be represented. Each weight multiplies the self-consistency between the respective vector

---

[486]For the term "coherence" in connectionism in general and in Smolensky in particular, see also, box 3.2.5.4 and the explanations in chap. 3.2.3, 3.2.5.2, 3.2.5.4, 6.1.3.

In mathematics and (mathematical) logic, the term "consistency" refers to the provable absence of contradictions in an axiom system, e.g. a logical calculus. Smolensky (1986a), however, uses the term "consistency" in the context of the theory of artificial neural networks. In my opinion, this theory knows no "hard" contradictions, but instead knows only "soft" constraint satisfaction, for example, when a value assignment to the variables which corresponds to the neuron vectors has a solution to the "Constraint Satisfaction Problem (CSP)" for a constraint net.
See also, box 3.2.5.4 and the comments in chap. 3.2.3, 3.2.5.2, 3.2.5.4, 6.1.3.

[487]In Smolensky (1986a), a "digraph" means a combination of two letters to form a single sound or phoneme, e.g. 'WA', which is represented by a neuron vector encoding the syllable 'WA', by activating the vector components of the vector representing the respective individual letters, e.g. 'W' and 'A'. The other vector components that would represent the other letters are deactivated.
See also Fig. 10.5.

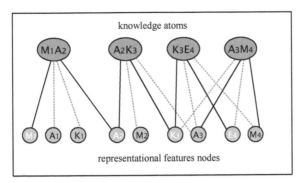

Figure 10.5: Schematic representation of the (perceptual) completion task: The task consists of correctly reproducing the partially hidden word 'MAKE', whereby the first node layer contains a sequence of the letters to be recognized. The second node layer contains the "knowledge atoms," which can represent in each case a sequence of two letters, e.g. the digraphs 'M1A2', 'A2K3', 'K3E4' and 'A3M4'. The indices specify the position of a letter in the word to be recognized. For example, if the first letter in the word is an 'M' and the second is an 'A', then there will be a maximum of correspondence with the knowledge atom, whose sequence of letters 'M1A2' corresponds best to that sequence. The atom will therefore have positive connection weights to the representational feature nodes of the first layer, which code this sequence of letters (solid lines). A certain knowledge vector, which shall encode the word 'MAKE', is generated by the network receiving a part of this vector as input, e.g. the feature vector, which encodes the sequence of letters 'M1' and 'A2', and the network then completes this vector to the searched knowledge vector, by interacting with all connection weights simultaneously. This is done in such a way that the state of the network that best matches the given input is found. This means, in this case, the knowledge atoms 'A2K3' and 'K3E4' will be activated most of all, because their letter sequence produces the highest degree of consistency with the partly hidden input and the already generated knowledge vector 'M1A2', in contrast to the knowledge atom 'A3M4' for example. In other words, the respective knowledge and feature vectors will generate the highest degree of consistency (following Smolensky 1986a).

of the knowledge atom and the vector consisting of the input features to be represented. The self-consistency is the similarity between the vector of the knowledge atom (the "knowledge vector", i.e. the vector, consisting of the connections to the input nodes of the first layer) and the "representational feature vector", which encodes the features of the system environment (i.e. the input patterns, also called the "representation vector") (see Fig. 10.5).

The theory of harmony in its mathematical form is presented by Smolensky as follows (Smolensky 1986a, Petitot 1994, Grauel 1992).
First, the representation vector is defined:

"At the center of any harmony theoretic model of a particular cognitive process is a set of *representational features* $r_1, r_2, \ldots$ These features constitute the cognitive system's representation of possible states of the environment with which it deals. (...)
A *representational state* of the cognitive system is determined by a collection of values for all the representational variables $\{r_i\}$. This collection can be designated by a list or vector of +'s and -'s: the representation vector r (Smolensky 1986a)."

Then the knowledge or information vector and the activation vector are defined:

"The representational features serve as a blackboard on which the cognitive system carries out its computations. The *knowledge* that guides those computations is associated with the second set of entities, the knowledge atoms. Each such atom α is characterized by a knowledge vector k_α, which is a list of +1, -1 and 0 values, one for each representation variable r_i. This list encodes a piece of knowledge that specifies what value each r_i should have: +1, -1, or unspecified (0).

Associated with knowledge atom α is its *activation variable, a_α.* This variable will also be taken to be binary: 1 will denote active; 0, inactive. (...) The list of $\{0,1\}$ values for the activations $\{a_\alpha\}$ comprises the *activation vector a_α.*
Knowledge atoms encode subpatterns of feature values which occur in the environment. The different frequencies with which various such patterns occur is encoded in the set of strengths, $\{\sigma_\alpha\}$, of the atoms (Smolensky 1986a)."

Finally, the harmony function is defined and its relation to probability theory established:

"A state of the cognitive system is determined by the values of the lower and upper level nodes. Such a state is determined by a pair (r,a) consisting of a representation vector r and an activation vector a. A harmony function assigns a real number $H_K(r,a)$ to each such state. The harmony function has as parameters, the set of knowledge vectors and their strengths: $\{(k_\alpha, \sigma_\alpha)\}$; I will call this the *knowledge base* K.
(...)
The harmony function[488] (...) is

$$H_K(r,a) = \sum_\alpha \sigma_\alpha a_\alpha h_K(r,k_\alpha). \tag{10.10}$$

Here, $h_K(r,k_\alpha)$ is the harmony contributed by activating atom α, given the current representation r. I have taken this to be

$$h_K(r,k_\alpha) = \frac{r \cdot k_\alpha}{|k_\alpha|} - \kappa. \tag{10.11}$$

---

[488] A simple case study of the harmony function is explained in Smolensky 1995. See also, the explanations in chap. 6.1.3.

The vector inner product[489] (...) is defined by

$$r \cdot k_\alpha = \sum_i r_i (k_\alpha)_i$$

(10.13)

and the norm (...) is defined by

$$|k_\alpha| = \sum_i |(k_\alpha)_i|$$

(10.14)

(Smolensky 1986a)."

According to Smolensky (1986a), the relationship between the harmony function and probability theory is as follows:

"(...) schemata are collections of knowledge atoms that become active in order to maximize harmony; inferences are also drawn to maximize harmony. This suggests that the probability of a possible state of the environment is estimated by computing its harmony: the higher the harmony, the greater the probability.
(...)
The relationship between the harmony function H and estimated probabilities is of the form

$$\text{probability} \propto e^{H/T}$$

(10.15)

where T is some constant that cannot be determined a priori.
This relationship between probability and harmony is mathematically identical to the relationship between probability and (minus) energy in statistical physics: the Gibbs[223] or Boltzmann[208] law. This is the basis of the isomorphism between cognition and physics, exploited by harmony theory. In statistical physics, H is called the *Hamiltonian function*; it measures the energy of a state of a physical system. In physics, T is the *temperature* of the system. In harmony theory, T is called the computational temperature (Smolensky 1983) of the cognitive system. When the temperature is very high, completions with high harmony are assigned estimated probabilities that are only slightly higher than those assigned to low harmony completions; the environment is treated as more random in the sense that all completions are estimated to have roughly equal probability. When the temperature is very low, only the completions with highest harmony are given non negligible estimated probabilities (Smolensky 1986a)."

---

[489] For the "inner product" ("scalar product") see e.g. Kallenrode 2005.
In Cartesian coordinates, the inner product of two vectors a and b can be computed as follows:

$$c = a \cdot b = \begin{pmatrix} a_x \\ a_y \\ a_z \end{pmatrix} \cdot \begin{pmatrix} b_x \\ b_y \\ b_z \end{pmatrix} = a_x b_x + a_y b_y + a_z b_z,$$

(10.12)

which means that the vector components of the vector a are multiplied by the corresponding vector components of the vector b, where c is a number (scalar).

In the context of a "(perceptual) completion task" (according to P.H. Lindsay and D.A. Norman [1972/1977]), the harmony theory, according to Smolensky, consists of the fact that the activation of the information atoms and their inference processes are mutually constrained.[490] This happens in such a way that the subassemblies of schemata (which are constituted by the activation of knowledge atoms), and the inference processes (which supplement the missing parts of the schema presentation as part of a probability estimation) are generated by finding the maximum self-consistent states of the system, which in turn are consistent with the sensory information (see Fig. 10.5).

10.3   FREE-ENERGY PRINCIPLE BY K. FRISTON

The so-called "Free-Energy Principle (FEP)"[491] of the British physicist, physician and neuroscientist, Karl John Friston is an information-theoretical measure which states that every adaptive change in a self-organized system leads to a minimization of "free energy"[492]. In a self-organized system, the entropy (Friston 2010a; see chap. 5) of its states of sensory information is minimized, so that the system can adopt a smaller number of neuronal states. This leads to a lower degree of probability for the occurrence of unexpected sensory data:

"Entropy is also the average self information or 'surprise'.
(...)
Entropy
The average surprise of outcomes sampled from a probability distribution or density. A density with low entropy means that, on average, the outcome is relatively predictable. Entropy is therefore a measure of uncertainty (Friston 2010a)."

---

[490] A case study of a completion task is presented in Smolensky 1986a, b.
A different application example of Ohm's law can be found e.g. in Riley and Smolensky 1984.
See the explanations in chap. 3.2.5.2.

[491] For basic information, see e.g. Friston and Stephan 2007, Friston 2009, 2010a, Friston et al. 2006.
For detailed information, see e.g. Friston et al. 2008, 2009, Friston 2010b, 2012, Friston and Ao 2012, Parr and Friston 2019.
For a brief introduction, see Maurer 2014a.
On the relationship of the Free Energy Principle to the "Lyapunov function" and to the "Harmony Theory" in the sense of Smolensky, see e.g. Friston et al. 2006, Friston and Stephan 2007.
With reference to the "Correlation Theory of Brain Function" according to von der Malsburg and the "Binding-By-Synchrony (BBS) Hypothesis" according to Singer et al., see e.g. Friston 2010a, 1997.
An information-theoretical analysis of the Free-Energy Principle can be found, for example, in Sengupta et al. 2013.

[492] The "free energy" F, also called the "Helmholtz free energy", is defined as:

$$F = E - TS, \tag{10.16}$$

where E denotes the internal, total energy of the system, T the absolute temperature and S the statistical entropy.
For an introduction to the term "free energy" in statistical mechanics, see e.g. Reichl 2009, Schwabl 2006, Gerthsen 1999, Moore 1998.
See also, Amit 1989, Müller et al. 1995.
See also, the explanations in chap. 5., Box 5.1.

Under the assumption that the neuronal-sensory information processes can be described with statistical models (in the sense of T. Bayes') on the basis of probability estimations ("Bayesian Brain Hypothesis")[493], so that the human brain can be interpreted as a statistical inference or Helmholtz machine,[494] Friston proposes that the quantitative concept of free energy derived from statistical physics provides a convincing theoretical information measure (Friston 2009, Friston and Stephan 2007). In mathematical notation according to Friston (2010a):

"The Bayesian brain hypothesis

$$\mu = \arg\min D_{KL}(q(\psi) \,\|\, p(\psi|\tilde{s})) \tag{10.17}$$

minimizing the difference between a recognition density and the conditional density on sensory causes."

Thus, in cognitive neuroscience, a self-organized biological agent can be described as an open non-equilibrium system relative to its system environment, based on Friston's generalized principle of minimization or optimization of free energy.[495] As part of its adaptation to specific, constantly changing environmental conditions, a (neuro-)biological agent attempts to adopt appropriate and meaningful states of order by reducing or suppressing free energy (in the form of prediction errors) in relation to action and perception. Based on neuronal probability distribution functions (in the sense of C.F. Gauss[496]) and stochastic gradient descent methods, this concept of free energy can be understood as a measure that describes how (neuro-)biological agents perform implicit statistical inferences in order to reduce the probability that they will face unexpected environmental facts (Friston et al. 2006, Friston and Stephan 2007, Friston 2009) (see chap. 3.2.5.3). Alternatively, this concept of free energy can be understood as a measure that describes how neurobiological agents accurately predict future environmental events with an increased degree of probability:

"We are open systems in exchange with the environment; the environment acts on us to produce sensory impressions and we act on the environment to change its states. This exchange rests upon sensory and effector organs (like photoreceptors and oculomotor muscles). If we change the environment or our relationship to it, sensory input

---

[493] See e.g. Friston 2010a, 2009, Kanai et al. 2014, Friston et al. 2009, Knill and Pouget 2004.

[494] See e.g. Dayan et al. 1995, Dayan and Hinton 1996.
On the relationship between the epistemic position H. von Helmholtz', in particular the concept of "unconscious inference," and the Bayes theorem, see e.g. Westheimer 2008.
For the term "Bayesian inference" see e.g. Pearl 1988, pp. 29-75.
See also, Stegmüller 1973.

[495] See e.g. Friston 2010a, Friston and Stephan 2007 with reference to Friston 2003, Friston et al. 2006.
For the term "non-equilibrium system", see e.g. Friston et al. 2006, Friston and Stephan 2007.
For more detailed information, see Maurer 2014a.

[496] Named after the German mathematician, astronomer, geodesist and physicist, Carl Friedrich Gauss.
For general information on the "Gaussian distribution," see e.g. Jaynes 2010.
See also, Applebaum 1996.

changes. Therefore, action can reduce free-energy (i.e. prediction errors) by chang-ing sensory input, whereas perception reduces free-energy by changing predictions. (...)

In summary, (i) agents resist a natural tendency to disorder by minimising a free-energy bound on surprise; (ii) this entails acting on the environment to avoid sur-prises, which (iii) rests on making Bayesian inferences about the world. In this view, the Bayesian brain ceases to be a hypothesis, it is mandated by the free-energy prin-ciple; free-energy is not used to finesse perception, perceptual inference is necessary to minimise free-energy (...). This provides a principled explanation for action and perception that jointly serve to suppress surprise or prediction error; (...) (Friston 2009)."

According to Friston, the mathematical definition of the free energy F of a system consisting of two terms, namely the "generative density" $p(\tilde{s}, \tilde{\psi} | m)$ and the "condi-tional density" (or "ensemble density") $q(\tilde{\psi} | \tilde{\mu})$ is[497]:

$$F = \text{energy} - \text{entropy} = - \langle \ln p(\tilde{s}, \tilde{\psi} | m) \rangle_q + \langle \ln q(\tilde{\psi} | \tilde{\mu}) \rangle_q, \qquad (10.18)$$

where m denotes the so-called "generative model" of the agent (Friston et al. 2012). This model includes the agent's active, adaptive actions a, which are, among other things, aimed at positively changing the sensory information in the environment. The variable $\tilde{\psi}$ stands for the external states, the hidden states and the environmental causes. The variable s stands for the externally conditioned states of the sensory re-ceptors, which are encoded using the internal system parameters $\tilde{\mu}$, such as neuronal activity, neuromodulation and neuronal connections, so that free energy is minimized or optimized (see Fig. 10.6):

"We will use $X : \Omega \rightarrow \mathbb{R}$ for real valued random variables and $x \in X$ for particular values. A probability density will be denoted by $p(x) = Pr\{x = X\}$ using the usual conventions and its entropy $H[p(x)]$ by $H(X)$. The tilde notation $\tilde{x} = (x, x', x'', ...)$ denotes variables in generalized coordinates of motion (...). Finally, $E[\cdot]$ denotes an expectation or average. For simplicity, constant terms will be omitted from equali-ties. In what follows, we would consider free energy minimization in terms of active inference: Active inference rests on the tuple $(\Omega, \Psi, S, A, R, q, p)$ that comprises the following:

– A *sample space* Ω or non-empty set from which random fluctuations or outcomes $\omega \in \Omega$ are drawn.

– *Hidden states* $\Psi : \Psi \times A \times \Omega \rightarrow \mathbb{R}$ that constitute the dynamics of states of the world that cause sensory states and depend on action.

– *Sensory states* $S : \Psi \times A \times \Omega \rightarrow \mathbb{R}$ that correspond to the agent's sensations and constitute a probabilistic mapping from action and hidden states.

---

[497]For detailed information, see e.g. Friston et al. 2012.
See also, Friston et al. 2006, Friston and Stephan 2007, Friston 2009, 2010a.
For the notation of the "Free Energy Principle" see e.g. Friston et al. 2012. See also, Friston and Stephan 2007.
The notation is supplemented by the introduction of the so-called "Markov Blanket" in Friston et al. 2014.

– *Action $A : S \times R \to \mathbb{R}$* that corresponds to action emitted by an agent and depends on its sensory and internal states.

– *Internal states $R : R \times S \times \Omega \to \mathbb{R}$* that constitute the dynamics of states of the agent that cause action and depend on sensory states.

– *Conditional density $q(\widetilde{\psi}) := q(\widetilde{\psi} | \widetilde{\mu})$* – an arbitrary probability density function over hidden states $\widetilde{\psi} \in \Psi$ that is parameterized by internal states $\widetilde{\mu} \in R$.

– *Generative density $p(\widetilde{s}, \widetilde{\psi} | m)$* – a probability density function over external (sensory and hidden) states under a generative model denoted by m. This model specifies the Gibbs[223] energy of any external states: $G(\widetilde{s}, \widetilde{\psi}) = -\ln p(\widetilde{s}, \widetilde{\psi} | m)$.

(...)

$\langle \cdot \rangle$ means the expectation under the density q."[497]

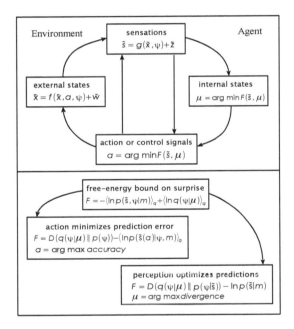

Figure 10.6: The schematic diagram shows the functional relationships between the various variables and parameters that define the "Free Energy Principle" and that model the exchange of a self-organized system, such as the human brain, with its environment. This includes the internal states of the brain $\mu(t)$ and the system variables describing the exchange with the environment (in the upper graphic segment): the sensory signals $\widetilde{s} = [s, s', s'', ...]^T$ and the actions $a(t)$. The internal brain states and actions minimize the free energy $F(\widetilde{s}, \mu)$. Free energy depends on two probability density terms: the term of ensemble probability density $q(\psi | \mu)$ and the term of generative probability density $p(\widetilde{s}, \psi | m)$, which describes the sensory patterns and their causes. An alternative expression to describe free energy is provided by the lower graphic segment: the actions of an agent reduce free energy by achieving increased accuracy in selecting those information patterns that were already expected. Conversely, optimally adapted brain states produce those representations that are the condition for the agent to avoid being confronted with unexpected, surprising sensory information (following Friston 2010a).

The necessary condition for an adaptive (neuro-)biological system is therefore the minimization of the uncertainty or "dispersion" of the information of the sensory receptors $\tilde{s}$, especially by means of appropriate action patterns a, affecting the environment and called the generative effector model m of the agent. The aim is to ensure a sustainable, homeostatic flow of equilibrium exchange with the environment so that surprising deviations from the system's predictions of environmental conditions can be minimized.[498] Mathematically noted, this dispersion of Shannon entropy corresponds to the probability density over the sensory states (see chap. 5.2). Under ergodic assumptions,[499] this entropy corresponds to the mean uncertainty or indefiniteness of the prediction of sensory information (so-called "self information") (Friston et al. 2012, Friston 2010a):

$$H(S) = E_t\left[L(\tilde{s}(t))\right] \tag{10.19}$$

$$L = -\ln p(\tilde{s}(t)\,|\,m). \tag{10.20}$$

This self-information $L(\tilde{s})$ is defined by the model of generative probability density, which means that the entropy of sensory states, i.e. the occurrence of prediction errors, can be minimized by the actions a of the (neuro-)biological system (Friston et al. 2012, Friston 2010a):

$$a(t) = \arg\min_{a\in A}\left\{L(\tilde{s}(t))\right\}.^{500} \tag{10.21}$$

This of course requires that the system's internal neuronal information states $\tilde{\mu}$ are optimally adapted to the environmental conditions via active Bayesian inference strategies (Friston et al. 2014, 2012).

This information-theoretical model has been further developed using the statistical concept of the "Markov Blanket."[501] According to Friston, it is to be assumed that any ergodic[499] dynamic system possessing such a Markov blanket separates or patitions the internal system states from external ones (Friston 2013, Friston et al. 2014). This separation minimizes the free energy of the system, such as to: (1) preserve its functional and structural integrity, (2) maintain a dynamic flux equilibrium,

---

[498] See Friston et al. 2014, Friston 2010a, Friston and Stephan 2007 with reference to Ashby 1947, Nicolis and Prigogine 1977, Haken 2004, Kauffman 1993, Evans and Searles 2002 and Evans 2003.

[499] See Friston 2013.
For the mathematical definition of the so-called "ergodicity," see e.g. Einsiedler and Ward 2011, Walters 1982.

[500] See Friston et al. 2012: "When Equation (10.21) is satisfied, the variation of entropy in Equation (10.19, 10.20) with respect to action is zero, which means sensory entropy has been minimized (at least locally). From a statistical perspective, surprise is called negative log evidence, which means that minimizing surprise is the same as maximizing the Bayesian model evidence for the agents generative model."

[501] For fundamental information on the concept of the so-called "Markov Blanket," see Pearl 1988.
For detailed information on the so-called "Markov Blanket," see e.g. Friston 2013, Kirchhoff et al. 2018.
For detailed description on the concept of the so-called "Markov Chains," see e.g. Maass 2015, Büsing et al. 2011, Reichl 2009. Named after the Russian mathematician Andrei A. Markov.
For an introduction, see e.g. Norris 1997, Griffiths et al. 2008.

and (3) constitute a simple form of autopoiesis which exhibits the general principle of biological self-organization, in other words *life*, as a necessary and emergent basic characteristic (Friston 2013, Friston et al. 2014, Maurer 2014a) (see chap. 2.3.1 (4)). Furthermore, this separation or partitioning of the internal system states leads to the situation in which these states represent the external information states according to probability theoretical criteria via a circular causality mechanism (Friston et al. 2014):

"(...) biological self-organization is not as remarkable as one might think – and is (almost) inevitable, given local interactions between the states of coupled dynamical systems. In brief, the events that 'take place within the spatial boundary of a living organism' (...) may arise from the very existence of a boundary or blanket, which itself is inevitable in a physically lawful world.

(...)

Under ergodic assumptions, the long-term average of surprise is entropy. This means that minimizing free energy – through selectively sampling sensory input – places an upper bound on the entropy or dispersion of sensory states. This enables biological systems to resist the second law of thermodynamics – or more exactly, the fluctuation theorem that applies to open systems far from equilibrium (...). However, because negative surprise is also evidence of the Bayesian model, systems that minimize free energy also maximize a lower bound on the evidence for an implicit model of how their sensory samples were generated. In statistics and machine learning, this is known as approximate Bayesian inference and provides a normative theory for the Bayesian brain hypothesis (...). In short, biological systems act on the world to place an upper bound on the dispersion of their sensed states while using those sensations to infer external states of the world. This inference makes the free energy bound a better approximation to the surprise that action is trying to minimize (...).

(...)

The ensuing (variational) free energy principle has been applied widely in neurobiology and has been generalized to other biological systems at a more theoretical level (...). The motivation for minimizing free energy has hitherto used the following sort of argument: systems that do not minimize free energy cannot exist, because the entropy of their sensory states would not be bounded and would increase indefinitely – by the fluctuation theorem (...). Therefore, biological systems must minimize free energy (Friston 2013)."

"In summary, for any ergodic random dynamical system, we have the following.

– The existence of a Markov blanket necessarily implies a partition of states into internal states, their Markov blanket (sensory and active states) and external or hidden states.

– This partition endows internal states with the apparent capacity to represent hidden states probabilistically, so that they appear to infer the hidden causes of sensory states (by minimizing a free-energy bound on log Bayesian evidence). By the circular causality induced by the Markov blanket, sensory states depend on active states, rendering inference active or embodied.

– Because active states change, but are not changed by, hidden states (...), they will appear to place an upper (free-energy) bound on the dispersion (entropy) of internal states and their Markov blanket. This means active states will appear to maintain the structural and functional integrity of the Markov blanket (Friston et al. 2014)."

In newer works (Bruineberg et al. 2018, Tani 2017, 2014, Tani et al. 2014), the FEP (the information-theoretic quantity of (variational) free-energy) can be regarded as a systematic analysis which describes the mutual and synchronized adaptation between embodied agents and their environments, "and to explain how agents perceive, act, learn, develop and structure their environment in order to optimize their fitness, or minimize their free-energy (Bruineberg et al. 2018)". In doing so, the FEP is applied to an agent's active construction of a niche over the time-scales of action, perception, learning and development in the context of active inference ("developmental niche construction"):

"The 'fit' between the agent and its environment can be improved, both by the agent coming to learn the structure of the environment and by the environment changing its structure in a way that better fits the agent. This gives rise to a continuous feedback loop, in which what the agent does changes the environment, which changes what the agent perceives, which changes the expectations of the agent, which in turn changes what the agent does (to change the environment). The interesting point here is that the minimum of free-energy is not (necessarily) at a point where the agent is maximally adapted to the statistics of a given environment, (...) but can better be conceptualized [as (author's note)] an attracting manifold within the joint agent environment state-space as a whole, which the system tends toward through mutual interaction." [The agent (author's note)] "can better be conceptualized as an attracting set of the *joint agent-environment system* (Bruineberg et al. 2018)."

Within this approach, the FEP attempts to resolve the tension between internalist and externalist positions in cognitive theory, e.g. the approach of "(radical) predictive processing" (A. Clark [2013, 2015], J. Hohwy [2013, 2016]) or "enactive views" of embodied cognition (A. Chemero [2011], S. Gallagher [2000], F. Varela et al. [1993]) in philosophy. "An ergodic dynamical interchange between 'internal' and 'external', rather than a cognitivist redominance of internal [or external; author's note] processing (Allen and Friston 2018) is decisive." The body-brain system, with its deep reciprocity, is embedded in the pattern of neural patterns which preconfigure the entity to best survive within its living world, and it specifies the types of behaviours and environments with which the system is likely to engage:

"Another way to say this is: the causal machinery of the brain and its representations are enslaved within the brain-body-environment loop of autopoiesis, which is reminiscent of the circular causality that underwrites the slaving principle in synergetics (Allen and Friston 2018)."

11 Epilogue: Discussion, Evaluation and Future Research

This concluding chapter offers a summary and an outlook on future research in the subject area of this book. First, fundamental considerations about the understanding of a new and fluent neurocognition are presented (chap. 11.1). Next, three promising architecture types are presented, which could, in the near future, further develop the solution of the binding problem by means of a phase synchronization mechanism (chap. 11.2.1-11.2.3). Furthermore, the state of the contemporary discussion is summarized and the main approaches to solving the binding problem of the most interesting neuroarchitectures are evaluated (chap. 11.3). This is followed by an outlook on future research in this field (chap. 11.4). Finally, some problems from the viewpoint of the philosophy of science and the philosophy of cognitive science are addressed and discussed (chap. 11.5).

11.1 BASIC CONSIDERATIONS ABOUT A FLUENT NEUROCOGNITION[502]

Based on the mathematics of nonlinear Dynamical System Theory (DST), including the Paradigm of Self-Organization (chap. 2), the above-discussed computational cognitive neuroarchitectures in modern connectionism, which are characterized by a high degree of neurobiological plausibilty, describe neurocognition as an inherently dynamical process (van Gelder and Port 1995). Thus, at its heart, cognition can be analyzed by convergent "fluent" and "transient" neurodynamics in abstract n-dimensional system state spaces in the form of nonlinear vector fields, vector streams or vector flows. "Fluent" means that the vectorial transformation processes have a highly flowing character with ongoing, continuous, and gradual transitions. "Transient" means that extremely fast, temporary and highly volatile vectorial information processing takes place in the cognitive neuroarchitectures described here: "In nonlinear dynamics the term 'transient' usually refers to the initial, self-limiting behavior of nonlinear systems that is observed before the system settles down into its attractor. (...) In other words, neuronal dynamics are not thought of as chaotic dynamics, played out on an invariant attractor, but as the succession of organized and struc

---

[502]This chapter is a largely adopted and partly revised version of the considerations in Maurer 2014a, 2016, 2017, 2018, 2019.

tured transients that ensue as the attractor itself changes (due to activity-dependent changes and modulation of synaptic connections) (Friston 1997)."

The models presented here, based on the integrative mechanism of temporal synchrony, contribute new insights in the service of constructing an integrated theory of cognition, and point toward modern neurophilosophy and cognitive science as a "Unified Science of the Mind/Brain" (Churchland 2007, Smith Churchland 2002): The Mind/Brain may be considered as one and the same nonlinear, complex dynamical system, in which information processing can be described with vector and tensor transformations and with attractors in multidimensional state spaces. This processual or dynamical perspective on cognition, including the dynamical binding mechanisms described above, has the advantage of more accurately modelling the fluent cognitive processes and the plasticity of the neural architecture (Smolensky 1988). As a result, neurocognition can be considered an organization of integrative system mechanisms which best explain the flow of neurocognitive information orchestrated in a recurrent network of positive and/or negative feedback loops in the subcortical and cortical areas, based on the so called "vectorial form" (Maurer 2014a, 2016, 2018, 2019). "Vectorial form" means that the computational transformation processes in the cognitive neuroarchitectures consist of (1) vectorial structures, e.g. semantic, syntactic or sensory concepts in the form of vectors or tensors, and (2) functions like vector additions, vector multiplications or tensor products.

The nature of this liquid or fluent vectorial form can be illustrated by means of a metaphor, referred to as the "Mountain Lake and Mountain Creek Metaphor" (Maurer 2014a, 2017, 2019), whereupon the nature of this neurocognitive information in the human brain (and therefore in the functioning of the human mind) can be best modeled by self-excited, self-amplifying and self-sustained waveforms superimposing on each other in flowing multiple-coupled feedback cycles (Kilpatrick 2015, Troy 2008a, b, Sandstede 2007, Werning 2012, Freeman 2000a, b, 1987, Kohonen 2001, Abeles 1991, Bienenstock 1995). Thus, the neural information storage and retrieval in long-term memory, for example, can be understood by means of computational adaptive resonance mechanisms in the dominant waveforms, or "modes" (Grossberg and Somers 1991), and by the warming up and annealing of oscillation modes by streams of informational processes in the context of computational "energy functions", as in "Harmony Theory" (Smolensky and Legendre 2006a).

The human neurocognitive system can be regarded as a nonlinear, dynamical and open non-equilibrium system (Glansdorff and Prigogine 1971, Nicolis and Prigogine 1977, von Bertalanffy 1950a, 1953, Schrödinger 1944/2012), which includes a non-equilibrium neurodynamic. In a continuous flow of information processing ("online and realtime computation" [Maass et al. 2002]) the system filters system-relative and system-relevant information from its highly ordered environment, and does so in a manner that integrates new information optimally into the informational structures constructed up to that time ("Free-Energy Principle" [Friston 2010a, Friston and Stephan 2007, Sporns 2011]). Thus, an internal neurocognitive concept consists of a dynamical process which filters out statistical prototypes from the sensory information in terms of coherent and adaptive n-dimensional vector fields. These prototypes serve as a basis for dynamic, probabilistic predictions or probabilistic hypotheses on prospective, new data (see the recently introduced approach of "predictive coding" in neurophilosophy [Clark 2013, Hohwy 2013]; chap. 10.3).

11.2 FUTURE RESEARCH WITH PHASE SYNCHRONIZATION MECHANISMS

In this chapter, three types of architecture are presented which, in my opinion, would be best suited to make a significant contribution in the near future to advancing the solution of the binding problem in the cognitive neurosciences based on phase-synchronous, integrative mechanisms.

11.2.1 DYNAMIC NEURAL FIELDS (DNF) ARCHITECTURES

Based on the basic ideas of H. Haken's Synergetics (chap. 2.3, 2.4.2), the German neuroinformatician, Gregor Schöner, developed the "Dynamic Field Theory (DFT)"[503] in developmental psychology and neuroinformatics against the background of the "Dynamic Neural Fields (DNF) Architectures" (Coombes et al. 2014; chap. 11.2.3).

This theory assumes that functionally relevant neural activity is generated by strongly recurrent neural networks, which require a temporal dimension: "Because spiking events in neural populations are not perfectly synchronized, the evolution of activity in strongly recurrent networks is best described in continuous time, asynchronously sampled by discrete spike times. Dynamical systems theory provides the mathematical language for doing so (Grossberg 1977)" (Schöner 2019; see also chap. 2). The required coupling mechanism in low-dimensional neural (attractor) dynamics which stabilize neural activation patterns (that are attractor states of the neural dynamics) against competing information for constructing stable neural representations, works as follows (Lomp et al. 2016): Subpopulations of neurons that form the same macrostate activation pattern "must, in effect, be excitatorily coupled to stabilize activation against decay", and subpopulations of "neurons that form part of competing activation patterns must, in effect, be inhibitorily coupled to stabilize activation against distractors. (...) This pattern of [recurrent (author's note)] connectivity within a population ('neural interaction') is the foundation of neural field theory (Schöner 2019)." Further, the basis of cognitive processes of higher cognition is the organized induction of dynamic instabilities (or bifurcations [chap. 2]) as the mechanism for (sensory detection) decision making and for autonomous sequential transitions between different activation representations:

"The detection decision itself arises from an instability, the *detection instability*, in which the resting state of a neural population becomes unstable (Schöner et al. 2016). The underlying mechanism is the threshold property of neural activity that makes neural dynamics nonlinear: Only neurons whose activation is above the firing threshold impact on the neurons to which they project. In a neural population, neural interaction only engages, therefore, once sufficient levels of activation have been reached.

---

[503]For a fundamental discussion, see e.g. Schöner et al. 2016.
For detailed information, see e.g. Schöner 2019, Lomp et al. 2016, Lipinsky et al. 2012, Spencer et al. 2009a, b, Johnson et al. 2009a, Spencer and Schöner 2003, Erlhagen and Schöner 2002.
For an introduction, see e.g. Schöner 2009, 2008, Calvo Garzón 2008.

The detection instability amplifies input signals into a macroscopic neural state. The input may be a uniform boost, a 'go' signal that does not specify a specific choice. The choice then arises from any inhomogeneity within the population, so that only regions in a population that are slightly closer to threshold than others may become activated. If these are discretely different regions, neural dynamics operate in a categorial regime that can be modeled by zero-dimensional fields or neural dynamic nodes. This may occur, for instance, at the categorization layer of deep feed-forward neural networks (Schöner 2019)."

Schöner stresses that, while the neural dynamics of low-dimensional fields of population activation generate complex forms of higher cognition (e.g. visual search, feature binding, and implement functions and relations), this emerged macroscopic neural dynamics of higher cognition "cannot be eliminated by 'reduction' to a more microscopic level. To the contrary, according to this hypothesis, the microscopic level is driven (or 'enslaved') by this slower, macroscopic level (Schöner 2019 with reference to Schöner et al. 2016)."

Finally, a Dynamic Field Approach to word learning has been presented (Samuelson and Faubel 2016) builds upon (1) a robotic object recognition system "CoRA" (that uses higher-dimensional label-feature fields and a shared label field with a strong WTA network ("fusion/decision layer") to bind visual features of objects via words (Faubel and Schöner 2008, Johnson et al. 2009b)), and (2) data from parent-child experiments (e.g. Samuelson et al. 2011) which indicate that shared space and the integration of timescales are the decisive mechanisms "by which names and objects are bound or mapped together" (Samuelson and Faubel 2016).

11.2.2   (SELF-ORGANIZED) DEEP LEARNING (DL) ARCHITECTURES

Since the early 2000s, a new subdiscipline of Machine Learning (ML) has emerged, socalled "Deep Learning (DL)",[504] developed by the British computer scientist and cognitive psychologist Geoffrey Hinton, his former post-doctoral fellow, the French neuroinformatician Yann LeCun, the Canadian computer scientist Yoshua Bengio and the German computer scientist Jürgen Schmidhuber. The traditional mathematical methods of pattern recognition in machine learning (in the form of statistical, selfadaptive algorithms) suffer from the course of dimensionality when scaling up to larger input signals such as images. Deep Learning tries to solve this with artificial neural networks by using multiple layers. This reduces the high number of dimensions to the (probably) most useful ones, the so-called "features", by using the Backpropagation (BP) algorithm (Schmidhuber 2015, Zell 2003; chap. 3.2.1, fn. 146):

"The conventional option is to hand design good feature extractors, which requires a considerable amount of engineering skill and domain expertise. But this can all be avoided if good features can be learned automatically, using a general-purpose learning procedure. This is the key advantage of deep learning.

A deep-learning architecture is a multilayer stack of simple modules, all (or most) of which are subject to learning, and many of which compute non-linear input-output

---

[504]For an fundamental discussion, see e.g. LeCun et al. 2015, Schmidhuber 2015, Goodfellow et al. 2016, Bengio 2009.
For detailed information, see e.g. Hinton 2014, Salakhutdinov and Hinton 2006, Hinton et al. 2006.
For an introduction, see e.g. Charniak 2019, Sejnowski 2018, 2020, LeCun et al. 2015.
For a critical view, see e.g. von der Malsburg 2020.

mappings. Each module in the stack transforms its input to increase both the selectivity and the invariance of the representation. With multiple non-linear layers, say a depth of 5 to 20, a system can implement extremely intricate functions of its inputs that are simultaneously sensitive to minute details (...) and insensitive to large irrelevant variations such as the background, pose, lighting and surrounding objects (LeCun et al. 2015)."

The so-called "(recurrent) Convolutional Neuronal Networks (CNN)" (LeCun et al. 2015, Schmidhuber 2015) represent a special, particularly powerful subclass of Deep Learning architectures, which are mainly applied for the classification of visual image data, e.g. handwritten zip code recognition (LeCun et al. 1989). CNN architectures have been so successful because they mimic the retinotopy of the biological system which allows them to share filter weights across the whole input and become equivariant to translations.

The German computational neuroscientist, Thomas Serre and the German neuroinformatician, David P. Reichert have shown how Singer's Binding-By-Synchrony Hypothesis and Fries' Communication Through Coherence Hypothesis could be incorporated into the Deep Learning approach to build richer, more versatile representations of sensory input (Reichert and Serre 2014; see chap. 4.4). The experiments are based on pretraining standard, real-valued deep Boltzmann Machines, as a multi-layer recurrent neural network, and converting them into complex-valued nets that, e.g., support the function which synchronizes individual objects in the image to distinct phases. This image comprises, for example, a version of the classic "bars problem" (Földiák 1990; chap. 4.4.3 (4.1), (4.2), 8.1.4), where binary images are created by randomly drawing horizontal and vertical bars. Thus, on first approach, it is shown how deep learning techniques can be used to ensure that the mechanism of phase synchronization supports the function "from gating or modulating neuronal interactions to establishing and signaling semantic grouping of neuronal representations (Reichert and Serre 2014)."

The Bulgarian computer scientist and cognitive scientist, Ivan I. Vankov and the Canadian psychologist, Jeffrey S. Bowers introduced a feed-forward (convolutional) DL neural network architecture, the so-called "Vector Approach to Representing Symbols (VARS)", to solve the combinatorial generalization problem for the purpose of representing symbols (Vankov and Bowers 2019). This architecture encodes complex symbolic structures of varying complexity ("variable binding problem") and visual objects ("feature binding problem") as a static, fixed size and numeric vector representation at the output layer. The model provides correct VARS representations of untrained role-filler bindings over 90% of the time.

Recently, the Dutch neuroscientist Martin Vinck, together with the German neurophysiologists Wolf Singer and Pascal Fries, and the Romanian neuroinformatician Andreea Lazar, used a self-supervised, generative feedforward Deep Neural Network (DNN) for object recognition (with an U-net architecture together with a VGG-16 Convolutional Neural Network (CNN)) (Uran et al. 2020). This DNN was trained "to predict small regions of natural images based on the spatial context (i.e. inpainting)." With this network predictions, "the spatial predictability of visual inputs into (macaque) V1 receptive fields (RFs) is determined, and distinguished low- from high-level predictability." These authors specifically analyzed how predictability modulates firing rates and neuronal synchronization patterns in gamma- (30–80Hz) and beta-bands (18–30Hz).

11.2.3   NEUR(-ON-)AL (WAVE) FIELD ARCHITECTURES[505]

Since the early 2000s, there has been growing interest in dynamical, (stochastic) "Neur(-on-)al (Wave) Field Architectures"[506] of the Wilson-Cowan and Amari type, which generate (1) travelling waves, (2) pulse (ring) waves, (3) spiral, spindle and rotating waves, (4) standing solitary (pulses) waves, (5) homogeneous (pulses) waves, (6) periodic wave trains and (7) phase synchronized waves. The Neural Field Theory (NFT) can be mathematically described by the standard integro-differential equation (IDE) for a scalar neural field whose integral term describes the (phase-synchronized) connectivity of a neuronal network: In many continuum models for the propagation of electrical activity in neural tissue, it is assumed that the synaptic input current is a function of the pre-synaptic firing rate function (Wilson and Cowan 1973). According to the American mathematician G. Bard Ermentrout, these infinite dimensional dynamical systems are, typically, variations on the form (Ermentrout 1998)

$$\frac{1}{\alpha}\frac{\partial u(x,t)}{\partial t} = -u + \int_{-\infty}^{\infty} dy w(y) f \circ u(x-y,t). \tag{11.1}$$

Here, $u(x,t)$ is interpreted as a neural field representing the local activity of a population of neurons at position $n \in \mathbb{R}$. The second term on the right represents the synaptic input, with $f \circ u$ interpreted as the firing rate function. There are several natural choices for the firing rate function. With a statistical mechanics approach to formulating mean-field neural equations, this all or nothing response is replaced by a smooth sigmoidal form (Wilson and Cowan 1972, Amari 1972). For an arbitrary firing rate response the model (11.1) is naturally written in the form

$$Qu(x,t) = \psi(x,t), \tag{11.2}$$

where $\psi(x,t)$ is given by the second term on the right hand side of (11.1) and $Q = (1 + \alpha^{-1}\partial t)$. It is convenient to write $u(x,t)$ in the form

$$\psi(x,t) = (w \otimes f)(x,t) \tag{11.3}$$

where $\otimes$ represents a spatial convolution which representing the synaptic connections of a spatially extended neuronal network

$$(w \otimes f)(x,t) = \int_{-\infty}^{\infty} w(y) f(x-y,t) dy. \tag{11.4}$$

Dealing with neural field models in a purely integral framework by integrating (11.2) one obtains

$$u = \eta * w \otimes f \circ u, \tag{11.5}$$

---

[505]This chapter is a largely adopted version of the considerations in Maurer 2019.

[506]For an fundamental discussion, see e.g. Wilson and Cowan 1972, 1973, Amari 1972, 1975, 1977. For detailed information, see e.g. Byrne et al. 2019, Kilpatrick 2015, Rougier and Detorakis 2013, Troy 2008a, b, Sandstede 2007.
For an introduction, see e.g. Coombes 2005, Ermentrout and Terman 2010, Coombes et al. 2014.
For an analysis of attention and internal predictions in the corticothalamic system by means of a Neural Field Theory (NFT) architecture, see e.g. Babaie-Janvier and Robinson 2019.

where the temporal convolution $*$ is defined by

$$(\eta * f)(x,t) = \int_0^t \eta(s)f(x,t-s)ds. \tag{11.6}$$

The distributed delay kernel $\eta(t)$ can be chosen so as to best describe the response of a given synapse.

Waves in the form of travelling fronts and pulses have now been observed in a variety of slice preparations (Golomb and Amitai 1997, Chervin et al. 1988, Traub et al. 1993, Wu et al. 1999, Richardson et al. 2005).

For simplicity, dynamical realisations of the neural field model as an integro-differential equation have typically been studied in idealised one spatial dimensional or two dimensional planar settings (Coombes 2005). New analysis of wave solutions in a delayed integro-differential equation, posed on a three dimensional sphere representing the physical domain of the neural field, have been made (Visser et al. 2017, Coombes 2005).

Recently, a first approach has been taken in the cognitive neurosciences and cognitive science to investigate the extent to which a new mathematical model of neuronal, phase-synchronized solitons in wave field theory is suitable for solving the binding problem (so-called "Neuro-Cognitive Soliton (NCS) Hypothesis" (Maurer 2019)), which can represent complex information structures in a neurocognitive wave field (such as visual scenes and compositional symbol structures in language processing). For example, a mathematical structure of the neural soliton will have to be developed for a coupling between the component solitons in the continuous soliton field by means of phase synchronization (Newell 1977, Kilpatrick 2015), so that more complex visual scenes or systematic and compositional symbol structures can be encoded by means of a dominant composite soliton.

11.3 DISCUSSION AND EVALUATION[507]

The cognitive neuroarchitectures of modern connectionism mentioned above, and the mathematics of nonlinear Dynamical System Theory (DST) (including Attractor Dynamics and the Paradigm of Self-Organization), can be regarded as a contribution towards building a deeper understanding of what neural or cognitive information really is. Furthermore, these new tools shed light on how the flow of informational elements are integrated into complex systemic structures, from the most basic perceptual representations generated by cell assemblies to the most complex cognitive representations, like symbol structures, generated by vector-based or oscillation-based representations: It is shown, in perception, how sensory object information, like the object's color or form, can be dynamically related or integrated into a neurally based representation of this perceptual object by means of a synchronization mechanism ("feature binding"), in, for example Werning's and Maye's Oscillatory Networks Architecture (chap. 8.1). In this cognitive neuroarchitecture, the coupled oscillators of different feature layers, which synchronize in phase, represent properties of the same object, like 'horizontal' and 'green' with reference to the same bar. Thus, this synchronization mechanism of an eigenmode analysis "binds" the features "together". In language processing, it is shown how semantic concepts and syntactic roles can be

---

[507]This chapter is a largely adopted and partly revised and extended version of the considerations in Maurer 2018.

dynamically related or integrated into neurally based systematic and compositional connectionist representations by means of a synchronization mechanism ("variable binding"). This solves the Fodor/Pylyshyn Challenge (chap. 3.1, 6.1.2), according to which the classical symbol-oriented model of cognition is characterized by: (1) a "combinatorial syntax and semantics of mental representations", and (2) mental operations in the sense of "structure sensitivity of processes", as in logical inferences. Thus, an adequate cognitive theory is characterized by the fact that cognitive processes are "causally sensitive" to the classical constituent structure of mental representations, so that the following closely related characteristics of human cognition can be explained: (1) productivity, (2) systematicity, (3) compositionality, and (4) inferential systematicity.

In connection with the Symbolism vs. Connectionism Debate in the 1980s and 1990s (chap. 6.1.2), the challenge for connectionism was to solve the systematicity and compositionality problems of mental representations by means of integrative and dynamic synchronization mechanisms, with regard to the "problem of variable binding". In other words, conditions both necessary and sufficient for an adequate structural language theory of connectionist neurocognition are the topic of concern. The classical symbolists Fodor, Pylyshyn and McLaughlin (Fodor and Pylyshyn 1988, Fodor and McLaughlin 1990, McLaughlin 1993a, Aizawa 2003), argued that it is not sufficient if only systematicity is performed in the network dynamics of a cognitive neuroarchitecture. This is because the connection weights processed in an artificial neural network by means of a learning procedure have to be considered as "nomologically arbitrary". On the contrary, the classical conception of systematicity is only truly explained if a causal mechanism is shown to be interrelating mental contents with nomological necessity and sufficiency. Thus, a system of mental representations is constructed based on symbolic constituent structures in the sense of Fodor's "Representational Theory of Mind", which can be interpreted as propositional attitudes (so-called "Language of Thought" (chap. 3.1.4.5)).

Rejecting this criticism, Chalmers (Chalmers 1993), and especially Hadley (Hadley 1994, 1997, 2003, Hadley and Hayward 1997), argue that, firstly, proponents of the classical symbol theory confuse nomological necessity with logical necessity, and, secondly, a complex composite vector can bear in a functional relation to its constituent vectors (as defined by van Gelder's "functional compositionality" [van Gelder 1991b, 1990a, Kralemann 2006]). In my opinion, however, a more compelling argument would involve appealing to Werning's (2012) definition of "formal compositionality", based on the mathematical concept of an algebraic structure. Under this definition, in the connectionist neuroarchitectures of the so-called "Vector Symbolic Architectures (VSA)" (chap. 6 [1], fn. 343), a vector-based semantic compositum is a homomorphic image of the syntactic structure of the language, such that the modern "Principle of Semantic Compositionality" (chap. 8.1.4) is fulfilled and thereby, a necessary condition for the criterion of systematicity. However, the "Principle of Semantic Constituency" (chap. 8.1.4) does not apply to the Tensor Product Representation within Smolensky's ICS architecture. This means that it is a neuroarchitecture with a non-symbolic, compositional semantics, as the part/whole relation in a vector-based constituent structure cannot always be preserved. On the other hand, in Plates' Holographic Reduced Representations (and therefore also in Eliasmith's and Stewart's Neural Engineering Framework), the Principle of Semantic Constituancy is fulfilled because of an algorithm of unbinding through which a syntactic part/whole relation can be (approximately) identified. Thus, these are neuroarchitectures with a symbolic, compositional semantics in the sense of the "Principle of Formal Compositionality" (Box 8.1.4.1; Werning 2012). The criticism of Fodor (1997) and McLaughlin (1993a) in the absence of an explicit physical presence of a constituent vector,[508] which is thus weakened, is also rejected by Clark (1992, 1989), in reference to the explicit or implicit character of cognitive information (Kirsh 1991). In contrast to the VSA architectures with their vector-based representations, the simulation model of the Oscillatory Networks (according to Werning and Maye [chap. 8.1]) operates with nonlinear oscillation functions. This model thereby connects the sensory perception of objects with a non-symbolic, compositional emulative neurosemantics for a monadic first-order predicate language, and does so with a high degree of neurobiological plausibility.

Since system-theoretical connectionism has succeeded in modeling the sensory objects that feature in perception as well as systematic and compositional representations in language processing, a convincing new theory of neurocognition which bridges the neuronal and the cognitive analysis level, has been developed. One of the unsolved core issues in the cognitive sciences is the mode of (hybrid) integration between connectionist-system-theoretical subsymbolic and logic and linguistic-based symbolic approaches. To what extent can new developments in the modeling and analysis of recurrent and self-organized ANN architectures (e.g. dynamical [stochastic] neuronal [Wave] Field Theories [chap. 11.2.3] of neural information processing) improve models from discrete mathematics through to continuous mathematics, operating both, on the basis of low-level processing of perceptual information, and high-level reasoning and symbol processing?

Thus, these integrative (synchronization) mechanisms can be regarded as substantially contributing towards bridging the gap between the discrete, abstract symbolic modeling of propositions in the mind, like in Fodor's "Language of Thought", and their continuous, numerical and dynamical modeling in the form of cognitive neuroarchitecture in connectionism.[509]

In cognitive neurorobotics, a promising approach has also been developed to bridge the gap between higher-order, symbolic cognition and lower-order, sensor-motor processes (Tani 2014, 2017, Tani et al. 2014; chap. 10.3 at the end). According to this approach, based on the principles of embodied cognition (chap. 1.1.1), compositionalty in higher-order cognition can be acquired by means of self-organizing, neurodynamic structures with circular causality, "via interactive learning between the top-down intentional process of acting on the physical world and the bottom-up recognition of perceptual reality (...) while sharing the same metric space (Tani 2014)". Within a dynamical, hierarchical cascade of "Recurrent Neural Networks

---

[508] See Fodor 1997: "The connection with (1) (...) the constituency relation is a part/whole relation: If C is a constituent of C*, then a token of C is a part of every token of C*. More precisely, constituency is a co-tokening relation; that is, if C is a constituent of C*, then it is metaphysically necessary that for every tokening of C* there is a corresponding tokening of C. (...) The connection with (2) (...) If R is constituency, then (2) says that the semantics of complex representations derives from the semantics of their parts."

[509] See e.g. Smolensky and Legendre 2006a and McLaughlin 1997: "(...) it is consistent with Classicism that mental representations are realized by activation patterns and that symbolic processes are implemented by matrix multiplication operations."

with Parametric Biases (RNNPB)" employed in the bound learning of pairs of linguistic and behavioral sequences, the constantly adapting activation vectors minimize the prediction error and, thus, construct "amodal, high level, dynamical representations that are both sensory and motor in nature (Tani 2014)". Thus, in the
robot experiments a central problem with regard to the cognitive competency for
compositional action generation becomes clear. While the bottom-up process modulates the whole behavioral flow by reflecting the perceptual reality as if the robot can
perform algebraic operations on behavioral primitives as concrete, distinct objects,
"the top-down intentional pathway attempts to generate the whole behavioral flow
proactively" by constructing continuous, "fluid and context sensitive concatenations
of primitives as delicate perceptual spatial-temporal patterns (Tani 2014)". Thus, this
can be called "fluid compositionality".

With regard to the Binding-By-Synchrony (BBS) mechanism (chap. 4.4), the following summary can be given (Singer and Lazar 2016; chap. 4.4.9): Although it is
not yet possible to speak of a unified theory of cortical code processing, it can be
stated that, in addition to the traditional strategy of analysing the discharge rate of
individual neurons ("labeled line code" [chap. 4.2.2]) in serial feed-forward processing, the additional strategy in recurrent neural networks processing must be used,
according to which "to a substantial degree (...) the precise temporal relations among
the discharge sequences of distributed nodes" are also relevant, e.g. for the definition
of relational constructs, both in signal processing and learning. The core of the BBS
hypothesis is "that the dynamic interactions within recurrently coupled oscillator networks (i) endow responses with the temporal structure required for the encoding of
context-sensitive relations, (ii) exhibit complex, high-dimensional correlation structures that reflect the signatures of an internal model stored in the weight distributions
of the coupling connections, and (iii) permit fast convergence toward stimulus specific substates that are easy to classify because they occupy well-segregated loci in
the high-dimensional state-space (Singer and Lazar 2016)". These neural states in
the state space can be best characterized as self-consistent (flow) equilibrium states
(chap. 2.3), which can be mathematically modeled as dynamic attractors (von der
Malsburg 2018), e.g. the convection cells in the Bénard system (chap. 2.3.1).

From the viewpoint of philosophy of science, however, it should be noted that this
generation of self-consistent structures by means of self-organized synchronization
mechanisms is correlative, rather than causal (Buzsáki 2019, Shea 2018, Thagard
2012; chap. 4.4.3 [4.3]). It is an unresolved question as to whether neuronal synchrony is a relevant causal mechanism for the phenomenon of (conscious) feature and
variable binding in perceptual and language processing or a statistical (cor-)relation,
and so, only a distal "marker" of this binding (chap. 4.4.8 [2]).

A complementary approach of a unified framework is presented by A. Kumar
(Hahn et al. 2019, 2013; chap. 9.6, 9.5): Neuronal oscillation-based communication can be divided into the sub-concept in which both the sender network and receiver network oscillate with the same frequency and phase (in a coherent manner)
("Communication Through Coherence (CTC) Hypothesis", 4.4.3 (5)) and into the
sub-concept in which the non-oscillatory receiver network is periodically activated
by the sender and generates an amplified oscillatory response through frequency
resonance ("Communication Through Resonance (CTR) Hypothesis", chap. 9.6) or

through phase synchrony ("Binding-By-Synchrony (BBS) Hypothesis", chap. 4.4.3). However, both the sub-concepts describe neuronal communication between populations of neurons with spike volleys represented in phase space, spanned by the number of spikes and their (phase) synchronization. "In both cases, synchronous spiking events are routed from a sending population to a receiving population, and the impact of a volley in the receiver is determined by common input synchrony generated in the sender. (...) The main difference between the two types of communication is in the speed of communication." The fast (synfire and gamma) communication mode (chap. 9.5) is possible when the transferred neural information is sufficiently strong and synchronous such that it is transmitted in a single wave. By contrast, slow (alpha and beta) oscillations in the CTC and CTR mechanisms require several oscillation cycles in the transmission of weak signals to achieve and establish neuronal communication. This can affect the phase, frequency and amplitude of faster gamma oscillations.

11.4 OUTLOOK ON FUTURE RESEARCH[510]

In this chapter a short outlook on future research will be given with reference to four topics:

(1) Symbolic versus sub-symbolic components in (hybrid) integrative cognitive neuroarchitectures:

Bridging the gap between different levels of description, explanation, representation, and computation in symbolic and sub-symbolic paradigms of neurocognitive systems modelling, one of the unsolved core issues in the cognitive sciences is the mode of (hybrid) integration between connectionist-system-theoretical subsymbolic and logic-linguistic-based symbolic approaches. To what extent can new developments in the modelling and analysis of recurrent, self-organized ANN architectures, e.g. wave field theories of neural information processing based on travelling waves and described by nonlinear oscillation functions (Kilpatrick 2015, Rougier and Detorakis 2013, Troy 2008a, b, Sandstede 2007, Coombes 2005; chap. 11.2.3), bring together models from discrete and continuous mathematics operating, both on the basis of low-level processing of perceptual information, and by performing high-level reasoning and symbol processing?

(2) Neurocognitive integration based on self-organized, cyclical (phase) synchronization mechanisms:

Self-organized phase synchronization mechanisms, as in the Binding-by-Synchrony Hypothesis are a key factor for the analysis of integrating information in neurocognition (chap. 4.4). This raises the question as to what extent the dynamic mode of combinations of synchronous process mechanisms can be used as a decisive criterion for a new concept of self-organization and emergence in neurocognition (see e.g. "Micro-Macro Link [MML] problem [Auyang 1998, Fromm 2005]; "Small-World

---

[510]This chapter is a totaly adapted version of the considerations in Maurer 2016.

Networks", "Connectome [Sporns 2011, Maurer 2018]) by cascading spreading activations in (upwards, downwards and sideways) feedback loops (in terms of multiple cyclic graph structures). In the "Theory of Dissipative Self-Organization" (chap. 2.3) one can consider the synergy of short-range, autocatalytic activation (excitation) through positive feedback cycles and long-range, crosscatalytic (lateral) inhibition through negative feedback cycles as one fundamental principle of pattern formation in neurobiological dynamical systems. According to this principle, which organizational structure of advanced cognitive neuroarchitectures would be preferable for an improved (abstract) pattern recognition (for example, the mixture of Oscillatory Networks with a Kohonen map)?

(3) Fluid or liquid perspective in modeling cognitive neuroarchitectures:

A special feature of the cognitive binding mechanisms in human-level intelligence is their fluid (or better: fluent) and transient character (chap. 11.1). What contribution can newer dynamic algorithmic methods ("Liquid Computing" [chap. 9.1], "Reservoir Computing" [chap. 9.3], "Deep [Machine] Learning" [chap. 11.2.2] or combination of models from connectionism and Dynamic System Theory, e.g. Dynamic Field Theory [DFT] [chap. 11.2.2, 3.2.6; Spencer et al. 2009]) make in the analysis and modeling of recurrent cognitive neuroarchitectures?

(4) Abstract neurocognitive systems incorporating embodied human-level cognition and intelligence:

A further rapprochement takes place between the dynamic system theory and (embodied) connectionism in "Cognitive Robotics", "Evolutionary Robotics", and "Developmental Robotics" (chap. 3.2.6, 7.3, 11.3). This raises the question as to what extent this progress towards a hybrid embodied approach made by robotics researchers can contribute new insights in solving the binding problem in embodied cognitive science (Barsalou 1999, Franklin 2013), with special consideration to these neurocognitive integrative mechanisms which have been implemented in robots and androids acting as agents in complex (developmental and social) situations.

11.5   IMPLICATIONS AND CONSEQUENCES FOR A PHILOSOPHY OF COGNITIVE SCIENCE[511]

The mathematics of nonlinear Dynamical System Theory (DST), including attractor dynamics and the paradigm of self-organization, can be regarded as a contribution towards building a deeper understanding of what neural or cognitive information really is. Furthermore, these new tools shed light on how the flow of informational elements are integrated into complex systematic structures, from the most basic perceptual representations, generated by cell assemblies, to the most complex cognitive representations, like symbol structures, generated by tensor products or oscillatory representations.

Thus, these integrative mechanisms can be regarded as a contribution towards bridging the gap between the discrete, abstract symbolic description of propositions

---

[511] This chapter is a partly adopted version of the considerations in Maurer 2014a, 2016, 2017, 2018.

in the mind, and their continuous, numerical implementation in neural networks in the brain. This may be regarded as a step toward an embodied, fully integrated theory of cognition.

The central issue in the Symbolism vs. Connectionism Debate is regarding which representational format is the most appropriate for the understanding of cognition. Van Gelder suggests "[t]he pivotal issue here is probably the role of time. (...) Details of timing (durations, rates, synchronies, etc.) are taken to be essential to cognition. Cognition is seen not as having a sequential (...) structure, but rather as a matter of continuous and continual coevolution. The sublety and complexity of cognition is found not at a time in elaborate static structures, but rather in time in the flux of change itself (van Gelder and Port 1995, van Gelder 1999d)." Following this, many authors, e.g., Smolensky, Elman, Petitot, Schöner, Tabor, Thomas, Pasemann, Mainzer, Bechtel, Abrahamsen, Horgan and Tienson, agree that "connectionism is perfectly compatible with the dynamical approach" because neural networks are themselves typically continuous, parallel, and non-linear dynamical systems (see the overview in Maurer 2014a). Thus, it remains difficult to distinguish between connectionist and dynamicist approaches. According to Eliasmith (1995), a decisive way in which dynamicists wish to distinguish themselves from the connectionist approach is by holding that there should be no representation in the cognitive neuroarchitecture. For dynamicists, a cognitive agent can be best captured with a system of differential equations which provides a scientifically tractable description of the agent's qualitative dynamics. In contrast to this, attempts have been made to merge connectionist models with the approach of Dynamic Systems Theory (Spencer et al. 2009) (e.g. in developmental psychology, with the Dynamic Field Approach and via Evolutionary Robotics [chap. 11.4, 11.2.1, 3.2.6]).

Thus, this tendency towards a dynamical, distributed representational format in modern connectionism also leads to a redefinition of the concept of an internal (mental) representation. Under connectionism, representation can be thought of as a statistical prototype described with vectors, which changes fluently over time, rather than as symbolic theory's fixed, static object. According to Pasemann (1996) and Roth (1992, 1994) (chap. 7.3), this means that the concept of internal representation should be used in terms of a "semantic configuration of coherent (synchronous) module dynamics". Therefore the classic conception of representations as static cannot be maintained, since a representation is an "expression of coherence between internal neurodynamic processes and the dynamics of the external environment, which is reflected in the changes in the receptor activities". Furthermore, individual neuromodules can fulfil different functions as a structural element due to their multifunctionality with different sensory information. At the same time, individual functions can be fulfilled by very different structural elements: "[R]epresentation thus loses the characteristic of being bound to specific static structural elements and having a structural system-intrinsic meaning. (...) If a representation appears as a semantic configuration in a cognitive process, then it can be assumed that it can never be identified as distinct, always equal partial dynamics. It will fulfil its function as transient dynamics in the form of an ever-changing dynamic process." This fluent internal neurocognitive information only becomes meaningful when it is "coupled" with external sensory information, as for example in an emulative neurosemantics (chap. 8.1.4).

Furthermore, this immanent fluent and transient dynamics in information processing in modern connectionism leads to a methodological rethink of the reduction problem in cognitive science. This new fluent perspective in cognitive science means that the researchers in philosophy of science make use of a mechanistic-systemic method ("mechanistic approach": Bechtel 2008, Craver 2007, Piccinini and Craver 2011, Kaplan and Craver 2011, Chemero and Silberstein 2008, Maurer 2014a; chap. 1.1.4): the BBS mechanisms and its modeling in the cognitive neuroarchitectures (based on nonlinear Dynamical System Theory), outlined above, describe and explain a phenomenon on multiple system levels and can be investigated both, under an analytical-mechanistic perspective, and under a synthetic-systemic perspective (Maurer 2014a). Viewed from an analytical-mechanistic perspective, a BBS phenomenon, such as feature and variable binding, can be broken down into its individual analytical vector components and vector operations and then examined. From a synthetic-systemic perspective, the corresponding system of non-linear differential equations with global order parameters can also be considered (Haken 1988a, b, 2004, Schöner 2019). It models macroscopic activation patterns that are generated through the global dynamics of large networks of neural populations. These dynamics of neural populations "form a privileged level of description" at which (higher) cognition and behaviour emerges, and "constitute the time courses of mental states, which are coupled to sensory information and ultimately drive muscles to bring about bodily movement " (Schöner 2019; chap. 11.2.1 at the end).

To conclude this book, I would like to raise a fundamental question: Would it not perhaps be more sensible, within the framework of a scientific analysis and an analysis in philosophy of science, to introduce, in addition to a theoretical model of reality viewed from a third-person perspective based on static, discrete *object* structures, the more fundamental analysis viewed from a first-person perspective based on dynamical, continuous and phase-synchronized *process* structures in a neurocognitive system (Maurer 2014a, 2016, 2017)? Based on the mechanism debate in philosophy of science (see above), one would have to define Binding-By-Synchrony (BBS) mechanisms that were at least correlative. These BBS mechanisms would then model the traditional assignment of object structures, such as object properties, to a particular object by means of algorithms in form of a system of linear and nonlinear differential equations with synchronization terms (so-called "process structures") (see e.g. Werning 2005c, 2012, Kilpatrick 2015). This would mean that the traditional assignment of attributes and substantial structural properties of an individual object to a "substance" would be substantiated by a temporal process structure, taking the form of nonlinear (probabilistic) functions with synchronization terms, within the framework of BBS mechanisms. This explains the "binding". It would therefore have to be taken into account that this would not be a causal but "only" a correlative explanation. In simple terms, from the perspective of a neurocognitive system, an object to be recognized and transferred into a logical predication (chap. 3.1.1, 8.1.4) only becomes an object when the neurocognitive synchronization mechanisms process the individual pieces of information correctly in such a way that a phase-synchronous, temporal "binding" of the object components is guaranteed.

From the viewpoint of Theoretical Neuroinformatics, Machine Learning, and Information Theory, this is done by converging the information flow (in the form of nonlinear, self-organized vector flows, vector streams and vector fields) into a (relatively) robust, dynamical attractor structure (von der Malsburg 2018). The dynamics of a coherent population of neurons thus strive for a "relatively stable, transient optimum of neural resonance" (Edelman 1987, Hahn et al. 2014, 2019, Varela 1995, 2006, Grossberg and Somers [1991]). The sensory piece of information set as invariant is selected system-relatively and system-relevantly, so that, during the transformation of the external information structure into internal neuronal information, its original "meaning" as environmental properties is "lost" and instead, a new system-internally constructed system-relative "meaning" is assigned to it. Each neuron is seen as a carrier of "semantic (micro-)information", and this "semantic elementary information" of all synchronously active neurons is then assembled within the framework of integrative mechanisms to form semantic symbols and symbol structures. Thus, in the context of a selective information process, a sensory stimulus -as transformed processual information- is only coded to further new information in the context of already existing (relational) structural information of the neurocognitive system itself (von der Malsburg 1994, McClelland et al. 2010). This processual or dynamic character of neural information processing has, in recent years been reflected in the tendency towards fluent or liquid mechanisms, models and cognitive neuroarchitectures (chap. 9.1, 11.1), which, in my opinion, could model the continuous, transient neural information flow, also with respect to the requirements of an "Embodied Cognition" or the "Brain-Body-Environment (BBE) interactions" (Bruineberg et al. 2018, Sporns 2011, Clark 2008, Varela and Thompson 2003, Thompson and Varela 2001, Beer 2000, Barsalou 1999, Brooks 1986, Braitenberg 1984; chap. 1.1.1, 1.4). The neurocognitive, structure-generating process mechanisms mentioned above are embedded in the mutual, circular-causal, and synchronized adaptation between embodied, active neurocognitive systems and their system environments, and this adaptation "can better be conceptualized [as (author's note)] an attracting manifold within the joint agent-environment state-space as a whole (Bruineberg et al. 2018)".

References

Abeles, M. 1982a. Local Cortical Circuits. An Electrophysiological Study. Springer-Verlag, Berlin, DE.

Abeles, M. 1982b. Role of the cortical neuron: integrator or coincidence detector? Israel Journal of Medical Sciences 18: 8392.

Abeles, M. 1991. Corticonics: neural Circuits of the Cerebral Cortex. Cambridge University Press, Cambridge, UK.

Abeles, M. 1994. Firing rates and well-timed events in the cerebral cortex. pp. 121-140. *In:* E. Domany, K. Schulten and J.L. van Hemmen [eds.]. Models of Neural Networks II. Chapter 3. Springer-Verlag, New York, USA.

Abeles, M. 2003. Synfire chains. pp. 1143-1146. *In:* A. Arbib [ed.]. The Handbook of Brain Theory and Neural Networks. 2nd Ed. The MIT Press, Cambridge, USA, London, UK.

Abeles, M. 2009. Synfire chains. pp. 829-832. *In:* L.R. Squire [ed.]. Encyclopedia of Neuroscience. Elsevier Academic Press, Amsterdam, NL, Heidelberg, DE.

Abeles, M., E. Vaadia, H. Bergman, Y. Prut, I. Haalman and H. Slovin. 1993. Dynamics of neuronal interactions in the frontal cortex of behaving monkeys. Concepts in Neuroscience 4: 131-158.

Abeles, M. and Y. Prut. 1996. Spatio-temporal firing patterns in the frontal cortex of behaving monkeys. Journal of Physiology Paris 90: 249-250.

Abeles, M., G. Hayon and D. Lehmann. 2004. Modeling compositionality by dynamic binding of synfire chains. Journal of Computational Neuroscience 17: 179201.

Abeles, M., M. Diesmann, T. Flash, T. Geisel, M. Herrmann and M. Teicher. 2013. Compositionality in neural control: an interdisciplinary study of scribbling movements in primates. Frontiers in Computational Neuroscience 7: 103.

Abraham, W.C. and A. Robins. 2005. Memory retention – the synaptic stability versus plasticity dilemma. Trends in Neurosciences 28: 73-78.

Abrahamsen, A. and W. Bechtel. 2006. Phenomena and mechanisms: putting the symbolic, connectionist, and dynamical systems debate in broader perspective. pp. 159-185. *In:* R. Stainton [ed.]. Contemporary Debates in Cognitive Science. Basil Blackwell, Oxford, UK.

Abrahman, F.D., R.H. Abrahman, C.D. Shaw and A. Garfinkel. 1990. A Visual Introduction to Dynamical System Theory for Psychology. Aerial Press, Santa Cruz, USA.

Abramowitz, M. and I.A. Stegun [eds.] 1972. Handbook of Mathematical Functions with Formulas, Graphs, and Mathematical Tables. 9th Pr. Dover, New York, USA.

Ackley, D.H., G.E. Hinton and T.J. Sejnowski. 1985. A learning algorithm for Boltzman machines. Cognitive Science 9: 147-169.

Adrian, E.D. and Y. Zotterman. 1926. The impulses produced by sensory nerve endings. Part II: The response of a single end organ. Journal of Physiology 61: 151-171.

Aertsen, A. and G.L. Gerstein. 1985. Evaluation of neuronal connectivity: sensitivity of cross-correlation. Brain Research 340: 341-354.

Aertsen, A., G.L. Gerstein, M.K. Harbib and G. Palm. 1989. Dynamics of neural firing correlation: modulation of "effective connectivity". Journal of Neurophysiology 61: 900-917.

Aertsen, A., E. Vaadia, M. Abeles, E. Ahissar, H. Bergman, B. Karmon, Y. Lavner, E. Margalit, I. Nelken and S. Rotter. 1991. Neural interactions in the frontal cortex of a behaving monkey: signs of dependence on stimulus context and behavioral state. Journal für Hirnforschung 32: 735-743.

Aertsen, A. and V. Braitenberg. [eds.] 1992. Information Processing in the Cortex. Experiments and Theory. Springer-Verlag, Berlin, DE, Heidelberg, DE.

Aertsen, A. and M. Arndt. 1993. Response synchronization in the visual cortex. Current Opinion in Neurobiology 3: 586-594.

Aertsen, A., M. Diesmann and M.-O. Gewaltig. 1996. Propagation of synchronous spiking activity in feedforward neural networks. Journal of Physiology Paris 90: 243-247.

Ainsworth, M., S. Lee, M.O. Cunningham, A.K. Roopun, R.D. Traub, N.J. Kopell and M.A. Whittington. 2011. Dual gamma rhythm generators control interlaminar synchrony in auditory cortex. The Journal of Neuroscience 31: 17040-17051.

Ainsworth, M., S. Lee, M.O. Cunningham, R.D. Traub, N.J. Kopell and M.A. Whittington. 2012. Rates and rhythms: a synergistic view of frequency and temporal coding in neuronal networks. Neuron 75: 572-583.

Aizawa, K. 2003. The Systematicity Arguments. Springer, New York, USA.

Aizawa, Y. 2006. Self-organization in nonlinear systems. pp. 43-57. In: Daiseion-ji e.V. /Wilhelm Gottfried Leibniz Gemeinschaft e.V. [ed.]. 2. Symposium zur Gründung der Deutsch-Japanischen Gesellschaft für integrative Wissenschaft, Verlag J.H. Röll, Bonn, DE. [German]

Ajjanagadde, V. and L. Shastri. 1989. Efficient inference with multiplace predicates and variables in a connectionist system, 396-403. *In* Proceedings of the Eleventh Conference of the Cognitive Science Society. Ann-Arbor, United States of America.

Albantakis, L. and G. Tononi. 2015. The intrinsic cause-effect power of discrete dynamical systems – from elementary cellular automata to adapting animats. Entropy 17: 5472-5502.

Alexiadou, A. 2013. Cognitive linguistics. pp. 63-66. *In:* A. Stephan and S. Walter [eds.]. Handbuch Kognitionswissenschaft. Metzler, Stuttgart,Weimar, DE. [German]

Allen, M. and K.J. Friston. 2018. From cognitivism to autopoiesis: towards a computational framework for the embodied mind. Synthese 195: 2459-2482.

Amari, S.-I. 1972. Characteristics of random nets of analog neuron-like elements. IEEE Transactions on Systems, Man and Cybernetics, SMC-2: 643657.

Amari, S.-I. 1975. Homogeneous nets of neuron-like elements. Biological Cybernetics 17: 211220.

Amari, S.-I. 1977. Dynamics of pattern formation in lateral inhibition type neural fields. Biological Cybernetics 27 7787.

Amirikian, B. and A.P. Georgopoulos. 2003. Motor cortex: coding and decoding of directional operations. pp. 690-696. *In:* A. Arbib [ed.]. The Handbook of Brain Theory and Neural Networks. 2nd Ed. The MIT Press, Cambridge, USA, London, UK.

Amit, D.J. 1989. Modeling Brain Function. TheWorld of Attractor Neural Networks. Cambridge University Press, Cambridge, UK.

Amit, D.J., H. Gutfreund and H. Sompolinsky. 1987. Statistical mechanics of neural networks near saturation. Annals of Physics 173: 30-67.

Anastasio, T.J. 2010. Tutorial on Neural Systems Modeling. Sinauer Associates, Sonderland, USA.

Anderson, B. 1999. Kohonen neural networks and language. Brain and Language 70: 86-94.

Anderson, J.A. 1972. A simple neural network generating an interactive memory. Mathematical Biosciences 14: 197-230.

Anderson, J.R. 1983. The Architecture of Cognition. Harvard University Press, Cambridge, USA.

Anderson, J.R. 1993. Production systems and the ACT-R theory. pp. 1-15. *In:* J.R. Anderson [ed.]. The Rules of the Mind. Erlbaum, Hillsdale, USA.

Anderson, J.R. 1998. Production systems and the ACT-R theory. pp. 59-76. *In:* P. Thagard [ed.]. Mind Readings. Introductory Selections on Cognitive Science. MIT Press, Cambridge, USA.

Anderson, J.R. 2002. ACT: A Simple Theory of Complex Cognition. pp. 49-68. *In:* T.A. Polk and C.M. Seifert [eds.]. Cognitive Modeling. The MIT Press. Cambridge, USA.

Anderson, J.R. 2007. How Can the Human Mind Occur in the Physical Universe? Oxford University Press, New York, USA.

Anderson, J.R. 2015. Cognitive Psychology and Its Implications. 8th Ed. Worth Publishers, New York, USA.

Anderson, J.R. and C. Lebiere. 1998. The Atomic Components of Thought. Lawrence Erlbaum, Mahwah, USA.

Anderson, J.R., D. Bothell, M.D. Byrne, S. Douglass, C. Lebiere and Y. Qin. 2004. An integrated theory of the mind. Psychological Review 111: 1036-1060.

Anderson, M.L. 2003. Embodied cognition: a field guide. Artificial Intelligence 149: 91-130.

Anderson, M.L. and D.R. Perlis. 2003. Symbol systems. pp. 281-287. *In:* L. Nadel [ed.]. Encyclopedia of Cognitive Science. Vol. 4. Natur Publishing Group. London, UK, New York, USA and Tokyo, JP.

Appeltant, L. 2012. Reservoir computing based on delay-dynamical systems. Ph.D. Thesis. Physics Department. Vrije Universiteit Brussel. Brussels, BE.

Applebaum, D. 1996. Probability and Information: An Integrated Approach. Cambridge University Press, Cambridge, UK.

Arbib, M.A. 2003. Dynamics and adaptation in neural networks. pp. 15-23. *In:* A. Arbib [ed.]. The Handbook of Brain Theory and Neural Networks. 2nd Ed. The MIT Press, Cambridge, USA, London, UK.

Argyris, J., G. Faust and M. Haase. 1995. The Exploration of Chaos: Textbook for Scientists and Engineers. Vieweg, Braunschweig,Wiesbaden, DE. [German]

Arndt, C. 2001. Information Measures. Information and its Description in Science and Engineering. Springer-Verlag, Berlin, DE.

Arrowsmith, D.K. and C.M. Place. 1990. An Introduction to Dynamical Systems. Cambridge University Press. Cambridge, UK.

Ashby, W.R. 1947. Principles of the self-organizing dynamic system. Journal of General Psychology 37: 125-128.

Ashby, W.R. 1952. Design for a Brain. Chapman and Hall, London, UK.

Ashby, W.R. 1962. Principles of self-organization. pp. 255-278. *In:* H. von Foerster and G.W. Zopf, Jr. [eds.]. Transactions of the University of Illinois Symposium. Pergamon Press, London, UK. (reprinted in Ashby, W.R. 2004.)

Ashby, W.R. 2004. Principles of the Self-Organizing System. E:CO Special Double Issue 6: 102-126.

Aswolinskiy, W. and G. Pipa. 2015. RM-SORN: a reward-modulated self-organizing recurrent neural network. Frontiers in Computational Neuroscience 9: 36.

Atallah, B.V. and M. Scanziani. 2009. Instantaneous modulation of gamma oscillation frequency by balancing excitation with inhibition. Neuron 62: 566-577.

Auyang, S.Y. 1998. Foundations of Complex-System Theories. Cambridge University Press, Cambridge, UK.

Aviel, Y., E. Pavlov, M. Abeles and D. Horn. 2002. Synfire chain in a balanced network. Neurocomputing 44: 285-292.

Aviel, Y., D. Horn and M. Abeles. 2004. Synfire waves in small balanced networks. Neurocomputing 58: 123-127.

Baas, N.A. 1997. Self-organization and higher order structures. pp. 71-81. *In:* F. Schweitzer [ed.]. Self-Organization of Complex Structures. From Individual to Collective Dynamics. Gordon & Breach, London, UK.

Babaie-Janvier, T. and P.A. Robinson. 2019. Neural field theory of corticothalamic attention with control system analysis. Frontiers in Human Neuroscience 12: 334.

Bacher, J., A. Pöge and K. Wenzig. 2010. Cluster Analysis. Application-oriented Introduction to Classification Methods. 3. Auflage. Oldenbourg Verlag, München, DE. [German]

Backhaus, K., B. Erichson, W. Plinke and R. Weiber. 2008. Multivariate Analysis Methods. An Application-oriented Introduction. 12. Auflage. Springer-Verlag, Berlin, DE, Heidelberg, DE. [German]

Baddeley, R. 2008. Introductory information theory and the brain. pp. 1-20. *In:* R. Baddeley, P. Hancock and P. Földiák [eds.]. Information Theory and the Brain. University Press, Cambridge, USA.

Bak, P., C. Tang and K. Wiesenfeld. 1987. Self-Organized Criticality. An Explanation of the 1/f Noise. Physical Review Letters 59: 381-384.

Bak, P. and K. Chen. 1991. Self-organized criticality. Spektrum der Wissenschaft 3: 62-71. [German]

Balaban, E., S. Edelman, S. Grillner, U. Grodzinski, E.D. Jarvis, J.H. Kaas, G. Laurent and G. Pipa. 2010. Evolution of dynamic coordination. pp. 59-82. *In:* C. von der Malsburg, W.A. Phillips and W. Singer [eds.]. Dynamic Coordination in the Brain. From Neurons to Mind. The MIT Press, Cambridge, USA.

Balakrishnan, R. and K. Ranganathan. 2012. A Textbook of Graph Theory. 2nd Ed. Springer, New York, USA.

Balduzzi, D. and G. Tononi. 2008. Integrated information in discrete dynamical systems: motivation and theoretical framework. PloS Computational Biology 4: e1000091.

Balduzzi, D. and G. Tononi. 2009. Qualia: the geometry of integrated information. PLoS Computational Biology 5: e1000462.

Banzhaf, W. 2009. Self-organizing systems. pp. 8040-8050. *In:* R.A. Meyers [ed.]. Encyclopedia of Complexity and Systems Science. Springer-Verlag, Heidelberg, DE.

Barandiaran, X. and A. Moreno. 2006. On what makes certain dynamical systems cognitive: a minimally cognitive organization program. Adaptive Behavior 14: 171-185.

Barlow, H.B. 1972. Single units and sensation: a neuron doctrine for perceptual psychology. Perception 1: 371-394.

Barnden, J.A. and M. Chady. 2003. Artificial intelligence and neural networks. pp. 113-117. *In:* A. Arbib [ed.]. The Handbook of Brain Theory and Neural Networks. 2nd Ed. The MIT Press, Cambridge, USA, London, UK.

Barsalou, L.W. 1992. Frames, concepts, and conceptual fields. pp. 21-74. *In:* A. Lehrer and E.F. Kittay [eds.]. Frames, Fields, and Contrasts: New Essays in Lexical and Semantic Organization. Erlbaum, Hillsdale, USA.

Barsalou, L.W. 1999. Perceptual symbol systems. Behavioral and Brain Sciences 22: 577609.

Bartels, A. 2009. Visual perception: converging mechanisms of attention, binding, and sequentation? Current Biology 19: R300-302.

Başar, E. and H. Haken. 1999. Brain Function and Oscillations: Integrative Brain Function. Neurophysiology and Cognitive Processes. Springer, Berlin, DE.

Başar-Eroğlu, C., E. Hoff, D. Struber and M.A. Stadler. 2003. Multistable phenomena in neurocognition research. pp. 349-364. *In:* G. Schiepek [ed.]. Neurobiologie der Psychotherapie. Studienausgabe. Schattauer, Stuttgart, DE. [German]

Bear, M.F., B.W. Connors and M.A. Paradiso. 2016. Neuroscience. Exploring the Brain. 4th Ed. Wolters Kluwer, Philadelphia, USA.

Bechtel, W. 1994. Connectionism. pp. 200-210. *In:* S. Guttenplan [ed.]. A Companion to the Philosophy of Mind. Blackwell Publishers, Oxford, UK, Cambridge, USA.

Bechtel, W. 1988. Connectionism and the philosophy of mind: an overview. *In:* T. Horgan and J. Tienson [eds.]. Spindel Conference 1987: Connectionism and the Philosophy of Mind. The Southern Journal of Philosophy. Special Issue on Connectionism and the Foundations of Cognitive Science. Supplement 26: 17-41. (reprinted in Bechtel, W. 1991.)

Bechtel, W. 1990. Multiple levels of inquiry in cognitive science. Psychological Research 52: 271-281.

Bechtel, W. 1991. Connectionism and the philosophy of mind: an overview. pp. 30-59. *In:* T. Horgan and J. Tienson [eds.]. Connectionism and the Philosophy of Mind. Kluwer Academic Publisher, Dordrecht, NL.

Bechtel, W. 1998. Representations and cognitive explanations: assessing the dynamicist challenge in cognitive science. Cognitive Science 22: 295-318.

Bechtel, W. 2006. Discovering Cell Mechanisms: The Creation of Modern Cell Biology. Cambridge University Press, Cambridge, UK.

Bechtel, W. 2008. Mental Mechanisms: Philosophical Perspectives on Cognitive Neuroscience. Routledge, London, UK.

Bechtel, W. 2009. Constructing a philosophy of science of cognitive science. Topics in Cognitive Science 1: 548-569.

Bechtel, W. and A.A. Abrahamsen. 1991. Connectionism and the Mind: An Introduction to Parallel Processing in Networks. Blackwell Publishers, Oxford, UK.

Bechtel, W. and A.A. Abrahamsen. 1993. Discovering Complexity: Decomposition and Localization as Strategies in Scientific Research. Princeton University Press, Princeton, USA.

Bechtel,W. and G. Graham [eds.]. 1998. A Companion to Cognitive Science. Blackwell Publisher, Malden, USA, Oxford, UK.

Bechtel, W., A. Abrahamsen and G. Graham. 1998. The life of cognitive science. pp. 1-104. *In:* W. Bechtel and G. Graham [eds.]. A Companion to Cognitive Science. Blackwell, Malden, USA, Oxford, UK.

Bechtel,W. and A.A. Abrahamsen. 2002. Connectionism and the Mind: Parallel Processing, Dynamics, and Evolution in Networks. 2nd Ed. Blackwell Publishers, Oxford, UK.

Bechtel, W. and A.A. Abrahamsen. 2005. Explanation: a mechanistic alternative. Studies in History and Philosophy of Biological and Biomedical Sciences 36: 421-441.

Bechtel, W. and M. Herschbach. 2010. Philosophy of the cognitive sciences. pp. 237-261. *In:* F. Allhoff [ed.]. Philosophy of the Sciences. Blackwell, Oxford, UK.

Beckermann, A. 1997. Introduction to Logic. Walter de Gruyter, Berlin, DE, New York, USA. [German]

Beckermann, A. 2008. Analytical Introduction to the Philosophy of Mind. 3. Auflage. De Gruyter, Berlin, DE. [German]

Beer, R.D. 1992a. Intelligence as Adaptive Behavior. An Experiment in Computational Neuroethology. Academic Press, Boston, USA.

Beer, R.D. 1992b. A dynamical systems perspective on autonomous agents. Technical Report CES-92-11, Department of Computer Engineering and Science, Case Western Reserve University, Cleveland, USA.

Beer, R.D. 1995. A dynamical systems perspective on agent-environment interaction. Artificial Intelligence 72: 173-215.

Beer, R.D. 1997. The dynamics of adaptive behavior: a research program. Robotics and Autonomous Systems 20: 257-289.

Beer, R.D. 2000. Dynamical approaches to cognitive science. Trends in Cognitive Sciences 4: 91-99.

Beer, R.D. 2008. The dynamics of brain-body-environment systems: a status report. pp. 99-120. *In:* P. Calvo and A. Gomilla [eds.]. Handbook of Cognitive Science. An Embodied Approach. 1st Ed. Elsevier, Amsterdam, NL.

Beer, R.D. 2014. Dynamical systems and embedded cognition. pp. 128-148. *In:* K. Frankish andW. Ramsey [eds.]. The Cambridge Handbook of Artificial Intelligence. Cambridge University Press, Cambridge, UK.

Bekolay, T., J. Bergstra, E. Hunsberger, T. DeWolf, T.C. Stewart, D. Rasmussen, X. Choo, A.R. Voelker and C. Eliasmith. 2014. Nengo: a python tool for building large-scale functional brain models. Frontiers in Neuroinformatics 7: 48.

Benchenane, K., P.H. Tiesinga and F.P. Battaglia. 2011. Oscillations in the prefrontal cortex: a gateway to memory and attention. Current Opinion in Neurobiology 21: 475-485.

Bengio, Y. 2009. Learning deep architectures for AI. Foundations and Trends in Machine Learning 2: 1-127.

Benker, H. 2003. Mathematical Optimization with Computer Algebra Systems. Introduction for Engineers, Natural Scientists and Economists using MATHEMATICA, MAPLE, MATHCAD, MATLAB and EXEL. Springer. Berlin, DE. [German]

Bennett, M.R. and P.M.S. Hacker. 2008. History of Cognitive Neuroscience. Wiley-Blackwell, Malden, USA.

Berger, A. 2001. Chaos and Chance. An Introduction to Stochastic Aspects of Dynamics. De Gruyter, Berlin, DE, New York, USA.

Berkeley, I.S.N. 1997. Some myths of connectionism. The University of Southwestern Louisiana, Lafayette, USA. [unpublished manuscript]

Berkeley, I.S.N. 2019. The curious case of connectionism. Open Philosophy 2: 190-205.

Bermúdez, J.L. 2014. Cognitive Science. An Introduction to the Science of the Mind. 2nd Ed. Cambridge University Press, Cambridge, UK.

Berwick, R.C., A.D. Friederici, N. Chomsky and J.J. Bolhuis. 2013. Evolution, brain and the nature of language. Trends in Cognitive Sciences 17: 89-98.

Besold, T.R. and K.-U. Kühnberger. 2013a. Connectionism, neural networks and parallel distributed processing. pp. 156-163. *In:* A. Stephan and S. Walter [eds.]. Handbuch Kognitionswissenschaft. Metzler, Stuttgart, Weimar, DE. [German]

Besold, T.R. and K.-U. Kühnberger. 2013b. Hybrid architectures. pp. 170-174. *In:* A. Stephan and S. Walter [eds.]. Handbuch Kognitionswissenschaft. Metzler, Stuttgart, Weimar, DE. [German]

Bhatti, M.A. 2000. Practical Optimization Methods with Mathematical Applications. Springer-Verlag, Berlin, DE.

Bialek, W., F. Rieke, R. de Ruyter van Steveninck and D. Warland. 1991. Reading a neural code. Science 252: 1854-1857.

Bibbig, A., H.J. Faulkner, M.A. Whittington and R.D. Traub. 2001. Self-organized synaptic plasticity contributes to the shaping of gamma and beta oscillations *in vitro*. The Journal of Neuroscience 21: 9054-9056.

Bibbig, A., R.D. Traub and M.A. Whittington. 2002. Long-range synchronization of gamma and beta oscillations and the plasticity of excitatory and inhibitory synapses: a network model. Journal of Neurophysiology 88: 1634-1654.

Bickhard, M.H. and L. Terveen. 1995. Foundational Issues in Artificial Intelligence and Cognitive Science: Impasse and Solution. Elsevier Scientific, New York, USA.

Biederlack, J., M. Castelo, S. Neuenschwander, D.W. Wheeler, W. Singer and D. Nikolić. 2006. Brightness induction: rate enhancement and neuronal synchronization as complementary codes. Neuron 52: 1073-1083.

Bienenstock, E. 1995. A model of neocortex. Network: Computation in Neural Systems 6: 179-224.

Bienenstock, E. 1996. Composition. pp. 269-300. *In:* A. Aertsen and V. Braitenberg [eds.]. Brain Theory – Biological Basis and Computational Theory of Vision. Elsevier, Amsterdam, NL, New York, USA.

Bienenstock, E. and C. von der Malsburg. 1987. A neural network for invariant pattern recognition. Europhysics Letters 4: 121-126.

Bienenstock, E., S. Geman and D. Potter. 1997. Compositionality, MDL priors, and object recognition. pp 838-844. *In:* M.C. Mozer, M.I. Jordan and T. Petsche [eds.]. Advances in Neural Information Processing Systems 9 (NIPS'1996), Denver, United States of America. MIT Press.

Billman, D. 1998. Representations. pp. 649-659. *In:* W. Bechtel and G. Graham [eds.]. A Companion to Cognitive Science. Blackwell Publisher, Malden, USA, Oxford, UK.

Birkhoff, G.D. 1927/1966. Dynamical Systems. 1st Pr. of Rev. Ed. AMS. Providence, USA.

Birkhoff, G. 1936a/1976a. The rise of modern algebra to 1936. pp. 41-63. *In:* J.D. Tarwater, J.T. White and J.D. Miller [eds.]. Men and Institutions in American Mathematics. Texas Tech Press, Lubbock, USA.

Birkhoff, G. 1936b/1976b. The rise of modern algebra, 1936 to 1950. pp. 65-85. *In:* J.D. Tarwater, J.T. White and J.D. Miller [eds.]. Men and Institutions in American Mathematics. Texas Tech Press, Lubbock, USA.

Bishop, R. 2008. Downward causation in fluid convection. Synthese 160: 229-248.

Bishop, R. 2012. Fluid convection, constraint and causation. Interface Focus 2: 4-12.

Bockhorst, T., F. Pieper, G. Engler, T. Stieglitz, E. Galindo-Leon, A.K. Engel. 2018. Synchrony surfacing: epicortical recording of correlated action potentials. European Journal of Neuroscience 48: 3583-3596.

Boden, M.A. 2006. Mind as Machine. A History of Cognitive Science. Clarendon Press, Oxford, UK.

Bogdan, M. 2017. Artificial neural networks and machine learning. Universität Leipzig, Leipzig, DE. [unpublished manuscript] [German]

Boltzmann, L. 1896. Lectures on Gas Theory. Barth Verlag, Leipzig, DE. [German]

Bonnans, J.F., J.C. Gilbert, C. Lemaréchal and C.A. Sagastizábal. 2003. Numerical Optimization. Theoretical and Practical Aspects. Springer-Verlag, Berlin, DE.

Borda, M. 2011. Fundamentals in Information Theory and Coding. Springer-Verlag, Berlin, DE.

Borst, A. and F.E. Theunissen. 1999. Information theory and neural coding. Nature Neuroscience 2: 947-957.

Borst, J.P. and J.R. Anderson. 2015. Using the cognitive architecture ACT-R in combination with fMRI data. pp. 339-352. *In:* B.U. Forstmann and E.-J. Wagenmakers [eds.]. An Introduction to Model-Based Cognitive Neuroscience. Springer, New York, USA.

Bortz, J. 1999. Statistics for Social Scientists. 5th Ed. Springer-Verlag, Berlin, DE. [German]

Bosch, S. 2006. Algebra. 6th Ed. Springer-Verlag. Berlin u.a., DE [German]

Bossert, M., R. Jordan and J. Freudenberger. 2002. Applied Information Theory. Universität Ulm. Ulm, DE. [German]

Bothe, H.-H. 1998. Neuro-fuzzy Methods. Introduction to Theory and Applications. Springer-Verlag, Berlin, DE. [German]

Bovier, A. and V. Gayrard. 1997. Statistical mechanics of neural networks: the Hopfield model and the Kac-Hopfield model. Markov Processes and Related Fields 3: 392-422.

Bowers, J.S. 2009. On the biological plausibilty of grandmother cells: implications for neural network theories in psychology and neuroscience. Psychological Review 116: 220-251.

Bowers, J.S. 2010. More on grandmother cells and the biological implausibility of PDP models of cognition: a reply to Plaut and McClelland (2010) and Quian Quiroga and Kreiman (2010). Psychological Review 117: 300-308.

Bracewell, R. 2000. Heaviside's Unit Step Function, $H(x)$. The Fourier Transform and its Applications. McGraw-Hill, New York, USA.

Bracholdt, S. 2009. Evaluation of cluster procedures. M.Sc. Thesis (Diplomarbeit), Fachbereich Informatik, Hochschule Mittweida, Mittweida, DE. [German]

Braitenberg, V. 1978. Cell assemblies in the cerebral cortex. pp. 171-188. *In:* R. Heim and G. Palm [eds.]. Theoretical Approaches to Complex Systems. Springer-Verlag, Berlin, DE.

Braitenberg, V. 1984. Vehicles. Experiments in Synthetic Psychology. MIT Press, Cambridge, USA.

Brama, H., S. Guberman, M. Abeles, E. Stern and I. Kanter. 2015. Synchronization among neuronal pools without common inputs: *in vivo* study. Brain Structure and Function 220: 3721-3731.

Brandl, J.L. 2013. Philosophy of mind and cognition. pp. 127-132. *In:* A. Stephan and S. Walter [eds.]. Handbuch Kognitionswissenschaft. Metzler, Stuttgart, Weimar, DE. [German]

Branke, J., M. Mnif, C. Müller-Schloer, H. Prothmann, U. Richter, F. Rochner and H. Schmeck. 2006. Organic computing – addressing complexity by controlled self-organization, 185-191. *In* Proceedings of the 2nd International Symposium on Leveraging Applications of Formal Methods, Verification and Validation (ISoLA 2006), Paphos, Cyprus. IEEE Press.

Braun, H., J. Feulner and R. Malaka. 1996. Practical Course Neural Networks. Springer-Verlag. Berlin, DE. [German]

Brause, R. 1995. Neuronal Nets. An Introduction to Neuroinformatics. B.G. Teubner, Stuttgart, DE. [German]

Brecht, M. and A.K. Engel. 1996. Cortico-tectal interactions in the cat visual system. pp. 395-399. *In:* C. von der Malsburg and W. von Seelen [eds.]. International Conference on Artificial Neural Networks (ICANN'96). Bochum, Germany, Springer-Verlag.

Brecht, M., W. Singer and A.K. Engel. 1998. Correlation analysis of corticotectal interactions in the cat visual system. Journal of Neurophysiology 80: 2394-2407.

Brecht, M., W. Singer and A.K. Engel. 1999. Patterns of synchronization in the superior colliculus of anesthetized cats. The Journal of Neuroscience 19: 3567-3579.

Brecht, M., W. Singer and A.K. Engel. 2004. Amplitude and direction of saccadic eye movements depend on the synchronicity of collicular population activity. Journal of Neurophysiology 92: 424-432.

Breedlove, S.M., M.R. Rosenzweig and N.V. Watson. 2017. Biological Psychology. An Introduction to Behavioral, Cognitive, and Clinical Neuroscience. 8th Ed. Sinauer Associates, Sunderland, USA.

Breidbach, O. 1996. Contours of a neurosemantic. pp. 9-29. *In:* G. Rusch, S.J. Schmidt and O. Breidbach [eds.]. Interne Repräsentationen – Neue Konzepteder Hirnforschung. Suhrkamp Verlag, Frankfurt/Main, DE. [German]

Bremer, M. and D. Cohnitz. 2004. Information and Information Flow. An Introduction. Ontos Verlag, Frankfurt am Main, DE.

Bressler, S.L. 2003. Event-related potentials. pp. 412-415. *In:* A. Arbib [ed.]. The Handbook of Brain Theory and Neural Networks. 2nd Ed. The MIT Press, Cambridge, USA, London, UK.

Brette, R. 2012. Computing with neural synchrony. PLoS Computational Biology 8: e1002561.

Briggs, J. and F.D. Peat. 1990. Turbulent Mirror: An Illustrated Guide to Chaos Theory and the Science of Wholeness. HarperCollins, New York, USA.

Brillouin, L. 1962. Science and Information Theory. Academic Press, London, UK.

Brin, M. and G. Stuck. 2002. Introduction to Dynamical Systems. Cambridge University Press, Cambridge, UK.

Bringsjord, S. and Y. Yang. 2003. Representations using formal logics. pp. 940-950. *In:* L. Nadel. [ed.]. Encyclopedia of Cognitive Science. Vol. 3. Natur Publishing Group. London, UK, New York, USA and Tokyo, JP.

Broadbent, D.E. 1958. Perception and Communication. Pergamon Press, Oxford, UK.

Broadbent, D.E. 1971. Cognitive psychology. British Medical Bulletin 27: 191-194.

Brockmeier, A.J., M.K. Hazrati, W.J. Freeman, J. Li, J.C. Principe. 2012. Locating spatial patterns of waveforms during sensory perception in scalp EEG, 2531-2534. *In* 2012 Annual International Conference of the IEEE Engineering in Medicine and Biology Society (EMBC), San Diego, United States of America, Institute of Electrical and Electronics Engineers (IEEE).

Brody, C.D. 1999. Correlations without synchrony. Neural Computation 11: 1537-1551.

Brook, A. [ed.] 2007. The Prehistory of Cognitive Science. Palgrave Macmillan, Basingstoke, UK.

Brooks, R.A. 1986. A robust layered control system for a mobile robot. IEEE Journal of Robotics and Automation 2: 14-23.

Brosch, M., R. Bauer and R. Eckhorn. 1995. Synchronous high-frequency oscillations in cat area 18. European Journal of Neuroscience 7: 86-95.

Brown, E.N., R.E. Kass and P.P. Mitra. 2004. Multiple neural spike train data analysis: state-of-the-art and future challenges. Nature Neuroscience 7: 456-461.

Bruineberg, J., E. Rietveld, T. Parr, L. van Maanen and K.J. Friston. 2018. Free-energy minimization in joint agent-environment systems: a niche construction perspective. Journal of Theoretical Biology 455: 161-178.

Brunel, N. and J.P. Nadal. 1998. Modeling memory: what do we learn from attractor neural networks? pp. 249-252. In Proceedings of Symposium: Memory, from Neuron to Cognition, Paris, France.

Bruner, J.S. 1957. On perceptual readiness. Psychological Review 64: 123-152.

Bruner, J.S., R.R. Olver, P.M. Greenfield et al. 1967. Studies in Cognitive Growth. Wile, New York, USA.

Brunet, N., M. Vinck, C.A. Bosman, W. Singer and P. Fries. 2014. Gamma or no gamma, that is the question. Trends in Cognitive Sciences 18: 507-509.

Bublak, P. and K. Finke. 2013. Neuropsychology. pp. 105-109. In: A. Stephan and S. Walter [eds.]. Handbuch Kognitionswissenschaft. Metzler, Stuttgart,Weimar, DE. [German]

Bucher, T.G. 1998. Introduction to Applied Logic. 2nd Ext. Ed. Walter de Gruyter, Berlin, DE, New York, USA. [German]

Buckner, C. and J. Garson. 2019. Connectionism. In: E.N. Zalta [ed.]. The Stanford Encyclopedia of Philosophy (Aug 16, 2019 Edition).

Büchel, C., H.-O. Karnath and P. Thier. 2012. Methods of cognitive neurosciences. pp. 9-34. In: H.-O. Karnath and P. Thier [eds.]. Kognitive Neurowissenschaften. 3rd Ed. Springer-Verlag, Heidelberg, DE. [German]

Büsing, L., J. Bill, B. Nessler and W. Maass. 2011. Neural dynamics as sampling: a model for stochastic computation in recurrent networks of spiking neurons. PLoS Computational Biology 7: e1002211.

Bullmore, E.T. and O. Sporns. 2012. The economy of brain network organization. Nature Review Neurosciences 13: 336-349.

Bunge, M. 1979. Treatise on Basic Philosophy. Vol. 4. Ontology II: A World of Systems. Reidel, Dordrecht, NE.

Burg, K., H. Haf, F. Wille and A. Meister. 2009. Higher Mathematics for Engineers. Volume III: Ordinary Differential Equations, Distributions, Integral Transformations. 5th Ed. Vieweg+Teubner, Wiesbaden, DE [German]

Burke Hubbard, B. 1997. Wavelets: The Mathematics of Small Waves. 1st Ed. Birkhäuser Verlag, Basel, CH. [German]

Burns, S.P., D. Xing, M.J. Shelley and R.M. Shapley. 2010. Searching for autocoherence in the cortical network with a time-frequency analysis of the local field potential. The Journal of Neuroscience 30: 4033-4047.

Burris, S. and H.P. Sankappanavar 1981/2012. A Course in Universal Algebra. University of Waterloo, CA.

Burrus, C.S., R.A. Gopinath and H. Guo. 1998. Introduction to Wavelets and Wavelet Transforms. A Primer. Prentice-Hall, Upper Saddle River, USA.

Burwick, T. 2014. The binding problem. WIREs Cognitive Science 5: 305-315.

Buzsáki, G. 2006. Rhythms of the Brain. Oxford University Press, Oxford, UK, New York, USA.

Buzsáki, G. 2019. The Brain from Inside Out. Oxford University Press, New York, USA.

Buzsáki, G., N. Logothetis and W. Singer. 2013. Scaling brain size, keeping timing: evolutionary preservation of brain rhythms. Neuron 80: 751-764.

Buzsáki, G. and W. Freeman. [eds.] 2015. SI: brain rhythms and dynamic coordination. Current Opinion in Neurobiology 31: 1-264.

Byrne, Á., D. Avitabile and S. Coombes. 2019. A next generation neural field model: the evolution of synchrony within patterns and waves. Physical Review E 99: 012313.

Calvo, P. and T. Gomila. [eds.] 2008. Handbook of Cognitive Science. An Embodied Approach. 1st Ed. Elsevier, Amsterdam, NL.

Calvo, P. and J. Symons [eds.] 2014. The Architecture of Cognition. Rethinking Fodor and Pylyshyn's Systematicity Challenge. MIT Press, Cambridge, USA, London, UK.

Calvo Garzón, F. 2003. Connectionist semantics and the collateral information challenge. Mind & Language 18: 77-94.

Calvo Garzón, F. 2008. Towards a general theory of antirepresentationalism. British Journal for the Philosophy of Science 59: 259-292.

Camazine, S. 2003. Self-organizing systems. pp. 1059-1062. In: L. Nadel [ed.]. Encyclopedia of Cognitive Science. Vol. 3. Natur Publishing Group. London, UK, New York, USA and Tokyo, JP.

Cao, R. 2010. Extended liquid computing in networks of spiking neurons. Report, Department of Neurophysiology, Max-Planck-Institute for Brain Research, Frankfurt/Main, DE: 19pp.

Capurro, R. 1978. Information. A Contribution to the Etymological and Historical Justification of the Concept of Information. Verlag Sauer, München, DE. [German]

Capurro, R. 1996. On the genealogy of information. pp. 259-270. *In:* K. Kornwachs and K. Jacoby [eds.]. Information: New Questions to a Multidisciplinary Concept. Akademie Verlag, Berlin, DE.

Capurro, R. 2000. Introduction to the Concept of Information. [unpublished manuscript] [German]

Capurro, R. and B. Hjørland. 2003. The concept of information. Annual Review of Information Science and Technology 37: 343-411.

Carpenter, G.A. 2011. Adaptive resonance theory. pp. 23-36. *In:* C. Sammut and G.I. Webb [eds.]. Encyclopedia of Machine Learning. Springer Science + Business Media, New York, USA.

Carpenter, G.A. and S. Grossberg. 1987a. A massively parallel architecture for a self-organizing neural pattern recognition machine. Computer Vision, Graphics, and Image Processing 37: 54-115.

Carpenter, G.A. and S. Grossberg. 1987b. ART 2: stable self-organization of pattern recognition codes for analog input patterns. Applied Optics 26: 4919-4930.

Carpenter, G.A. and S. Grossberg. 1988. The ART of adaptive pattern recognition by a self-organizing neural network. Computer 21: 77-88.

Carpenter, G.A. and S. Grossberg. 1990a. Self-organizing neural network architectures for real-time adaptive pattern recognition. pp. 455-478. *In:* S.F. Zornetzer, J. Davis and C. Lau [eds.]. An Introduction to Neural and Electronic Networks. Academic Press, San Diego, USA.

Carpenter, G.A. and S. Grossberg. 1990b. Adaptive resonance theory. Neural network architectures for self-organizing pattern recognition. pp. 383-389. *In:* R. Eckmiller, G. Hartmann and G. Hauske [eds.]. Parallel Processing in Neural Systems and Computers. Elsevier Science Inc., Amsterdam, NL.

Carpenter, G.A. and S. Grossberg. 1990c. ART 3: hierarchical search using chemical transmitters in self-organizing pattern recognition architectures. Neural Networks 3: 129-152.

Carpenter, G.A. and S. Grossberg. 1991. Pattern Recognition by Self-Organizing Neural Networks. MIT Press, Cambridge, USA.

Carpenter, G.A., S. Grossberg and D.B. Rosen. 1991a. Fuzzy ART: fast stable learning and categorization of analog patterns by an adaptive resonance system. Neural Networks 4: 759-771.

Carpenter, G.A., S. Grossberg and D.B. Rosen. 1991b. ART 2-A: an adaptive resonance algorithm for rapid category learning and recognition. Neural Networks 4: 493-504.

Carpenter, G.A., S. Grossberg and D.B. Rosen. 1991c. A neural network realization of fuzzy ART. Technical Report, CAS/CNS-91-021, Boston University Boston, USA: 16pp.

Carpenter, G.A., S. Grossberg and J.H. Reynolds. 1991d. ARTMAP: supervised realtime learning and classification of nonstationary data by a self-organizing neural network. Neural Networks 4: 565-588.

Carpenter, G.A. and S. Grossberg. 2002. A self-organizing neural network for supervised learning, recognition, and prediction. pp. 289-314. *In:* T.A. Polk and C.M. Seifert [eds.]. Cognitive Modeling. MIT Press, Cambridge, USA.

Carpenter, G.A. and S. Grossberg. 2003. Adaptive resonance theory. pp. 87-90. *In:* A. Arbib [ed.]. The Handbook of Brain Theory and Neural Networks. 2*nd* Ed. The MIT Press, Cambridge, USA, London, UK.

Cassenaer, S. and G. Laurent. 2007. Hebbian STDP in mushroom bodies facilitates the synchronous flow of olfactory information. Nature 448: 709-713.

Castelo-Branco, M., S. Neuenschwander and W. Singer. 1998. Synchronization of visual responses between the cortex, lateral geniculate nucleus, and retina in the anesthetized cat. The Journal of Neuroscience 18: 6395-6410.

Casti, J.L. 1977. Dynamical System and their Applications. Linear Theory. Academic Press, New York, USA.

Casti, J.L. 1985. Nonlinear System Theory. Academic Press, Orlando, USA, London, UK.

Cha, S.-H. 2007. Comprehensive survey on distance/similarity measures between probability density functions. International Journal of Mathematical Models and Methods in Applied Sciences 4: 300-307.

Chaitin, G.J. 1975. Randomness and mathematical proof. Scientific American 232: 47-52.

Chalmers, D.J. 1993. Connectionism and compositionality: why Fodor and Pylyshyn were wrong. Philosophical Psychology 6: 305-319.

Chalmers, D. 1995. Facing up to the problem of consciousness. Journal of Consciousness Studies 2: 200-219.

Chapman, B., K.R. Zahs and M.P. Stryker. 1991. Relation of cortical cell orientation selectivity to alignment of receptive fields of the geniculocortical afferents that arborize within a single orientation column in ferret visual cortex. Journal of Neuroscience 11: 1347-1358.

Charniak, E. 2019. Introduction to Deep Learning. The MIT Press, Cambridge, USA.

Chemero, A. 2011. Radical Embodied Cognitive Science. MIT Press. Cambridge, USA.

Chemero, A. and M. Silberstein 2008. After the philosophy of mind: replacing scholasticism with science. Philosophy of Science 75; 1-27.

Chen, K., Q. Huang, H. Palangi, P. Smolensky, K.D. Forbus and J. Gao. 2019. Natural- to formal-language generation using tensor product representations.

In Thirty-Third Conference on Neural Information Processing Systems (NeurIPS'2019), Vancouver, Canada.

Chen, K., Q. Huang, H. Palangi, P. Smolensky, K.D. Forbus and J. Gao. 2020. Mapping natural-language problems to formal-language solutions using structured neural representations. *In* Proceedings of the 37th International Conference on Machine Learning, Vienna, Austria.

Chervin, R.D., P.A. Pierce and B.W. Connors. 1988. Periodicity and directionality in the propagation of epileptiform discharges across neortex. Journal of Neurophysiology 60: 16951713.

Chomsky, N. 1957. Syntactic Structures. Mouton Publishers, Den Haag, NL, Paris, FR.

Chomsky, N. 1965. Aspects of the Theory of Syntax. MIT Press, Cambridge, USA.

Chomsky, N. 1968. Language and Mind. Harcourt, Brace and World, New York, USA.

Chomsky, N. 1980. Rules and representations. Behavioral and Brain Sciences 3: 1-62.

Chomsky, N. 2013. Problems of projection. Lingua 130: 33-49.

Chrisley, R.L. 2000. Fluid architecture: connectionist systematicity. [unpublished manuscript] From: https://www.researchgate.net/publication/2353715.

Chrisley, R. and T. Ziemke.2003. Embodiment. pp. 1102-1108. *In:* L. Nadel. [ed.]. Encyclopedia of Cognitive Science. Vol. 1. Natur Publishing Group. London, UK, New York, USA and Tokyo, JP.

Chu, D., R. Strand and R. Fjelland. 2003. Theories of complexity. Common denominators of complex systems. Complexity 8: 19-30.

Churchland, P.M. 1989. A Neurocomputational Perspective: The Nature of Mind and the Structure of Science. The MIT Press, Bradford Books, Cambridge, USA.

Churchland, P.M. 1995. The Engine of Reason, the Seat of the Soul. MIT Press, Cambridge, USA.

Churchland, P.M. 2007. Neurophilosophy at Work. Cambridge University Press, New York, USA.

Clark, A. 1989. Microcognition: Philosophy, Cognitive Science, and Parallel Distributed Processing. A Bradford Book. The MIT Press, Cambridge, USA, London, UK.

Clark, A. 1992. The presence of a symbol. Connection Science 4: 193-205.

Clark, A. 1993. Associative Engines. Connectionism, Concepts, and Representational Change. The MIT Press, Cambridge, USA, London, UK.

Clark, A. 1997a. Being there: Putting Brain, Body and World together again. MIT Press, Cambridge, USA.

Clark, A. 1997b. The dynamical challenge. Cognitive Science 21: 461-481.

Clark, A. 1998. Embodied, situated, and distributed cognition. pp. 506-517. *In:* W. Bechtel and G. Graham [eds.]. A Companion to Cognitive Science. Blackwell Publisher, Malden, USA, Oxford, UK.

Clark, A. 1999. An embodied cognitive science? Trends in Cognitive Science 3: 345-351.

Clark, A. 2001. Mindware. An Introduction to the Philosophy of Cognitive Science. Oxford University Press, New York, USA, Oxford, UK.

Clark, A. 2008. Supersizing the Mind. Embodiment, Action, and Cognitive Extension. Oxford University Press, Oxford, UK.

Clark, A. 2013. Whatever next? Predictive brains, situated agents, and the future of cognitive science. Behavioral and Brain Sciences 36: 181-204.

Clark, A. 2015. Radical predictive processing. The Southern Journal of Philosophy 53: 3-27.

Clark, A. and D.J. Chalmers. 1998. The extended mind. Analysis 58: 7-19.

Clark, J.W. 1988. Statistical mechanics of neural networks. Physics Reports 158: 91-157.

Cleeremans, A. [ed.] 2003. The Unity of Consciousness: Binding, Integration, and Dissociation. Oxford University Press, Oxford, UK.

Cohen, M.A. and S. Grossberg. 1983. Absolute stability of global pattern formation and parallel memory storage by competitive neural networks. IEEE Transactions on Systems, Man, and Cybernetics 13: 815-826.

Cohen-Tannoudji, C., B. Diu and F. Laloë. 2010. Quantum Mechanics. Vol. 2. 4th Ed. Walter de Gruyter, Berlin, DE, New York, USA. [German]

Conklin, J. and C. Eliasmith. 2005. An attractor network model of path integration in the rat. Journal of Computational Neuroscience 18: 183-203.

Coolen, A.C.C. 2001a. Statistical Mechanics of Recurrent Neural Networks I – Statics. pp. 553-618. *In:* F. Moss and S. Gielen [eds.]. Handbook of Biological Physics. Vol. 4. Neuro-Informatics and Neural Modelling. Gulf Professional Publishing, Elsevier, Houston, USA.

Coolen, A.C.C. 2001b. Statistical Mechanics of Recurrent Neural Networks II – Dynamics. pp. 619-684. *In:* F. Moss and S. Gielen [eds.]. Handbook of Biological Physics. Vol. 4. Neuro-Informatics and Neural Modelling. Gulf Professional Publishing, Elsevier, Houston, USA.

Coombes, S. 2005. Waves, humps, and patterns in neural field theories. Biological Cybernetics 91: 93108.

Coombes, S., P. Beim Graben, R. Potthast and J.J. Wright [eds.] 2014. Neural Fields: Theory and Applications. Springer, Berlin, DE, Heidelberg, DE.

Copeland, B.J. [ed.] 2004. The Essential Turing: Seminal Writings in Computing, Logic, Philosophy, Artificial Intelligence, and Artificial Life plus The Secrets of Enigma. Clarendon Press, Oxford University Press, Oxford, UK.

Cosmelli, D., J.-P. Lachaux and E. Thompson. 2007. Neurodynamics of consciousness. pp. 729-770. *In:* P.D. Telazo, M. Moscovitch and E. Thompson [eds.]. The Cambridge Handbook of Consciousness. Chapter 26. Cambridge University Press, Cambridge, UK.

Cottrell, G.W. 2003. Attractor networks. pp. 253-262. *In:* L. Nadel. [ed.]. Encyclopedia of Cognitive Science. Vol. 1. Natur Publishing Group. London, UK, New York, USA and Tokyo, JP.

Cottrell, G.W. 2016. Computational Cognitive Neuroscience (CCNBook). Wiki Textbook. 3rd (partial) Ed.

Cover, T.M. and J.A. Thomas. 2006. Elements of Information Theory. 2nd Ed. Wiley-Interscience, Hoboken, USA.

Craver, C.F. 2007. Explaining the Brain. Mechanisms and the Mosaic Unity of Neuroscience. Oxford University Press, Oxford, UK.

Craver, C.F. and W. Bechtel. 2006. Mechanism and mechanistic explanation. *In:* S. Sarkar and J. Pfeifer [eds.]. Philosophy of Science: An Encyclopedia. Routledge, New York, USA.

Craver, C.F. and L. Darden. 2013. In Search of Mechanisms. Discoveries across the Life Sciences. University of Chicago, Chicago, USA, London, UK.

Crick, F. and C. Koch. 1990. Towards a neurobiological theory of consciousness. Seminars in the Neurosciences 2: 263-275.

Crick, F. and C. Koch. 2003. A framework for consciousness. Nature Neuroscience 6: 119-126.

Csicsvari, J., D.A. Henze, B. Jamieson, K.D. Harris, A. Sirota, P. Barthó, K.D. Wise and G. Buzsáki. 2003. Massively parallel recording of unit and local field potentials with silicon-based electrodes. Journal of Neurophysiology 90: 1314-1323.

Cummins, R. 1975. Functional analysis. Journal of Philosophy 72: 741-764.

Cummins, R. 1983. The Nature of Psychological Explanation. MIT Press, Cambridge, USA and London, UK.

Cutland, N.J. 1980. Computability: An Introduction to Recursive Function Theory. Cambridge University Press, Cambridge.

Dalenoort, G.J. 1989a. The paradigm of self-organization: studies of autonomous systems. pp. 1-22. *In:* G.J. Dalenoort [ed.]. The Paradigm of Self-Organization. Current Trends in Self-Organization. Gordon & Breach Science Publishers, Yverdon, CH.

Dalenoort, G.J. 1989b. Mechanisms of self-organization. pp. 298-308. *In:* G.J. Dalenoort [ed.]. The Paradigm of Self-Organization. Current Trends in Self-Organization. Gordon & Breach Science Publishers, Yverdon, CH.

Dalenoort, G.J. [ed.] 1989c. The Paradigm of Self-Organization. Current Trends in Self-Organization. Gordon & Breach Science Publishers, Yverdon, CH.

Daugman, J. 2013. Information theory and coding. Computer science tripos, Part II. Michaelmas Term 2013/14. Lecture notes and exercises. Cambridge University, Cambridge, UK. [unpublished manuscript]

Davalo, E. and P. Naït. 1991. Neural Networks. MacMillan, London, UK.

Davis, J.J., R. Kozma and W.J. Freeman. 2013. Neurophysiological evidence of the cognitive cycle and the emergence of awareness. pp. 149-157. *In:* A. Daigaku [ed.]. International Joint Conference on Awareness Science and Technology and Ubi-Media Computing (iCAST-UMEDIA), Aizuwakamatsu, Japan. Institute of Electrical and Electronics Engineers (IEEE).

Dawson, M.R.W. 2001. Understanding Cognitive Science. Blackwell Publishers, Malden, USA, Oxford, UK.

Dawson, M.R.W. 2003. Computer modeling of cognition: levels of analysis. pp. 635-638. *In:* L. Nadel [ed.]. Encyclopedia of Cognitive Science. Vol. 1. Natur Publishing Group. London, UK, New York, USA, and Tokyo, JP.

Dawson, M.R.W. and D.A. Medler. 2010. Alberta's Dictionary of Cognitive Science.

Dayan, P., G.E. Hinton and R.M. Neal. 1995. The Helmholtz machine. Neural Computation 7: 889-904.

Dayan, P. and G.E. Hinton. 1996. Varieties of Helmholtz machines. Neural Networks 9: 1385-1403.

Dayan, P. and L.F. Abbott. 2001. Theoretical Neuroscience. Computational and Mathematical Modeling of Neural Systems. The MIT Press, Cambridge, USA, London, UK.

Debener, S., C.S. Herrmann, C. Kranczioch, D. Gembris and A.K. Engel. 2003. Top-Down attentional processing enhances auditory evoked gamma band activity. Neuroreport 14: 683-686.

deCharms, R.C. and M.M. Merzenich. 1996. Primary cortical representation of sounds by the coordination of action-potential timing. Nature 381: 610-612.

Dechter, R. 1999. Constraint satisfaction. pp. 195-197. *In:* R.A. Wilson and F.C. Keil [eds.]. The MIT Encyclopedia of the Cognitive Sciences. The MIT Press, Cambridge, USA, London, UK.

Dechter, R. and F. Rossi. 2003. Constraint satisfaction. pp. 793-800. *In:* L. Nadel [ed.]. Encyclopedia of Cognitive Science. Vol. 1. Natur Publishing Group. London, UK, New York, USA and Tokyo, JP.

Deco, G., G. Tononi, M. Boly and M.L. Kringelbach. 2015. Rethinking segregation and integration: contributions of whole-brain modelling. Nature Reviews Neuroscience 16: 430-439.

Dekkers, R. 2017. Applied Systems Theory. 2nd Ed. Springer International Publishing, Cham, CH.

Delörme, A., L. Perrinet and S.J. Thorpe. 2001. Networks of integrate-and-fire neurons using rank order coding B: spike timing dependent plasticity and emergence of orientation selectivity. Neurocomputing. Vol. 38: 539-545.

Denis, M. 2004. Representation. pp. 321-323. *In:* O. Houdé [ed.]. Dictionary of Cognitive Science. Neuroscience, Psychology, Artificial Intelligence, Linguistic, and Philosophy. Psychology Press, New York, USA, Hove, UK.

Dennett, D.C. 1978. Brainstorms. Philosophical Essays on Mind and Psychology. MIT Press, Cambridge, USA.

Dennett, D.C. 1990. Quining qualia. pp. 519-547. *In:* W.G. Lycan [ed.]. Mind and Cognition. A Reader. Blackwell, Oxford, UK.

Der, R. and J.M. Herrmann. 2002. Script dynamical systems and autonomous agents. Part I: theory of dynamical systems. Institute for Informatics, University of Leipzig, Leipzig, DE. [unpublished manuscript]

Derthick, M. 1990. Mundane reasoning by settling on a plausible model. Artificial Intelligence 46: 107-158.

Desimone, R., T.D. Albright, C.G. Gross and C. Bruce. 1984. Stimulus-selective properties of inferior temporal neurons in the macaque. The Journal of Neuroscience 4: 2051-2062.

Desimone, R. and L.G. Ungerlieder. 1989. Neural mechanisms of visual processing in monkeys. pp. 267-299. *In:* F. Boller and J. Grafman [eds.]. Handbook of Neuropsychology. Vol. 2. Chap. 1. Elsevier, Amsterdam, NL.

Devaney, R.L. 1994. An Introduction to Chaotic Dynamical Systems. 2nd Ed. Addison-Wesley, New York, USA.

Diesmann, M., M.-O. Gewaltig and A. Aertsen. 1996. Characterization of synfire activity by propagating pulse packets. pp. 59-64. *In:* J.M. Bower [ed.]. Computational Neuroscience: Trends in Research 1995. Academic Press, San Diego, USA.

Diesmann, M., M.-O. Gewaltig and A. Aertsen. 1999. Stable propagation of synchronous spiking in cortical neural networks. Nature 402: 529-533.

Diesmann, M., M.-O. Gewaltig, S. Rotter and A. Aertsen. 2001. State space analysis of synchronous spiking in cortical neural networks. Neurocomputing 38-40: 565-571.

Dietrich, E. 1999. Algorithm. pp. 11-12. *In:* R.A. Wilson and F.C. Keil [eds.]. The MIT Encyclopedia of the Cognitive Sciences. The MIT Press, Cambridge, USA, London, UK.

Dieudonné, J.A. 1970. The work of Nicolas Bourbaki. American Mathematical Monthly 77: 134-145.

Dilger, W. 2003/2004. Neurocognition. Lecture manuscript. Technische Universität Chemnitz, Chemnitz, DE. [unpublished manuscript] [German]

Dinsmore, J. 1992. Thunder in the gap. pp. 1-23. *In:* J. Dinsmore [ed.]. The Symbolic and Connectionist Paradigms: Closing the Gap. Lawrence Erlbaum Associates, Publishers, Hillsdale, USA.

Dixon, J.A., J.G. Holden, D. Mirman and D.G. Stephen 2012. Multifractal dynamics in the emergence of cognitive structure. Topics in Cognitive Science 4: 51-62.

Dolan, C.P. and P. Smolensky. 1989a. Implementing a connectionist production system using tensor products. pp. 265-272. *In:* D. Touretzky, G.E. Hinton and T.J. Sejnowski [eds.]. Proceedings of the 1988 Connectionist Models Summer School, San Mateo, United States of America. Morgan Kaufmann.

Dolan, C.P. and P. Smolensky. 1989b. Tensor product production system: a modular architecture and representation. Connection Science 1: 53-68.

Dominey, P.F. 1995. Complex sensory-motor sequence learning based on recurrent state representation and reinforcement learning. Biological Cybernetics 73: 265-274.

Dominey, P.F., M. Hoen, J.-M. Blanc and T. Lelekov-Boissard. 2003. Neurological basis of language and sequential cognition: evidence from simulation, aphasia, and ERP studies. Brain and Language 86: 207-225.

Dominey, P.F., M. Hoen and T. Inui. 2006. A neurolinguistic model of grammatical construction processing. Journal of Cognitive Neuroscience 18: 2088-2107.

Dong, Y., S. Mihalas, F. Qiu, R. von der Heydt and E. Niebur. 2008. Synchrony and the binding problem in macaque visual cortex. Journal of Vision 8: 1-16.

Dorffner, G. 1991. Connectionism. From Neural Networks to a "Natural" AI. B.G. Teubner, Stuttgart, DE. [German]

Dorffner, G. 1997. Radical connectionism – a neural bottom-up approach to AI. pp. 93-132. *In:* G. Dorffner [ed.]. Neural Networks and a New Artificial Intelligence. International Thomson Computer Press, London, UK, Boston, USA.

Doursat, R. and J. Petitot. 2005. Dynamical systems and cognitive linguistics: toward an active morphodynamical semantics. Neural Networks 18: 628-638.

Dreyfus, H.L. and S.E. Dreyfus. 1986. Mind over Machine: The Power of Human Intuition and Expertise in the Era of the Computer. Basil Blackwell, Oxford, UK.

Duch, W. 1994. A solution to the fundamental problems of cognitive sciences. UMK – KMK – TR 1/94 Report, Nicholas Copernicus University, Toruń, PL: 16pp.

Dürscheid, C. 2005. Syntax. Foundations and Theories. 3rd Ed. Westdeutscher Verlag, Wiesbaden, DE. [German]

Dummit, D.S. and R.M. Foote. 2004. Abstract Algebra. 3rd Ed. Wiley, New York, USA.

Duncan, J. and G. Humphreys. 1989. Visual search and stimulus similarity. Psychological Review 96: 433-458.

Dupuy, J.-P. 2009. On the Origins of Cognitive Science. The Mechanization of the Mind. MIT Press, Cambridge, USA.

Dyer, M.G. 1991. Connectionism versus symbolism in high-level cognition. pp. 382-416. *In:* T. Horgan and J. Tienson [eds.]. Connectionism and the Philosophy of Mind. Kluwer Academic Publisher, Dordrecht, NL.

Ebeling, W. 1982. Physics of Self-Organization and Evolution. Akademie-Verlag, Berlin, DDR. [German]

Ebeling, W. 1989. Chaos – Order – Information. Self-Organization in Nature and Technology. Verlag Harri Deutsch, Frankfurt am Main, DE. [German]

Ebeling, W., H. Engel and H. Herzel. 1990. Self-Organization in Time. Akademie-Verlag, Berlin, DDR. [German]

Ebeling, W., J. Freund and F. Schweitzer. 1995. Entropy – Information – Complexity. SFB 230. Universität Tübingen, Stuttgart, DE. [German]

Ebeling, W., J. Freund and F. Schweitzer. 1998. Complex Structures: Entropy and Information. Teubner Verlag. Stuttgart, Leipzig, DE. [German]

Eckhorn, R., R. Bauer, W. Jordan, M. Brosch, M. Kruse, M. Munk and H.J. Reitboeck. 1988. Coherent oszillations: a mechanism for feature linking in the visual cortex? Multiple electrode and correlations analyses in the cat. Biological Cybernetics 60: 121-130.

Eckhorn, R., H.J. Reitboeck, M. Arndt and P. Dicke. 1989. A neural network for feature linking via synchronous activity: results from cat visual cortex and from simulations. pp. 255-272. *In:* R.M.J. Cotterill [ed.]. Models of Brain Function. Cambridge University Press, Cambridge, UK.

Eckhorn, R., T. Schanze, M. Brosch,W. Salem and R. Bauer. 1992. Stimulus-specific synchronisations in cat visual cortex: multiple microelectrode and correlation studies from several cortical areas. pp. 47-80. *In:* E. Başar and T. Bullock [eds.]. Induced Rhythms in the Brain. Springer-Verlag, New York, USA.

Eckhorn, R., A. Bruns, M. Saam, A. Gail, A. Gabriel and H.J. Brinksmeyer. 2001. Flexible cortical gammaband correlations suggest neural principles of visual processing. Visual Cognition 8: 519-530.

Eckhorn, R., A. Gail, A. Bruns, A. Gabriel, B. Al-Shaikhli and M. Saam. 2007. Phase coupling supports associative visual processing – Physiology and related models. Chaos and Complexity Letters 2: 169-187.

Edelman, G.M. 1987. Neural Darwinism: The Theory of Neuronal Group Selection. Basic Books, New York, USA.

Edelman, G.M. and G. Tononi. 2000. A Universe of Consciousness: How Matter Becomes Imagination. Basic Books, New York, USA.

Egan, F. 2012. Representationalism. pp. 250-272. In: E. Margolis, R. Samuels and S. Stich [eds.]. The Oxford Handbook of Philosophy of Cognitive Science. Oxford University Press, Oxford, UK.

Eguchi, A., J.B. Isbister, N. Ahmad and S. Stringer. 2018. The emergence of polychronization and feature binding in a spiking neural network model of the primate ventral visual system. Psychological Review 125: 545-571.

Eigen, M. 1971. Molecular self-organization and the early stages of evolution. Quarterly Reviews of Biophysics 4: 149-212.

Eigen, M. and P. Schuster. 1977. The hypercycle. A principle of natural self-organization. Part A: emergence of the hypercycle. Naturwissenschaften 64: 541-565.

Eigen, M. and P. Schuster. 1979. The Hypercycle. A Principle of Natural Self-organization. Springer-Verlag, Berlin, Heidelberg, DE.

Eilenberger, G. 1990. Complexity. A new paradigm in the natural sciences. pp. 71-134. In: H. von Ditfurth and E.P. Fischer [eds.]. Mannheimer Forum 1989/90. Ein Panorama der Naturwissenschaften. Piper, M"unchen, DE. [German]

Einsiedler, M. and T. Ward. 2011. Ergodic Theory with a View towards Number Theory. Springer-Verlag, London, UK.

Eliasmith, C. 1995. Mind as a dynamical system. M.A. Thesis, Faculty of Philosophy, University of Waterloo. Ontario, CA.

Eliasmith, C. 1996. The third contender: a critical examination of the dynamicist theory of cognition. Philosophical Psychology 9: 441-463. (reprinted in Eliasmith 1998a.)

Eliasmith, C. 1997. Structure without symbols: providing a distributed account of low-level and high-level cognition, 3-6. In The 89th Annual Meeting of the Southern Society for Philosophy and Psychology, Atlanta, United States of America.

Eliasmith, C. 1998a. The third contender: a critical examination of the dynamicist theory of cognition. pp. 303-336. In: P. Thagard [ed.]. Mind Readings: Introductory Selections in Cognitive Science. MIT Press. Cambridge, USA.

Eliasmith, C. 1998b. Dynamical models and van Gelder's dynamicism: two different things. Commentary. *In:* T. van Gelder: The Dynamical Hypothesis in Cognitive Science. Bahavioral and Brain Sciences 21: 615-628.

Eliasmith, C. 2002. The myth of the Turing machine: the failing of functionalism and related theses. Journal of Experimental & Theoretical Artificial Intelligence 14: 1-8.

Eliasmith, C. 2003. Neural engineering. Unraveling the complexities of neural systems. IEEE Canadian Review 43: 13-15.

Eliasmith, C. 2005. A unified approach to building and controlling spiking attractor networks. Neural Computation 17: 1276-1314.

Eliasmith, C. 2007. Computational neuroscience. pp. 313-338. *In:* P. Thagard [ed.]. Philosophy of Psychology and Cognitive Science. Elsevier, Amsterdam, NE.

Eliasmith, C. 2009. Neurocomputational models. Theory and applications. pp. 346-369. *In:* J. Bickle [ed.]. Oxford Handbook of Philosophy of Neuroscience. Oxford University Press, Oxford, UK.

Eliasmith, C. 2010. How we ought to describe computation in the brain. Studies in History and Philosophy of Science 41: 313-320.

Eliasmith, C. 2012. The complex systems approach: rhetoric or revolution. Topics in Cognitive Science 4: 7277.

Eliasmith, C. 2013. How to Build a Brain. A Neural Architecture for Biological Cognition. Oxford University Press, Oxford, UK.

Eliasmith, C. 2015. On the eve of artificial minds. pp. 1-17. *In*: T. Metzinger and J.M. Windt [eds.]. Open MIND. MIND Group, Frankfurt am Main, DE.

Eliasmith, C., M.B. Westover and C.H. Anderson. 2002. A general framework for neurobiological modeling: an application to the vestibular system. Neurocomputing 46: 1071-1076.

Eliasmith, C. and C.H. Anderson. 2003. Neural Engineering: Computation, Representation, and Dynamics in Neurobiological Systems. MIT Press, Cambridge, USA.

Eliasmith, C. and W. Bechtel. 2003. Symbolic versus subsymbolic. pp. 288-295. *In:* L. Nadel. [ed.]. Encyclopedia of Cognitive Science. Vol. 4. Natur Publishing Group. London, UK, New York, USA and Tokyo, JP.

Eliasmith, C., T.C. Stewart, X. Choo, T. Bekolay, T. DeWolf, Y. Tang and D. Rasmussen. 2012. A Large-Scale Model of the Functioning Brain. Science 338: 1202-1205.

Eliasmith, C. and O. Trujillo. 2013. The use and abuse of large-scale brain models. Current Opinion in Neurobiology 25: 1-6.

Eliasmith, C., J. Gosmann and X. Choo. 2016. BioSpaun: a large-scale behaving brain model with complex neurons. arXiv: 1602.05220.

El-Laithy, K. and M. Bogdan. 2009. Synchrony state generation in artificial neural networks with stochastic synapses. pp. 181-190. *In:* C. Alippi, M.M. Polycarpou, C.G. Panayiotou and G. Ellinas [eds.]. Proceedings of the 19th International Conference, Artificial Neural Networks (ICANN 2009), Part I, Limassol, Cyprus. Springer.

El-Laithy, K. and M. Bogdan. 2010a. Predicting spike-timing of a thalamic neuron using a stochastic synaptic model. pp. 357-362. *In:* M. Verleysen [ed.]. Proceedings of the 18th European Symposium on Artificial Neural Networks, Computational Intelligence and Machine Learning (ESANN 2010), Bruges, Belgium.

El-Laithy, K. and M. Bogdan. 2010b. A Hebbian-based reinforcement learning framework for spike-timing-dependent synapses. pp. 160-169. *In:* K. Diamantaras, W. Duch and L.S. Iliadis [eds.]. Proceedings of the 20th International Conference on Artificial Neural Networks (ICANN'2010), Part II, Thessaloniki, Greece. Springer.

El-Laithy, K. and M. Bogdan. 2011a. Synchrony state generation: an approach using stochastic synapses. Journal of Artificial Intelligence and Soft Computing Research 1: 17-25.

El-Laithy, K. and M. Bogdan. 2011b. A hypothetical free synaptic energy function and related states of synchrony. pp. 40-47. *In:* T. Honkela [ed.]. Proceedings of the 21th International Conference on Artificial Neural Networks and Machine Learning (ICANN'2011), Part II, Espoo, Finland. Springer.

El-Laithy, K. and M. Bogdan. 2011c. A reinforcement learning framework for spiking networks with dynamic synapses. Journal of Computational Intelligence and Neuroscience 2011: 10.1155/2011/869348.

El-Laithy, K. and M. Bogdan. 2011d. On the capacity of transient internal states of synchrony in liquid state machines. pp. 56-63. *In:* T. Honkela [ed.]. Proceedings of the 21th International Conference on Artificial Neural Networks and Machine Learning (ICANN'2011), Part II, Espoo, Finland. Springer.

El-Laithy, K. and M. Bogdan. 2014. Synaptic energy drives the information processing mechanisms in spiking neural networks. Mathematical Biosciences and Engineering 11: 233-256.

El-Laithy, K. and M. Bogdan. 2017. Enhancements on the modified stochastic synaptic model: the functional heterogeneity. pp. 389-396. *In:* A. Lintas, S. Rovetta, P.F.M.J. Verschure and A.E.P. Villa [eds.] Proceedings of the 26th International Conference on Artificial Neural Networks and Machine Learning (ICANN'2017), Alghero, Italy. Springer.

Elman, J.L. 1990. Finding structure in time. Cognitive Science 14: 179-211.

Elman, J.L. 1998. Connectionism, artificial life, and dynamical systems. pp. 488-505. *In:* W. Bechtel and G. Graham [eds.]. A Companion to Cognitive Science. Blackwell Publisher, Malden, USA, Oxford, UK.

Elman, J.L. 2005. Connectionist models of cognitive development: where next? Trends in Cognitive Sciences 9: 111-117.

Elman, J.L., E.A. Bates, M.H. Johnson, A. Karmiloff-Smith, D. Parisi and K. Plunkett. 1998. Rethinking Innateness. A Connectionist Perspective on Development. MIT Press, Cambridge, USA.

Elstner, D. 2010. Information as a process. TripleC – Cognition, Communication, Cooperation 8: 310-350. [German]

Engel, A.K. 1996a. Temporal Coding in Neural Networks: Evidence for Coherent Activity in the Visual System. LIT Verlag, Münster, DE. [German]

Engel, A.K. 1996b. Principles of perception: The visual system. pp. 181-207. *In:* G. Roth and W. Prinz [eds.]. Kopf-Arbeit. Gehirnfunktionen und kognitive Leistungen. Spektrum Akademischer Verlag, Heidelberg, DE. [German]

Engel, A.K. 2005. Neuronal synchronization and perceptual awareness. pp. 16-41. *In:* C.S. Herrmann, M. Pauen, J.W. Rieger and S. Schicktanz [eds.]. Bewusstsein – Philosophie, Neurowissenschaften, Ethik. Wilhelm Fink Verlag, München, DE. [German]

Engel, A.K. 2009. Gamma oscillations. pp. 321-327. *In:* P. Wilken, A. Cleeremans and T. Bayne [eds.]. Oxford Companion to Consciousness. Oxford University Press, Oxford, UK.

Engel, A.K. 2012. Neural foundations of feature integration. pp. 67-77. *In:* H.-O. Karnath and P. Thier [eds.]. Kognitive Neurowissenschaften. 3rd Ed. Springer-Verlag, Heidelberg, DE. [German]

Engel, A.K., P. König, C.M. Gray and W. Singer. 1990a. Stimulus-dependent neuronal oscillations in cat visual cortex: inter-columnar interaction as determined by cross-correlation analysis. European Journal of Neuroscience 2: 588-606.

Engel, A.K., P. König, C.M. Gray and W. Singer. 1990b. Synchronization of oscillatory responses: a mechanism for stimulus-dependent assembly formation in cat visual cortex. pp. 105-108. *In:* R. Eckmiller, G. Hartmann and G. Hauske [eds.]. Parallel Processing in Neural Systems and Computers. Elsevier Science Inc., New York, USA.

Engel, A.K., A.K. Kreiter, P. König and W. Singer. 1991a. Synchronization of oscillatory neuronal responses between striate and extrastriate visual cortical areas of the cat. Proceedings of the National Academy of Sciences of the United States of America 88: 6048-6052.

Engel, A.K., P. König, A.K. Kreiter and W. Singer. 1991b. Interhemispheric synchronization of oscillatory neuronal responses in cat visual cortex. Science 252: 1177-1179.

Engel, A.K., P. König and W. Singer. 1991c. Direct physiological evidence for scene segmentation by temporal coding. Proceedings of the National Academy of Sciences of the United States of America 88: 9136-9140.

Engel, A.K., P. Kvnig, A.K. Kreiter, T.B. Schillen and W. Singer. 1992. Temporal coding in the visual cortex: new vistas on integration in the nervous System. Trends in Neuroscience 15: 218-226.

Engel, A.K., P. König and W. Singer. 1993. Formation of representational states in the brain. Spektrum der Wissenschaften 9: 42-47. [German]

Engel, A.K. and P. König. 1996. The construction of neuronal representations in the visual system. pp. 122-152. In: G. Rusch, S.J. Schmidt and O. Breidbach [eds.]. Interne Repräsentationen – Neue Konzepte der Hirnforschung. Suhrkamp Verlag, Frankfurt/M., DE. [German]

Engel, A.K. and W. Singer. 1997. Neuronal foundations of Gestalt perception. pp. 66-73. In: [Spektrum der Wissenschaft Verlag]. Spektrum der Wissenschaften. Dossier 4/97 "Kopf und Computer". Spektrum Akademischer Verlag. Heidelberg, DE. [German]

Engel, A.K. and P. König. 1998. The neurobiological paradigm of perception. A critical survey. pp. 157-194. In: P. Gold and A.K. Engel [eds.]. Der Mensch in der Perspektive der Kognitionswissenschaften. Suhrkamp, Frankfurt/M., DE. [German]

Engel, A.K., M. Brecht, P. Fries and W. Singer. 1998. Temporal binding and the construction of visual object representations. pp. 193-200. In: U. Kotkamp and W. Krause [eds.]. Intelligente Informationsverarbeitung. Deutscher Universit "atsverlag, Wiesbaden, DE. [German]

Engel, A.K., P. Fries, P. König, M. Brecht and W. Singer. 1999a. Temporal binding, binocular rivalry, and consciousness. Consciousness and Cognition 8: 128-151.

Engel, A.K., P. Fries, P. König, M. Brecht and W. Singer. 1999b. Does time help to understand consciousness. Consciousness and Cognition 8: 260-268.

Engel, A. and W. Singer. 2001. Temporal binding and the neural correlates of sensory awareness. Trends in Cognitive Sciences 5: 16-25.

Engel, A. and C. Van den Broeck. 2001. Statistical Mechanics of Learning. Cambridge University Press, Cambridge, UK.

Engel, A., P. Fries and W. Singer. 2001. Dynamic predictions: oscillations and synchrony in top-down processing. Nature Reviews Neuroscience 2: 704-716.

Engel, A.K., D. Senkowski and T.R. Schneider. 2012. Multisensory integration through neural coherence. pp. 115-130. In: M.M. Murray and M.T. Wallace [eds.]. The Neural Bases of Multisensory Processes, CRC Press. Boca Raton, USA.

Engel, A.K., A. Maye, M. Kurthen and P. König 2013a. Wheres the action? The pragmatic turn in cognitive science. Trends in Cognitive Sciences 17: 202-209.

Engel, A.K., C. Gerloff, C.C. Hilgetag and G. Nolte. 2013b. Intrinsic coupling modes: multiscale interactions in ongoing brain activity. Neuron 80: 867-886.

Engel, A.K., K. Friston and D. Kragic [eds.] 2016. The Pragmatic Turn – Towards Action-Oriented Views in Cognitive Science. MIT Press, Cambridge, USA.

Engelkamp, J. and T. Pechmann. 1993. Critical remarks on the concept of mental representation. pp. 7-16. In: J. Engelkamp and T. Pechmann [eds.]. Mentale Repräsentation. Huber Verlag, Bern, CH. [German]

Engelkamp, J. and H.D. Zimmer 2006. Textbook of Cognitive Psychology. Hogrefe, Göttingen, DE, Bern, CH, Wien, AT. [German]

Erk, K. and L. Priese 2000. Theoretical Computer Science. A Comprehensive Introduction. Springer, Berlin, DE. [German]

Erk, K. and L. Priese 2008. Theoretical Computer Science. A Comprehensive Introduction. 3rd Ed. Springer, Berlin, DE. [German]

Ermentrout, B. 1994. An introduction to neural oscillators. pp. 79-110. In: F. Ventriglia [ed.]. Neural Modeling and Neural Networks. Pergamon Press, Oxford, UK.

Ermentrout, B. 1998. Neural networks as spatio-temporal pattern-forming systems. Reports on Progress in Physics 61: 353-430.

Ermentrout, B. and N. Kopell. 1984. Frequency plateaus in a chain of weakly coupled oscillators. Siam Journal on Mathematical Analysis 15: 215-237.

Ermentrout, G.B. and D.H. Terman. 2010. Mathematical Foundations of Neuroscience. Springer-Verlag, New York, USA, London, UK.

Erlhagen, W. and G. Schöner. 2002. Dynamic field theory of movement preparation. Psychological Review 109: 545-572.

Evans, D.J. 2003. A non-equilibrium free-energy theorem for deterministic systems. Molecular Physics 101: 1551-1554.

Evans, D.J. and D.J. Searles. 2002. The fluctuation theorem. Advances in Physics 51: 1529-1585.

Everitt, B., S. Landau and M. Leese. 2001. Cluster Analysis. 4th Ed. Edward Arnold, London, UK.

Eysenck, M.W. and M.T. Keane 2010. Cognitive Psychology: A Student's Handbook. 6th Ed. Psychology Press, Hove, UK.

Ezawa, H. 1979. Einsteins contribution to statistical mechanics. pp. 69-88. In: P.C. Aichelburg and R.U. Sexl [eds.]. Albert Einstein. His Influence on Physics, Philosophy and Politics. Vieweg+Teubner, Braunschweig, DE.

Fang, F., H. Boyaci and D. Kersten. 2009. Border ownership selectivity in human early visual cortex and its modulation by attention. Journal of Neuroscience 29: 460-465.

Farmer, S.F. 1998. Rhythmicity, synchronization and binding in human and primate motor systems. Journal of Physiology 509: 3-14.

Faubel, C. and G. Schöner. 2008. Learning to recognize objects on the fly: a neurally based dynamic field approach. Neural Networks 21: 562-576.

Favela, L.H. and J. Martin 2017. "Cognition" and dynamical cognitive science. Minds and Machines 27: 331-355.

Feige, B., A. Aertsen and R. Kristeva-Feige. 2000. Dynamic synchronization between multiple motor areas and muscle activity in phasic voluntary movements. Journal of Neurophysiology 84: 2622-2629.

Feldman, J. 2013. The neural binding problem(s). Cognitive Neurodynamics 7: 1-11.

Feldman, J.A. 1982. Dynamic connections in neural networks. Biological Cybernetics 46: 27-39.

Feldman, J.A. 1989. A connectionist model of visual memory. pp. 49-81. In: G.E. Hinton and J.A. Anderson [eds.]. Parallel Models of Associative Memory. Erlbaum, Hillsdale, USA.

Feldman, J.A. and D.H. Ballard. 1982. Connectionist models and their properties. Cognitive Science 6: 205-254.

Feldman, J.A. and L. Shastri. 2003. Connectionism. pp. 680-687. In: L. Nadel. [ed.]. Encyclopedia of Cognitive Science. Vol. 1. Natur Publishing Group. London, UK, New York, USA, and Tokyo, JP.

Feltz, B. 2006. Self-organization, selection and emergence in the theories of evolution. pp. 341-360. In: B. Feltz, M. Crommelinck and P. Goujon [eds.]. Self-Organization and Emergence in Life Sciences. Springer-Verlag, Dordrecht, NL.

Ferber, J. 1999. Multi-Agent Systems: An Introduction to Distributed Artificial Intelligence. Addison Wesley Longman Publishing, Boston, USA.

Fernandes, T. and C. von der Malsburg. 2015. Self-organization of control circuits for invariant fiber projections. Neural Computation 27: 1005-1032.

Fernando, C. and S. Sojakka. 2003. Pattern recognition in a bucket. pp. 588-597. In: W. Banzhaf, J. Ziegler, T. Christaller, P. Dittrich and J.T. Kim [eds.] 2003. Advances in Artificial Life. 7th European Conference (ECAL 2003), Dortmund, Germany, Springer.

Fetzer, J.H. 2002. Computers and Cognition. Why Minds are not Machines. Kluwer, Dordrecht, NL.

Fickel, U. 2007. Temporal patterns of neuronal activity. Stimulus-coupled and intrinsically generated components. Ph.D. Thesis. Universität Hamburg, Hamburg, DE. [German]

Fieguth, P. 2017. An Introduction to Complex Systems. Springer International Publishing Switzerland, Cham, CH.

Finger, H. and P. König. 2014. Phase synchrony facilities binding and segmentation of natural images in a coupled neural oscillator network. Frontiers in Computational Neuroscience 7: 195.

Fischer, B. 2005. A model of the computations leading to a representation of auditory space in the midbrain of the barn owl. Ph.D. Thesis, Washington University, St. Louis, USA.

Fischer, H. and H. Kaul. 2008. Mathematics for Physicists 2: Ordinary and Partial Differential Equations, Mathematical Fundamentals of Quantum Mechanics. 3rd Ed. Teubner, Wiesbaden, DE. [German]

Fischer, H. and H. Kaul. 2011. Mathematics for Physicists 1: Basic Course. 7th Ed. Teubner, Wiesbaden, DE. [German]

Fitzhugh, R. 1961. Impulses and physiological states in theoretical models of nerve membrane. Biophysical Journal 1: 445-466.

Fletcher, R. 1987. Practical Methods of Optimization. 2nd Ed. Wiley, Chichester, UK.

Floridi, L. 2010. Information. A Very Short Introduction. Oxford University Press, Oxford, UK.

Flusberg, S.J. and J.L. McClelland. 2017. Connectionism and the emergence of mind. pp. 69-89. In: S.E.F. Chipman [ed.]. The Oxford Handbook of Cognitive Science. Oxford University Press, Oxford, UK.

Fodor, J.A. 1976. The Language of Thought. Harvester Press. Sussex, UK.

Fodor, J.A. 1981a. Three cheers for propositional attitudes. pp. 100-123. In: J.A. Fodor [ed.]. Representations. MIT Press, Cambridge, USA.

Fodor, J.A. 1981a. Propositional Attitudes. pp. 177-203. In: J.A. Fodor [ed.]. Representations. MIT Press, Cambridge, USA.

Fodor, J.A. 1983. The Modularity of Mind. MIT Press, Cambridge, USA.

Fodor, J.A. 1987. Psychosemantics. MIT Press, Cambridge, USA.

Fodor, J.A. 1990. A theory of content, I: the problem. pp. 51-87. In: J.A. Fodor [ed.]. A Theory of Content and other Essays. MIT Press, Cambridge, USA.

Fodor, J.A. 1997. Connectionism and the problem of systematicity (continued): why Smolensky's solution still doesn't work. Cognition 62: 109-119.

Fodor, J.A. 2008. LOT 2: The Language of Thought Revisited. Oxford University Press, New York, USA.

Fodor, J.A. and Z.W. Pylyshyn. 1988. Connectionism and cognitive architecture: a critical analysis. Cognition 28: 3-71.

Fodor, J.A. and B.P. McLaughlin. 1990. Connectionism and the problem of systematicity: why Smolensky's solution doesn't work. Cognition 35: 183-204.

Földiák, P. 1990. Forming sparse representations by local anti-Hebbian learning. Biological Cybernetics 64: 165-170.

Földiák, P. 2003. Sparse coding in the primate cortex. pp. 1064-1068. *In:* A. Arbib [ed.]. The Handbook of Brain Theory and Neural Networks. 2nd Ed. The MIT Press, Cambridge, USA, London, UK.

Forbes, A.R. 1964. An item analysis of the advanced matrices. British Journal of Educational Psychology 34: 1-14.

François, C. 1999. Systemics and cybernetics in a historical perspective. Systems Research and Behavioral Science 16: 203-219.

Frankish, K. and W. Ramsey [eds.]. 2012. The Cambridge Handbook of Cognitive Science. Cambridge University Press, Cambridge, UK.

Franklin, S. 2013. LIDA: A systems-level architecture for cognition, emotion, and learning. IEEE Transactions on Autonomous Mental Development 6: 1941.

Freeman, W.J. 1972. Waves, pulses and the theory of neural masses. Progress in Theoretical Biology 2: 87-165.

Freeman, W.J. 1975. Mass Action in the Nervous System. Examination of the Neurophysiological Basis of Adaptive Behavior through the EEG. Academic Press, New York, USA.

Freeman, W.J. 1978. Spatial properties of an EEG event in the olfactory bulb and cortex. Electroencephalography and Clinical Neurophysiology 44: 586-605.

Freeman, W.J. 1987. Simulation of chaotic EEG patterns with a dynamic model of the olfactory system. Biological Cybernetics 56: 139-150.

Freeman, W.J. 1995. Societies of Brains. A Study in the Neuroscience of Love and Hate. Lawrence Erlbaum Associates, Hillsdale, USA.

Freeman, W.J. 2000a. How Brains Make up their Minds. Columbia University Press, New York, USA.

Freeman, W.J. 2000b. [ed.] 2000. Neurodynamics: An Exploration of Mesoscopic Brain Dynamics. Springer, London, UK.

Freeman, W.J. 2003a. A neurobiological theory of meaning in perception. Part 1. Information and meaning in nonconvergent and nonlocal brain dynamics. International Journal of Bifurcation and Chaos 13: 2493-2511.

Freeman, W.J. 2003b. A neurobiological theory of meaning in perception. Part 2. Spatial patterns of phase in gamma EEG from primary sensory cortices reveal the properties of mesoscopic wave packets. International Journal of Bifurcation and Chaos 13: 2513-2535.

Freeman, W.J. 2005. A field-theoretic approach to understanding scale-free neocortical dynamics. Biological Cybernetics 92: 350-359.

Freeman, W.J. 2013. Chaotic neocortical dynamics. pp. 271-284. *In:* A. Adamatzky and G. Chen [eds.]. Chaos, Cnn, Memristors and Beyond: A Festschrift For Leon Chua. World Scientific, Singapore, SG.

Freeman, W.J. 2015. Mechanism and significance of global coherence in scalp EEG. Current Opinion in Neurobiology 31: 199-205.

Freeman, W.J. and W. Schneider. 1982. Changes in spatial patterns of rabbit EEG with conditioning to odors. Psychophysiology 19: 44-56.

Freeman, W.J. and G. Viana Di Prisco. 1986. EEG spatial pattern differences with discriminated odors manifest chaotic and limit cycle attractors in olfactory bulb of rabbits. pp. 97-119. *In:* G. Palm and A. Aertsen [eds.]. Brain Theory. Springer, Berlin, DE.

Freeman, W.J. and R. Quian Quiroga. 2013. Wavelets. pp. 49-64. *In:* W.J. Freeman and R. Quian Quiroga: Imaging Brain Function with EEG. Advanced Temporal and Spatial Analysis of Electroencephalographic Signals. Springer, New York, USA.

Frege, G. 1879/1964. Begriffsschrift: a formula language, modeled on that of arithmetic, of pure thought. pp. VII-88. *In:* I. Angelelli [ed.]. G. Frege: Begriffsschrift und andere Aufsätze. 2. Auflage. Wissenschaftliche Buchgesellschaft, Darmstadt, DE. [German]

Frege, G. 1891/1994. Function and concept. pp. 18-39. *In:* G. Frege (G. Patzig [ed.]). Funktion, Begriff und Bedeutung. Fünf logische Studien. 7. Auflage. Vandenhoeck & Ruprecht, Göttingen, DE. [German]

Frege, G. 1892/1994a. On sense and reference. pp. 40-65. *In:* G. Patzig [ed.]. Funktion, Begriff und Bedeutung. Fünf logische Studien. 7. Auflage. Vandenhoeck & Ruprecht, Göttingen, DE. [German]

Frege, G. 1892/1994b. On concept and object. pp. 66-80. *In:* G. Patzig [ed.]. Funktion, Begriff und Bedeutung. Fünf logische Studien. 7. Auflage. Vandenhoeck & Ruprecht, Göttingen, DE. [German]

Frege, G. 1918-1919. The thought. A logical inquiry. Beiträge zur Philosophie des deutschen Idealismus 1: 58-77. (reprinted in Frege 1923/1976.) [German]

Frege, G. 1923/1976. The thought. A logical inquiry. pp. 30-53. *In:* G. Patzig [ed.]. Logische Untersuchungen. 2. Auflage. Vandenhoeck & Ruprecht, Göttingen, DE. [German]

Frege, G. 1923-1926. Logical Investigations. Third part: Compound thoughts. Beiträge zur Philosophie des deutschen Idealismus 3: 36-51. (reprinted in Frege 1923/1976.) [German]

Frege, G. 1923/1976. Logical Investigations. Third part: Compound thoughts. pp. 72-91. *In:* G. Patzig [ed.]. Logische Untersuchungen. 2nd Ed. Vandenhoeck & Ruprecht, Göttingen, DE. [German]

Freiwald, W.A., A.K. Kreiter and W. Singer. 1995. Stimulus dependent intercolumnar synchronization of single unit responses in cat area 17. Neuroreport 6: 2348-2352.

Freiwald, W.A., A.K. Kreiter and W. Singer. 2001. Synchronization and assembly formation in the visual cortex. pp. 111-140. *In:* M.A.L. Nicolelis [ed.]. Advances in Neural Population Coding. Elsevier, Amsterdam, NL.

French, R.M. 2003. Catastrophic forgetting in connectionist networks. pp. 431-435. *In:* L. Nadel. [ed.]. Encyclopedia of Cognitive Science. Vol. 1. Natur Publishing Group. London, UK, New York, USA, and Tokyo, JP.

Fresco, N. 2014. Physical Computation and Cognitive Science. Springer, Berlin, DE.

Freund, A.M., M.-T. Huett and M. Vec. 2006. Self-organization: Aspects of concept and method transfer. pp. 12-32. *In:* M. Vec, M.-T. Huett and A.M. Freund [eds.]. Selbstorganisation. Ein Denksystem für Natur und Gesellschaft. Böhlau, Köln, DE. [German]

Frey, T. and M. Bossert, M. 2008. Signal and System Theory. 2nd corr. Ed. Vieweg+Teubner Verlag. Wiesbaden, DE. [German]

Friedenberg, J. 2009. Dynamical Psychology. Complexity, Self-Organization and Mind. ISCE Publishing.

Friedenberg, J. and G. Silverman. 2012. Cognitive Science. An Introduction to the Study of Mind. 2nd Ed. SAGE, Los Angeles, USA.

Friederici, A.D. and S.M.E. Gierhan. 2013. The language network. Current Opinion in Neurobiology 23: 250-254.

Friederici, A.D. and W. Singer. 2015. Grounding language processing on basic neurophysiological principles. Trends in Cognitive Sciences 19: 329-338.

Friedrich, R.W., C.J. Habermann and G. Laurent. 2004. Multiplexing using synchrony in the zebrafish olfactory. Nature Neuroscience 7: 862-871.

Frien, A., R. Eckhorn, R. Bauer, T. Woelbern and H. Kehr. 1994. Stimulus-specific fast oscillations at zero phase between visual areas V1 and V2 of awake monkey. Neuroreport 5: 2273-2277.

Fries, P. 2005. A mechanism for cognitive dynamics: neuronal communication through neuronal coherence. Trends in Cognitive Sciences 9: 474-480.

Fries, P. 2015. Rhythms for cognition: communication through coherence. Neuron 88: 220-235.

Fries, P., P.R. Roelfsema, A.K. Engel, P. König and W. Singer. 1997. Synchronization of oscillatory responses in visual cortex correlates with perception in interocular rivalry. Proceedings of the National Academy of Sciences of the United States of America 94: 12699-12704.

Fries, P., J.H. Reynolds, A.E. Rorie and R. Desimone. 2001. Modulation of oscillatory neuronal synchronization by selective visual attention. Science 291: 1560-1563.

Fries, P., J.-H. Schröder, P.R. Roelfsema, W. Singer and A.K. Engel. 2002. Oscillatory neuronal synchronization in primary visual cortex as a correlate of stimulus selection. The Journal of Neuroscience 22: 3739-3754.

Fries, P., D. Nikolić and W. Singer. 2007. The gamma cycle. Trends in Neurosciences 30: 309-316.

Friese, U., J. Daume, F. Göschl, P. König, P. Wang and A.K. Engel. 2016. Oscillatory brain activity during multisensory attention reflects activation, disinhibition, and cognitive control. Scientific Reports 6: 32775.

Friston, K.J. 1995. Neuronal transients. Proceedings of the Royal Society of London Series B 261: 401-405.

Friston, K.J. 1997. Another neural code? Neuroimage 5: 213-220.

Friston, K. 2003. Learning and inference in the brain. Neural Networks 16: 1325-1352.

Friston, K. 2009. The free-energy principle: A rough guide to the brain? Trends in Cognitive Sciences 13: 293-301.

Friston, K. 2010a. The free-energy principle: a unified brain theory. Nature Reviews Neuroscience 11: 127-138.

Friston, K. 2010b. Is the free-energy principle neurocentric? Nature Reviews Neuroscience 11: 605.

Friston, K. 2012. The history of the future of the Bayesian brain. NeuroImage 62: 1230-1233.

Friston, K. 2013. Life as we know it. Journal of the Royal Society Interface 10: 20130475.

Friston, K., J. Kilner and L. Harrison. 2006. A free energy principle for the brain. Journal of Physiology Paris 100: 70-87.

Friston, K. and K.E. Stephan. 2007. Free-energy and the brain. Synthese 159: 417-458.

Friston, K.J., N. Trujillo-Barreto and J. Daunizeau. 2008. DEM: a variational treatment of dynamic systems. NeuroImage 41: 849-885.

Friston, K., K.E. Stephan and S. Kiebel. 2009. Free-energy, value and neuronal systems. pp. 266-302. In: D. Heinke and E. Mavritsaki [eds.]. Computational Modelling in Behavioural Neuroscience. Closing the Gap between Neurophysiology and Behaviour. Psychology Press, Hove, UK.

Friston, K. and P. Ao. 2012. Free-energy, value and attractors. Computational and Mathematical Methods in Medicine 2012: 1-27.

Friston, K., M. Breakstear and G. Deco. 2012. Perception and self-organized instability. Frontiers in Computational Neuroscience 6: 1-19.

Friston, K., B. Sengupta and G. Auletta. 2014. Cognitive dynamics: from attractors to active inference. Proceedings of the IEEE 102: 427-444.

Fritzke, B. 1992. Growing cell structures – A self-organizing neural network model. Ph.D. Thesis. Universität Erlangen-Nürnberg. Erlangen, DE. [German]

Fromkin, V.A. [ed.] 2001. Linguistics. An Introduction to Linguistic Theory. Blackwell, Malden, USA.

Fromm, J. 2005. Ten questions about emergence. Complexity Digest 40: 0509049.

Fusella, P.V. 2013. Dynamic systems theory in cognitive science. Major elements, applications, and debates surrounding a revolutionary meta-theory. Dynamical Psychology 03/2012-2013.

Fuster, J.M. 2003. Cortex and Mind. Unifying Cognition. Oxford University Press, Oxford, UK.

Gabbiani, F. 2003. Rate coding and signal processing. pp. 941-945 In: M.A. Arbib [ed.]. The Handbook of Brain Theory and Neural Networks. 2nd Ed. The MIT Press. Cambridge, USA, London, UK.

Gärdenfors, P. 2000. Conceptual Spaces. The Geometry of Thought. The MIT Press, Cambridge, USA.

Gallagher, S. 2000. Philosophical conceptions of the self: implications for cognitive science. Trends in Cognitive Sciences: 4: 1421.

Gallistel, C.R. and A.P. King. [eds.] 2009. Memory and the Computational Brain. Why Cognitive Science Will Transform Neuroscience. Wiley-Blackwell, Chichester, UK.

Gardner, H. 1985. The Mind's New Science. A History of the Cognitive Revolution. Basic Books, New York, USA.

Gardner, H. 1986. The Mind's New Science. A History of the Cognitive Revolution. 3rd Pr. Basic Books, New York, USA.

Garson, J.W. 1994. No representations without rules: the prospects for a compromise between paradigms in cognitive science. Mind & Language 9: 25-37.

Gautrais, J. and S. Thorpe. 1998. Rate coding versus temporal order coding: a theoretical approach. BioSystems 48: 57-65.

Gayler, R.W. 1998. Multiplicative binding, representation operators, and analogy [Abstract of Poster]. In: K. Holyoak, D. Gentner and B. Kokinov [eds.]. Advances in Analogy Research: Integration of Theory and Data from the

Cognitive, Computational, and Neural Sciences. New Bulgarian University Press, Sofia, BG.

Gayler, R.W. 2003. Vector symbolic architectures answer Jackendoff's challenges for cognitive neuroscience. pp. 133-138. *In:* P. Slezak [ed.]. The 4th ICCS International Conference on Cognitive Science and the 7th ASCS Australasian Society for Cognitive Science Conference (ICCS/ASCS), Sydney, Australia.

Gayler, R.W. 2006. Vector symbolic architectures are a viable alternative for Jackendoff's challenges. Commentary on: F. van der Velde and M. de Kamps: Neural blackboard architectures of combinatorial structures in cognition. Behavioral and Brain Sciences 29: 78-79.

Gayler, R.W. and R. Wales. 1998. Connections, binding, unification, and analogical promiscuity. pp. 181-190. *In:* K. Holyoak, D. Gentner and B. Kokinov [eds.]. Advances in Analogy Research: Integration of Theory and Data from the Cognitive, Computational, and Neural Sciences. New Bulgarian University Press, Sofia, BG.

Gazzaniga, M.S., R.B. Ivry and G.R. Mangun. 2018. The Cognitive Neurosciences. The Biology of the Mind. 5nd Ed. W.W. Norton, New York, USA.

Gemoll, W. and K. Vretska. 2006. Gemoll. Greek-German School and Concise Dictionary. 10th Ed. Oldenbourg Schulbuchverlag. München, DE. [German]

Genç, E., J. Bergmann, W. Singer and A. Kohler. 2015. Surface area of early visual cortex predicts individual speed of traveling waves during binocular rivalry. Cerebral Cortex 25: 1499-1508.

Georgopoulos, A.P., J. Kalaska, R. Caminiti and J. Massey. 1982. On the relations between the direction of two-dimensional arm movements and gell discharge in primate motor cortex. The Journal of Neuroscience 2: 1527-1537.

Georgopoulos, A.P., R. Caminiti, J. Kalaska and J. Massey. 1983. Spatial coding of movement: a hypothesis concerning the coding of movement direction by motor control populations. Experimental Brain Research Supplement 7: 327-336.

Georgopoulos, A.P., A.B. Schwartz and R.E. Kettner. 1986. Neuronal population coding of movement direction. Science 233: 1416-1419.

Georgopoulos, A.P., R.E. Kettner and A.B. Schwartz. 1988. Primate motor cortex and free arm movements to visual targets in three-dimensional space. II. Coding of the direction of the movement by a neuronal population. The Journal of Neuroscience 8: 2928-2937.

Georgopoulos, A.P., J.T. Lurito, M. Petrides, A.B. Schwartz and J.T. Massey. 1989. Mental rotation of the neuronal population vector. Science 243: 234-236.

Gershenson, C. and F. Heylighen. 2003. When can we call a system selforganizing? pp. 606-614. *In:* W. Banzhaf, T. Christaller, P. Dittrich, J.T. Kim and J. Ziegler [eds.]. Proceedings of the 7th European Conference on Advances in Artificial Life (ECAL 2003), Dortmund, Germany. Springer-Verlag.

Gerstein, G.L., P. Bedenbaugh and A. Aertsen. 1989. Neuronal assemblies. IEEE Transactions on Biomedical Engineering 36: 4-14.

Gerstner, W. 1999. Spiking neurons. pp. 3-54. *In:* W. Maass and C.M. Bishop [eds.]. Pulsed Neural Networks. MIT Press, Cambridge, USA.

Gerstner,W. and W.M. Kistler. 2002. Spiking Neuron Models. Single Neurons, Populations, Plasticity. Cambridge University Press, Cambridge, UK.

Gerthsen, C. 1999. Gerthsen Physics. 20th Ed. Springer, Berlin, DE. [German]

Ghahramani, Z. 2003. Information theory. pp. 551-555. *In:* L. Nadel. [ed.]. Encyclopedia of Cognitive Science. Vol. 2. Natur Publishing Group. London, UK, New York, USA and Tokyo, JP.

Gibbs, Jr., R.W. 2007. Embodiment and Cognitive Science. Cambridge University Press, Cambridge, UK.

Gibbs, R.W. and G. Van Orden 2012. Pragmatic choice in conversation. Topics in Cognitive Science 4: 7-20.

Gilmore, R. 1980. Catastrophe Theory for Scientists and Engineers. Wiley, New York, USA.

Glansdorff, P. and I. Prigogine. 1971. Thermodynamic Theory of Structure, Stability and Fluctuations. Wiley-Interscience, London, UK.

Glaser, W.R. 1993. Representation for man and machine. pp. 40-50. *In:* J. Engelkamp and T. Pechmann [eds.]. Mentale Repräsentation. Huber Verlag, Bern, CH. [German]

Glaser, W.R. 2006. Information theory. pp. 741-747. *In:* J. Funke and P.A. Frensch [eds.]. Handbuch der Allgemeinen Psychologie – Kognition. Band 5. Hogrefe, Göttingen, DE. [German]

Glass, L. 2001. Synchronization and rhythmic processes in physiology. Nature 410: 277-284.

Gleick, J. 1987. Chaos: Making a New Science. Pergamon Press, Elmsford, USA.

Glennan, S. 2008. Mechanisms. pp. 376-384. *In:* S. Psillos and M. Curd [eds.]. The Routledge Companion to Philosophy of Science. Routledge Taylor & Francis Group, London, UK, New York, USA.

Gloy, K. 1998a. Systems theory – the new paradigm? pp. 227-242. *In:* K. Gloy, W. Neuser and P. Reisinger [eds.]. Systemtheorie. Philosophische Betrachtungen und ihre Anwendungen. Bouvier Verlag, Bonn, DE. [German]

Gloy, K. 1998b. Roots and application areas of systems theory. Critical questions. pp. 5-12. *In:* K. Gloy, W. Neuser and P. Reisinger [eds.]. Systemtheorie.

Philosophische Betrachtungen und ihre Anwendungen. Bouvier Verlag, Bonn, DE. [German]

Göbel, E. 1998. Theory and Design of Self-Organization. Duncker und Humblodt, Berlin, DE. [German]

Gödel, K. 1932/1986. On the intuitionistic propositional calculus. pp. 223-225. *In:* S. Feferman [ed.]. Kurt Gödel. Collected Works. Vol. I. Publications 1929-1936. Oxford University Press, New York, USA, Clarendon Press, Oxford, UK.

Goebel, R. 1994. Synchronous oscillations in visual systems and in neural network models. pp. 312-313. *In:* I. Duwe, F. Kurfess, G. Paass, G. Palm, H. Ritter and S. Vogel [eds.]. Konnektionismus und Neuronale Netze. Beiträge zur Herbstschule (HeKoNN'94). GMD-Studien. Nr. 242, Münster, Germany. [German]

Goel, P. and B. Ermentrout. 2002. Synchrony, stability, and firing patterns in pulse coupled oscillators. Physica D 163: 191-216.

Göschl, F., U. Friese, J. Daume, P. König and A.K. Engel. 2015. Oscillatory signatures of crossmodal congruence effects: an EEG investigation employing a visuotactile pattern matching paradigm. Neuroimage 116: 177-186.

Götschl, J. 2006. Self-organisation: New foundations for a uniform understanding of reality. pp. 35-65. *In:* M. Vec, M.-T. Huett and A.M. Freund [eds.]. Selbstorganisation. Ein Denksystem für Natur und Gesellschaft. Böhlau, Köln, DE. [German]

Gold, P. 1998. Philosophical aspects of artificial intelligence. pp. 49-97. *In:* A. Engel and P. Gold [eds.]. Der Mensch in der Perspektive der Kognitionswissenschaft. Suhrkamp Verlag, Frankfurt am Main, DE. [German]

Gold, P. and Engel, A.K. 1998. Why cognitive sciences? pp. 9-16. *In:* A. Engel and P. Gold [eds.]. Der Mensch in der Perspektive der Kognitionswissenschaft. Suhrkamp Verlag, Frankfurt am Main, DE. [German]

Goldstein, H., C.P. Poole Jr. and J.L. Safko. 2001. Classical Mechanics. 3rd Ed. Pearson, Essex, GB.

Golomb, D. and Y. Amitai. 1997. Propagating neuronal discharges in neocortical slices: Computational and experimental study. Journal of Neurophysiology 78: 11991211.

Gómez Ramírez, J.D.G. 2014. A New Foundation for Representation in Cognitive and Brain Science: Category Theory and the Hippocampus. Springer, Dordrecht, NE.

Goodfellow, I., Y. Bengio and A. Courville. 2016. Deep Learning: Adaptive Computation and Machine Learning. MIT Press, Cambridge, USA, London, UK.

Gore, P.A., Jr. 2000. Cluster analysis. pp. 297-321. *In:* H.E.A. Tinsley and S.D. Brown [eds.]. Handbook of Applied Multivariate Statistics and Mathematical Modeling. Academic Press, San Diego, USA.

Goschke, T. and D. Koppelberg 1990. Connectionist representation, semantic compositionality, and the instability of concept structure. Psychological Research 52: 253-270.

Gosmann, J. and C. Eliasmith. 2016. Optimizing semantic pointer representations for symbol-like processing in spiking neural networks. PLoS ONE 11(2): e0149928.

Gottwald, S. 2001. A Treatise on Many-Valued Logics. Research Studies Press, Baldock, UK.

Grassberger, P. 1989a/2012. Randomness, information, and complexity. *In:* F. Ramos-Gomes [ed.]. Proceedings of the Fifth Mexican School on Statistical Physics. World Scientific.

Grassberger, P. 1989b. Problems in quantifying self-generated complexity. Helvetica Physica Acta 62: 489-511.

Grauel, A. 1992. Neural Networks. Fundamentals and Mathematical Modeling. BI Wissenschaftsverlag, Mannheim, DE. [German]

Graupe, D. 2008. Principles of Artificial Networks. 2*nd* Ed. World Scientific, New Jersey, USA.

Gray, C.M. 1994. Synchronous oscillations in neuronal systems: mechanisms and functions. Journal of Computational Neuroscience 1: 11-38.

Gray, C.M. and W. Singer. 1989. Stimulus-specific neuronal oscillations in orientation columns of cat visual cortex. Proceedings of the National Academy of Sciences of the United States of America 86: 1698-1702.

Gray, C.M., P. König, A.K. Engel and W. Singer. 1989. Oscillatory responses in cat visual cortex exhibit inter-columnar synchronization which reflects global stimulus properties. Nature 338: 334-337.

Gray, C.M., A.K. Engel, P. König and W. Singer. 1992. Mechanisms underlying the generation of neuronal oscillations in cat visual cortex. pp. 29-45. *In:* E. Başar and T.H. Bullock [eds.]. Induced Rhythms in the Brain. Birkhäuser, Boston, USA, Basel, CH, Berlin, DE.

Gray, R.M. 2009. Entropy and Information Theory. Springer-Verlag, New York, USA.

Gray, W.D. 2012. Great debate on the complex systems approach to cognitive science. Topics in Cognitive Science 4: 2.

Green, D.W. and Others. 1996. Cognitive Science. An Introduction. Blackwell, Oxford, UK.

Grewendorf, G., F. Hamm and W. Sternefeld. 1993. Linguistic Knowledge. An Introduction to Modern Theories of Grammatical Description. Suhrkamp, Frankfurt am Main, DE. [German]

Griffiths, T.L., C. Kemp and J.B. Tenenbaum. 2008. Bayesian models of cognition. pp. 59-100. *In:* R. Sun [ed.]. The Cambridge Handbook of Computational Psychology. Cambridge University Press, Cambridge, UK.

Grillet, P.A. 2007. Abstract Algebra. 2nd Ed. Springer, New York, USA.

Groeben, N. and B. Scheele. 1977. Arguments for a Psychology of the Reflective Subject. Paradigm Shift from the Behavioral to the Epistemological View of Man. Dr. Dietrich Steinkopff Verlag, Darmstadt, DE. [German]

Gross, C.G. 2002. Genealogy of the "Grandmother Cell". The Neuroscientist 8: 512-518.

Gross, C.G., C.E. Rocha-Miranda and D.B. Bender. 1972. Visual properties of neurons in inferotemporal cortex of the macaque. Journal of Neurophysiology 35: 96-111.

Grossberg, S. 1968a. A prediction theory for some nonlinear functional-differential equations, I: learning of lists. Journal of Mathematical Analysis and Applications 21: 643-694.

Grossberg, S. 1968b. A prediction theory for some nonlinear functional-differential equations, II: learning of patterns. Journal of Mathematical Analysis and Applications 22: 490-522.

Grossberg, S. 1970. Neural pattern discrimination. Journal of Theoretical Biology 27: 291-337.

Grossberg, S. 1972. Neural expectation: cerebellar and retinal analogs of cells fired by learnable or unlearned patterns classes. Kybernetik 10: 49-57.

Grossberg, S. 1976a. On the development of feature detectors in the visual cortex with applications to learning and reaction-diffusion systems. Biological Cybernetics 21: 145-159.

Grossberg, S. 1976b. Adaptive pattern classification and universal recoding: I. Parallel development and coding of neural feature detectors. Biological Cybernetics 23: 121-134.

Grossberg, S. 1976c. Adaptive pattern classification and universal recoding: II. Feedback, expectation, olfaction, and illusions. Biological Cybernetics 23: 187-202.

Grossberg, S. 1977. Pattern formation by the global limits of a nonlinear competitive interaction in n dimensions. Journal of Biology V4: 237256.

Grossberg, S. 1980. How does a brain build a cognitive code? Psychological Review 87: 1-51.

Grossberg, S. 1987. Competitive learning: from interactive activation to adaptive resonance. Cognitive Science 11: 23-63.

Grossberg, S. [ed.] 1988. Neural Networks and Natural Intelligence. MIT Press, Cambridge, USA.

Grossberg, S. 1997. Principles of cortical synchronization. Commentary on: W.A. Phillips and W. Singer: In search of common foundations for cortical computation. The Behavioral and Brain Sciences 20: 689-690.

Grossberg, S. 2017. Towards solving the hard problem of consciousness: the varieties of brain resonances and the conscious experiences that they support. Neural Networks 87: 38-95.

Grossberg, S. and D. Somers. 1991. Synchronized oscillations during cooperative feature linking in a cortical model of visual perception. Neural Networks 4: 453-466.

Grossberg, S. and M. Versace. 2008. Spikes, synchrony, and attentive learning by laminar thalamocortical circuits. Brain Research 1218: 278-312.

Grush, R. 2001. The architecture of representation. pp. 349-368. In: W. Bechtel, P. Mandik, J. Mundale and R.S. Stufflebeam [eds.]. Philosophy and the Neurosciences. A Reader. Wiley-Blackwell. Oxford, UK.

Grush, R. 2004. The emulation theory of representation: motor control, imagery, and perception. Behavioral and Brain Sciences 27: 377-442.

Guckenheimer, J. and P. Holmes. 1990. Nonlinear Oscillations, Dynamical Systems and Bifurcations of Vector Fields. Revised and corrected 3rd Printing. Springer, New York, USA.

Guesgen, H.W. 2000. Constraints. pp. 267-287. In: G. Görz, C.-R. Rollinger and J. Schneeberger [eds.]. Handbuch der Künstlichen Intelligenz. 3rd Ed. Oldenbourg Verlag, München, DE, Wien, AT. [German]

Guesgen, H.W. and J. Hertzberg. 1992. A Perspective of Constraint-Based Reasoning. An Introductory Tutorial. Springer-Verlag, Berlin, DE.

Gutfreund, H. 1990. From statistical mechanics to neural networks and back. Physica A: Statistical Mechanics and its Applications 163: 373-385.

Hadley, R.F. 1994. Systematicity in connectionist language learning. Mind and Language 9: 247-272.

Hadley, R.F. 1997. Cognition, systematicity and nomic necessity. Mind and Language 12: 137-153.

Hadley, R.F. 2003. Systematicity of generalizations in connectionist networks. p. 1152. In: M.A. Arbib [ed.]. The Handbook of Brain Theory and Neural Networks. 2nd Ed. The MIT Press. Cambridge, USA, London, UK.

Hadley, R.F. and M.B. Hayward. 1995. Strong semantic systematicity from unsupervised connectionist learning. pp. 358-363. *In:* J.D. Moore and J.F. Lehman [eds.]. Proceedings of the Seventeenth Annual Conference of the Cognitive Science Society. Pittsburgh, United States of America. Psychology Press.

Hadley, R.F. and M.B. Hayward. 1997. Strong semantic systematicity from Hebbian connectionist learning. Minds and Machines 7: 1-37.

Händle, F. and S. Jensen. 1974. Introduction by the editors. pp. 7-50. *In:* F. Händle and S. Jensen [eds.]. Systemtheorie und Systemtechnik. Nymphenburger Verlagshandlung, M¨unchen, DE. [German]

Häuslein, A. 2003. System Analysis. Basics, Techniques, Quotations. VDE Verlag, Berlin, Offenbach, DE. [German]

Häussler, A.F. and C. von der Malsburg. 1983. Development of retinotopic projections. An analytical treatment. Journal of Theoretical Neurobiology 2: 47-73.

Hahn, G., A.F. Bujan, Y. Frégnac, A. Aertsen and A. Kumar. 2013. Synfire chains and gamma oscillations: two complementary modes of information transmission in cortical networks. BMC Neuroscience 14 (Suppl. 1): 226.

Hahn, G., A.F. Bujan, Y. Frégnac, A. Aertsen and A. Kumar. 2014. Communication through resonance in spiking neuronal networks. Plos Computational Biology 10: e1003811.

Hahn, G., A. Ponce-Alvarez, G. Deco, A. Aertsen and A. Kumar. 2019. Portraits of communication in neuronal networks. Nature Reviews Neuroscience 20: 117-127.

Hair, J.F., W. Black, B. Babin, R. Anderson and R. Tatham. 2010. Multivariate Data Analysis. A Global Perspective. 7th Ed. Pearson, Upper Saddle River, USA.

Haken, H. 1983. Synergetics. An Introduction. Nonequilibrium Phase Transitions and Self-Organization in Physics, Chemistry, and Biology. 3rd Ed. Springer-Verlag. Berlin, Heidelberg, DE.

Haken, H. 1988a. Development lines of synergetics I. Naturwissenschaften 75: 163-172. [German]

Haken, H. 1988b. Development lines of synergetics II. Naturwissenschaften 75: 225-234. [German]

Haken, H. 2000. Information and Self-Organization. A Macroscopic Approach to Complex Systems. 2nd Ed. Springer-Verlag. Berlin, DE, Heidelberg, DE.

Haken, H. 2004. Synergetics. Introduction and Advanced Topics. Springer-Verlag, Berlin, Heidelberg, DE.

Haken, H. 2008. Brain Dynamics. An Introduction to Models and Simulations. 2nd Ed. Springer-Verlag. Berlin, DE, Heidelberg, DE.

Hall, A.D. and R.E. Fagen. 1968. Definition of system. pp. 81-92. *In:* W. Buckley [ed.]. Modern System Research for the Behavioral Scientist. Aldine Publishing Company, Chicago, USA.

Hammer, B. 2013. Neuroinformatics. pp. 52-55. *In:* A. Stephan and S. Walter [eds.]. Handbuch Kognitionswissenschaft. Metzler, Stuttgart, Weimar, DE. [German]

Hammer, B. and T. Villmann. 2003. Mathematical aspects of neural networks. pp. 59-72. *In:* Proceedings of the 11th European Symposium on Artificial Networks (ESANN'2003), Bruges, Belgium.

Hansen, V.L. 2016. Functional Analysis. Entering Hilbert Space. 2nd Ed. World Scientific, New Jersey, USA.

Hanson, S.J. 1999. Connectionist neuroscience: representional and learning issues for neuroscience. pp. 401-427. *In:* E. Lepore and Z.W. Pylyshyn [eds.]. What is Cognitive Science? Blackwell Publishers, Malden, USA, Oxford, UK.

Hardcastle, V.G. 1994. Psychology's binding problem and possible neurobiological solutions. Journal of Consciousness Studies 1: 76-79.

Hardcastle, V.G. 1997. Consciousness and the neurobiology of perceptual binding. Seminars in Neurology 17: 163-170.

Hardcastle, V.G. 1998. The binding problem. pp. 555-565. *In:* W. Bechtel and G. Graham [eds.]. A Companion to Cognitive Science. Blackwell Publisher, Malden, USA, Oxford, UK.

Hardcastle, V.G. 1999. On being importantly necessary for consciousness. Consciousness and Cognition 8: 152-154.

Harel, D. 2004. Algorithmics. The Spirit of Computing. 3rd Ed. Addison-Wesley, Harlow, UK.

Harnish, R.M. [ed.] 2002. Minds, Brains, and Computers. An Historical Introduction to the Foundations of Cognitive Science. Blackwell Publishers, Malden, USA.

Harré, R. 2002. Cognitive Science. A Philosophical Introduction. SAGE, London, UK, Los Angeles, USA.

Hartley, R.V.L. 1928. Transmission of information. Bell System Technical Journal 7: 535-563.

Hartline, H.K. 1949. Inhibition of activity of visual receptors by illuminating nearby retinal areas in the limulus eye. Federation Proceedings 8: 69.

Haselager, P.,A. de Groot and H. Van Rappard 2003. Representationalism vs. antirepresentationalism. A debate for the sake of appearance. Philosophical Psychology 16: 5-23.

Haslwanter, T. 2016. An Introduction to Statistics with Python. With Applications in the Life Sciences. Springer International Publishing, Cham, CH.

Hatfield, G. 1991. Representation and rule-instantiation in connectionist systems. pp. 90-112. *In:* T. Horgan and J. Tienson [eds.]. Connectionism and the Philosophy of Mind. Kluwer Academic Publisher, Dordrecht, NE.

Haugeland, J. 1985. Artificial Intelligence: The Very Idea. 7th Ed. The MIT Press. A Bradford Book, Cambridge, USA.

Haun, M. 1998. Simulation of Neural Networks. A Practice-Oriented Introduction. Expert Verlag, Renningen-Malmsheim, DE. [German]

Haykin, S. 1999. Neural Networks: A Comprehensive Foundation. 2nd Ed. Prentice Hall, Upper Saddle River, USA.

Haykin, S. 2012. Cognitive Dynamic Systems. Perception-Action Cycle, Radar, and Radio. Cambridge University Press, Cambridge, UK.

Hayon, G., M. Abeles and D. Lehmann. 2005. A model for representing the dynamics of a system of synfire chains. Journal of Computational Neuroscience 18: 41-53.

Hebb, D.O. 1949. The Organization of Behavior. A Neuropsychological Theory. Wiley-Interscience, New York, USA.

Hebb, D.O. 1960. The american revolution. American Psychologist 14: 735-745.

Heidelberger, M. 1990. Self-organisation in the 19th century. pp. 67-104. *In:* W. Krohn and G. Küppers [eds.]. Selbstorganisation. Aspekte einer wissenschaftlichen Revolution. Vieweg, Braunschweig und Wiesbaden, DE. [German]

Heine, J. 2009. Topology and Functional Analysis. Oldenbourg, München, DE, Wien, AT. [German]

Helm, G. 1991. Symbolic and Connectionist Models of Human Information Processing. A Critical Juxtaposition. Springer-Verlag, Berlin, Heidelberg, DE. [German]

Helm, G. 1998. Computers can think. pp. 132-155. *In:* A. Engel and P. Gold [eds.]. Der Mensch in der Perspektive der Kognitionswissenschaft. Suhrkamp Verlag, Frankfurt am Main, DE. [German]

Hermes, D., K.J. Miller, B.A. Wandell and J. Winawer. 2015. Stimulus dependence of gamma oscillations in human visual cortex. Cerebral Cortex 25: 2951-2959.

Herrmann, C. 2002. Importance of 40 Hz oscillations for cognitive processes. Habilitationsschrift, Fakultät für Biowissenschaften, Pharmazie und Psychologie, Universität Leipzig, Max-Planck-Institut für Kognitions- und Neurowissenschaften, Sächsisches Digitalzentrum, Dresden, DE, Leipzig, DE. [German]

Herrmann, C.S., M.H.J. Munk and A.K. Engel. 2004. Cognitive functions of gammaband activity: memory match and utilization. Trends in Cognitive Sciences 8: 347-355.

Herrmann, M., J. Hertz and A. Prügel-Bennett. 1995. Analysis of synfire chains. Network: Computation in Neural Systems 6: 403-414.

Herrmann, T. 1993. Mental representation—a term in need of explanation. pp. 17-30. *In:* J. Engelkamp and T. Pechmann [eds.]. Mentale Repräsentation. Huber Verlag, Bern, CH. [German]

Hertz, J. 1998. Modelling synfire processing. pp. 135-144. *In:* K.Y.M.Wong, I. King and D.Y. Yeung [eds.]. Theoretical Aspects of Neural Computation. A Multi-Disciplinary Perspective. International Workshop (TANC'97) Hong Kong. Springer-Verlag, Singapore, SG.

Hertz, J. and A. Prügel-Bennett. 1996. Learning synfire chains: turning noise into signal. International Journal of Neural Systems 7: 445-450.

Herzog, M.H., M. Esfeld and W. Gerstner. 2007. Consciousness & the small network argument. Neural Networks 20: 1054-1056.

Heudin, J.-C. 2006. Artificial life and the sciences of complexity: history and future. pp. 227-247. *In:* B. Feltz, M. Crommelinck and P. Goujon [eds.]. Self-Organization and Emergence in Life Sciences. Springer-Verlag, Dordrecht, NL.

Heylighen, F. 2003. The science of self-organization and adaptivity. pp. 253-280. *In:* L.D. Kiel [ed.]. The Encyclopedia of Life Support Systems. Vol. 5. EOLSS Publishers, Oxford, UK.

Heylighen, F. and C. Joslyn. 2001. Cybernetics and second-order cybernetics. pp. 155-170. *In:* R.A. Meyers [ed.]. Encyclopedia of Physical Science & Technology. Vol. 4. 3rd Ed. Academic Press, New York, USA.

Hilario, M. 1997. An overview of strategies for neurosymbolic integration. pp. 13-35. *In:* R. Sun and F. Alexandre [eds.]. Connectionist-Symbolic Integration: From Unified to Hybrid Approaches. Lawrence Erlbaum, Mahwah, USA.

Hinrichsen, D. 1981/1988. Introduction to mathematical systems theory. Lecture Notes for a Joint Course at the Universities of Warwick and Bremen. Zentraldruckerei der Universität Bremen, Bremen, DE.

Hinrichsen, D. and A.J. Pritchard. [eds.] 2010. Mathematical Systems Theory I. Modeling, State Space Analysis, Stability and Robustness. Springer, Berlin, DE.

Hinton, G.E. 1989. Connectionist learning procedures. Artificial Intelligence 40: 185-234.

Hinton, G.E. 1990. Mapping part-whole hierarchies into connectionist networks. Artificial Intelligence 46: 47-76.

Hinton, G.E. 2014. Where do features come from? Cognitive Science 38. 10781101.

Hinton, G.E. and J.A. Anderson [eds.] 1981. Parallel Models of Associative Memory. Lawrence Erlbaum Associates, Hillsdale, USA.

Hinton, G.E. and T.J. Sejnowski. 1986. Learning and relearning in Boltzmann Machines. pp. 282-317. *In:* D.E. Rumelhart and J.L. McClelland [eds.]. Parallel Distributed Processing: Explorations in the Microstructure of Cognition. Vol. 1: Foundations. MIT Press. A Bradford Book, Cambridge, USA.

Hinton, G.E., J.L. McClelland and D.E. Rumelhart. 1986. Distributed representations. pp. 77-109. *In:* D.E. Rumelhart and J.L. McClelland [eds.]. Parallel Distributed Processing: Explorations in the Microstructure of Cognition. Vol. 1: Foundations. MIT Press. A Bradford Book, Cambridge, USA.

Hinton, G.E., S. Osindero and Y.-W. Teh. 2006. A fast learning algorithm for deep belief nets. Neural Computation 18: 1527-1554.

Hipp, J.F., A.K. Engel and M. Siegel. 2011. Oscillatory synchronization in large-scale cortical networks predicts perception. Neuron 69: 387-396.

Hirsch, M.W. and S. Smale. 1974. Differential Equations, Dynamical Systems, and Linear Algebra. Academic Press, New York, USA.

Hölldobler, S. 2004. Computational logic. Working Material. Fakultät für Informatik. International Center For Computational Logic. Technische Universität Dresden, Dresden, DE. [unpublished manuscript]

Hölscher, C. 2009. How could populations of neurons encode information. pp. 3-17. *In:* C. Hölscher and M. Munk [eds.]. Information Processing by Neuronal Populations. Cambridge University Press, Cambridge, UK.

Hoffmann, K.-P. and C. Wehrhahn. 2001. Central visual systems. pp. 407-428. *In:* J. Dudel, R. Menzel and R.F. Schmidt [eds.]. Neurowissenschaft. Vom Molekül zur Kognition. 2nd Ed. Springer-Verlag, Berlin, DE. [German]

Hofstadter, D.R. 1985. Metamagical Themas: Questing for the Essence of Mind and Pattern. Basic Books, New York, USA.

Hofstadter, D.R. 2007. I am a Strange Loop. Basic Books, New York.

Hohwy, J. 2013. The Predictive Mind. Oxford University Press, Oxford, UK.

Hohwy, J. 2016. The self-evidencing brain. Noûs 50: 259285.

Holcombe, A.O. 2010. The binding problem. pp. 205-208. *In:* E.B. Goldstein [ed.]. The Sage Encyclopedia of Perception. Vol. 1. SAGE Publications, Thousand Oaks, USA.

Holthausen, K. 1995. Neural networks and information theory. Ph.D. Thesis, Universität Münster, Münster, DE. [German]

Holthausen, K. and O. Breidbach. 1997. Self-organized feature maps and information theory. Network: Computation in Neural Systems 8: 215-227.

Holyoak, K.J. and P. Thagard. 1989. Analogical mapping by constraint satisfaction. Cognitive Science 13: 295-355.

Holzmann, G. 2008. Echo state networks with filter neurons and a delay&sum readout with applications in audio signal processing. M.Sc. Thesis. Institute for Theoretical Computer Science. Graz University of Technology, Graz, AT.

Hooker, C. 2011. Introduction to philosophy of complex systems: A. Part A: Towards a framework for complex systems. pp. 3-90. *In:* C. Hooker [ed.]. Philosophy of Complex Systems. Handbook of the Philosophy of Science. Vol. 10. Elsevier, New York, USA.

Hopcroft, J.E., R. Motwani and R.D. Ullman 2006. Introduction to Automata Theory, Languages, and Computation. 3rd Ed. Addison-Wesley, Boston, USA.

Hopfield, J.J. 1982. Neural networks and physical systems with emergent collective computational properties. Proceedings of the National Academy of Sciences of the United States of America 79: 2554-2558. (reprinted in: Hopfield 1988.)

Hopfield, J.J. 1988. Neural networks and physical systems with emergent collective computational properties. pp. 460-464. *In:* J.A. Anderson and E. Rosenfeld [eds.]. Neurocomputing: Foundations of Research. Chapter 27. MIT Press, Cambridge, USA.

Hopfield, J.J. 1995. Pattern recognition computation using action potential timing for stimulus representation. Nature 376: 33-36.

Hopfield, J.J. and C.D. Brody. 2000. What is a moment? "Cortical" sensory integration over a brief interval. Proceedings of the National Academy of Sciences of the United States of America 97: 13919-13924.

Horgan, T. and J. Tienson. [eds.] 1988. Spindel Conference 1987: Connectionism and the Philosophy of Mind. The Southern Journal of Philosophy 26 Supplement: Special Issue on Connectionism and the Foundations of Cognitive Science. pp. 1-193.

Horgan, T. and J. Tienson. 1989. Representation without rules. Philosophical Topics 17: 147-174.

Horgan, T. and J. Tienson. 1990. Soft laws. pp. 256-279. *In:* P.A. French, T.E. Uehling, Jr. and H.K. Wettstein [eds.]. Midwest Studies in Philosophy. Volume XV. The Philosophy of the Human Sciences. University of Notre Dame Press, Notre Dame, USA.

Horgan, T. and J. Tienson [eds.] 1991a. Connectionism and the Philosophy of Mind. Kluwer Academic Publisher, Dordrecht, NE.

Horgan, T. and J. Tienson. 1991b. Settling into a new paradigm. pp. 241-260. *In:* T. Horgan and J. Tienson [eds.]. Connectionism and the Philosophy of Mind. Kluwer Academic Publisher, Dordrecht, NE.

Horgan, T. and J. Tienson. 1992a. Structured representations in connectionist systems? pp. 195-228. *In:* S. Davis [ed.]. Connectionism: Theory and Practice. Oxford University Press, New York, USA, Oxford, UK.

Horgan, T. and J. Tienson. 1992b. Cognitive systems as dynamical systems. Topoi 11: 27-43.

Horgan, T. and J. Tienson. 1994a. A nonclassical framework for cognitive science. Synthese 101: 305-345.

Horgan, T. and J. Tienson. 1994b. Representations don't need rules: reply to James Garson. Mind & Language 9: 38-55.

Horgan, T. and J. Tienson. 1996. Connectionism and the Philosophy of Psychology. The MIT Press, Cambridge, USA.

Horgan, T. and J. Tienson. 1998. Rules. pp. 660-670. *In:* W. Bechtel and G. Graham [eds.]. A Companion to Cognitive Science. Blackwell Publisher, Malden, USA, Oxford, UK.

Horgan, T. and J. Tienson. 1999. Rules and representations. pp. 724-726. *In:* R.A. Wilson and F.C. Keil [eds.]. The MIT Encyclopedia of the Cognitive Sciences. The MIT Press, Cambridge, USA, London, UK.

Horgan, T. and J. Tienson. 2006. Cognition needs syntax but not rules. pp. 147-158. *In:* R. Stainton [ed.]. Contemporary Debates in Cognitive Science. Basil Blackwell, Oxford, UK.

Hotton, S. and J. Yoshimi 2011. Extending dynamical systems theory to model embodied cognition. Cognitive Science 35: 444-479.

Houdé, O. [ed.] 2004. Dictionary of Cognitive Science. Neuroscience, Psychology, Artificial Intelligence, Linguistic, and Philosophy. Psychology Press, New York, USA, Hove, UK.

Houghton, G. [ed.] 2005. Connectionist Models in Cognitive Psychology. Psychology Press, Hove, UK.

Houng, A.Y. 2003. Philosophical issues about levels of analysis. pp. 852-855. *In:* L. Nadel. [ed.]. Encyclopedia of Cognitive Science. Vol. 3. Natur Publishing Group. London, UK, New York, USA and Tokyo, JP.

Hoyningen-Huene, P. 1998. Formal Logic. A Philosophical Introduction. Philipp Reclam jun., Stuttgart, DE. [German]

Hoyningen-Huene, P. 2007. Reduction and emergence. pp. 177-198. *In:* A. Bartels [ed.]. Wissenschaftstheorie. Ein Studienbuch. Mentis Verlag, Paderborn, DE. [German]

Huang, Q., P. Smolensky, X. He, L. Deng and D. Wu. 2017. A neural-symbolic approach to design of CAPTCHA. arXiv preprint arXiv:1710.11475.

Huang, Q., P. Smolensky, X. He, L. Deng and D. Wu. 2018. Tensor product generation network for deep NLP modeling, 1263-1273. Proceedings of the 2018 Conference of the North American Chapter of the Association for Computational Linguistics: Human Language Technologies (NAACL 2018),

Vol. 1, New Orleans, United States of America. Association for Computational Linguistics.

Hubel, D.H. and T.N. Wiesel. 1959. Receptive fields of single neurones in the cat's striate cortex. Journal of Physiology 148: 574-591.

Hubel, D.H. and T.N. Wiesel. 1965. Receptive fields and functional architecture in two nonstriate visual areas (18 and 19) of the cat. Journal of Neurophysiology 28: 229-289.

Huber, L. 2000. How the new gets into the brains. Emergence and chaos in neuronal processes. pp. 157-174. *In:* L. Huber [ed.]. Wie das Neue in die Welt kommt. Phasenübergänge in Natur und Kultur. WUV, Wien, AT. [German]

Hülsmann, M., C.Wycisk, R. Agarwal and J. Grapp. 2007. Prologue to Autonomous Cooperation – the Idea of Self-Organization as its Basic Concepts. pp. 23-44. *In:* M. Hülsmann and K. Windt [eds.]. Understanding Autonomous Cooperation and Control in Logistics. Springer-Verlag, Berlin, Heidelberg, DE.

Huett, M.-T. 2006. What is self-organization and what is its use in understanding nature? pp. 91-105. *In:* M. Vec, M.-T. Huett and A.M. Freund [eds.]. Selbstorganisation. Ein Denksystem für Natur und Gesellschaft. Böhlau, Köln, DE. [German]

Huett, M.-T. and C. Marr. 2006. Self-organization as metatheory. pp. 106-126. *In:* M. Vec, M.-T. Huett and A.M. Freund [eds.]. Selbstorganisation. Ein Denksystem für Natur und Gesellschaft. Böhlau, Köln, DE. [German]

Hull, C.L. 1943. Principles of Behavior. Appleton-Century-Crofts, New York, USA.

Hummel, J. 1999. Binding problem. pp. 85-86. *In:* R.A. Wilson and F.C. Keil [eds.]. The MIT Encyclopedia of the Cognitive Sciences. The MIT Press, Cambridge, USA, London, UK.

Hummel, J.E. and K.J. Holyoak. 1997. Distributed representation of structure: a theory of analogical access and mapping. Psychological Review 104: 427-466.

Hummel, J.E. and K.J. Holyoak. 2003. A symbolic-connectionist theory of relational inference and generalization. Psychological Review 110: 220-264.

Huppert, B. and W. Willems. 2010. Linear Algebra. With Numerous Applications in Cryptography, Coding Theory, Mathematical Physics and Stochastic Processes. 2nd Ed. Vieweg+Teubner, Wiesbaden, DE. [German]

Huyck, C.R. and P.J. Passmore. 2013. A review of cell assemblies. Biological Cybernetics 107: 263-288.

Ihringer, T. 1993. General Algebra. 2nd Ed. Teubner, Stuttgart, DE. [German]

Iida, F., R. Pfeifer, L. Steels and Y. Kuniyoshi [eds.] 2004. Embodied Artificial Intelligence. International Seminar, Dagstuhl Castle, Germany, July 7-11, 2003. Springer, Berlin, Heidelberg, DE.

Ikegaya, Y., G. Aaron, R. Cossart, D. Aronov, I. Lampl, D. Ferster and R. Yuste. 2004. Synfire chains and cortical songs: temporal modules of cortical activity. Science 304: 559564.

Imboden, D.M. and S. Koch. 2008. System Analysis. Introduction to the Mathematical Modeling of Natural Systems. 1st Ed. 3rd corr. Iss. Springer. Berlin, DE. [German]

Isbister, J.B., A. Eguchi, N. Ahmad, J.M. Galeazzi, M.J. Buckley and S. Stringer. 2018. A new approach to solving the feature-binding problem in primate vision. Interface Focus 8: 20180021.

Izhikevich, E.M. 2006. Polychronization: computation with spikes. Neural Computation 18: 245-282.

Izhikevich, E.M., J.A. Gally and G.M. Edelman. 2004. Spike-timing dynamics of neuronal groups. Cerebral Cortex 14: 933-944.

Jackendoff, R. 2002. Foundations of Language. Brain, Meaning, Grammar, Evolution. Oxford University Press, Oxford, UK.

Jacob, S.N., D. Hähnke and A. Nieder. 2018. Structuring of abstract working memory content by fronto-parietal synchrony in primate cortex. Neuron 99: 588-597.

Jacobs, A.M. and M.J. Hofmann. 2015. Neurocognitive modeling. Freie Universität Berlin, Berlin, DE. [unpublished manuscript] [German]

Jacobs, A.M., F. Hutzler and V. Engl. 2006. On the trail of the spirit. Neurocognitive methods for measuring learning and memory processes. Zeitschrift für Erziehungswissenschaft 9: 71-86. [German]

Jaeger, H. 1996. Dynamic systems in cognitive science. Kognitionswissenschaft 5: 152-157. [German]

Jaeger, H. 2001/2010. The "echo state" approach to analysing and training recurrent neural networks – with an erratum note. GMD Report 148, GMD – German National Research Center for Information Technology, Sankt Augustin, DE: 47pp.

Jaeger, H. 2002/2008. Tutorial on training recurrent neural networks, Covering BPPT, RTRL, EKF and the echo state network approach. GMD Report 159, GMD – German National Research Center for Information Technology, Sankt Augustin, DE: 46pp.

Jaeger, H., W. Maass and J. Principe. 2007a. Special issue on echo state networks and liquid state machines: editorial. Neural Networks 20: 287-289.

Jaeger, H., M. Lukoševičus, D. Popovici and U. Siewert. 2007b. Optimization and applications of echo state networks with leaky integrator neurons. Neural Networks 20: 335-352.

Jäncke, L. 2017. Textbook Cognitive Neurosciences. 2nd Ed. Hogrefe, Göttingen, DE. [German]

Jänich, K. 2005. Topology. 8th Ed. Springer-Verlag, Berlin, Heidelberg, DE. [German]

Jagadeesh, B., H.S. Wheat and D. Ferster. 1993. Linearity of summation of synaptic potentials underlying direction selectivity of simple cells of the cat visual cortex. Science 262: 1901-1904.

Janich, P. 2006. What is Information? Suhrkamp Verlag, Frankfurt am Main, DE. [German]

Janssen, T.M.V. 2011. Compositionality. pp. 495-554. *In:* J. van Benthem and A. ter Meulen [eds.]. Handbook of Logic and Language. 2nd Ed. Elsevier, Amsterdam, NL.

Jantsch, E. 1979/1980. The Self-Organizing Universe: Scientific and Human Implications of the Emerging Paradigm of Evolution. Pergamon, Oxford, UK, Elmsford, USA.

Jantsch, E. 1980. The unifying paradigm behind autopoiesis, dissipative structures, hyper- and ultracycles. pp. 81-87. *In:* M. Zeleny. [ed.]. Autopoiesis, Dissipative Structure, and Spontaneous Social Orders. Westview Press, Boulder, USA.

Jantsch, E. 1981. Autopoiesis: a central aspect of dissipative self-organization. pp. 63-88. *In:* M. Zeleny [ed.]. Autopoiesis: A Theory of the Living Organizations. North Holland, New York, USA.

Jantsch, E. 1989. System, system theory. p. 332. *In:* H. Seiffert and G. Radnitzky [eds.]. Handlexikon zur Wissenschaftstheorie. Ehrenwirth Verlag, München, DE. [German]

Jaynes, E.T. 2010. Probability Theory: The Logic of Science. 7th Ed. Cambridge University Press, Cambridge, UK.

Jetschke, G. 1989. Mathematics of Self-Organization. Qualitative Theory of Nonlinear Dynamical Systems and Structures far from Equilibrium in Physics, Chemistry and Biology. Vieweg, Braunschweig, DE. [German]

Jha, D. 2005. Use Reentrant Functions for Safer Signal Handling. IBM Corporation. Developer-Works. Technical Topics. Linux. Technical Library. [unpublished technical manuscript: https://www.ibm.com/developerworks/library/l-reent/lreent-pdf.pdf]

Jia, X., D. Xing and A. Kohn. 2013a. No consistent relationship between gamma power and peak frequency in macaque primary visual cortex. The Journal of Neuroscience 33: 1725.

Jia, X., S. Tanabe and A. Kohn. 2013b. Gamma and the coordination of spiking activity in early visual cortex. Neuron 77: 762-774.

Johnson, J.S., J.P. Spencer and G. Schöner. 2009a. A layered neural architecture for the consolidation, maintenance, and updating of representations in visual working memory. Brain Research 1299: 17-32.

Johnson, J.S., J.P. Spencer, S.J. Luck and G. Schöner. 2009b. A dynamic neural field model of visual working memory and change detection. Psychological Science 20: 568-577.

Jones, G. and F.E. Ritter. 2003. Production systems and rule-based inference. pp. 741-747. *In:* L. Nadel. [ed.]. Encyclopedia of Cognitive Science. Vol. 3. Natur Publishing Group. London, UK, New York, USA and Tokyo, JP.

Jordan, M.I. 1986. Attractor dynamics and parallelism in a connectionist sequential machine, 531-546. *In* Cognitive Science Society (U.S.) [ed.] Proceedings of the 8th Conference of the Cognitive Science Society. Amherst, Unites States of America. Lawrence Erlbaum.

Jost, J., K. Holthausen and O. Breidbach. 1997. On the mathematical foundations of a theory of neural representation. Theory in Biosciences 116: 125-139.

Kallenrode, M.-B. 2005. Computational Methods of Physics. Mathematical Guide to Experimental Physics. 2nd Ed. Springer-Verlag, Berlin, DE. [German]

Kalman, R.E. 1960a. Contributions to the theory of optimal control. Boletin de la Sociedad Matematica Mexicana 5: 102-119.

Kalman, R.E. 1960b. A new approach to linear filtering and prediction problems. ASME Journal of Basic Engineering 82: 35-45.

Kampis, G. 1991. Self-Modifying Systems in Biology and Cognitive Science: A New Framework for Dynamics, Information and Complexity. Pergamon Press, Oxford, UK.

Kanai, R., Y. Komura, S. Shipp and K. Friston. 2014. Cerebral hierarchies: predictive processing, precision and the pulvinar. Philosophical Transactions of the Royal Society of London. B Biological Sciences 370: 20140169.

Kandel, E.R., J.H. Schwartz, T.M. Jessell, S.A. Siegelbaum, A.J.Huds-Peth [eds.] 2013. Principles of Neural Science. 5th Ed. McGraw-Hill Medical. New York, USA, Toronto, CA.

Kanerva, P. 1990. Sparse Distributed Memory. 2nd Ed. MIT Press, Cambridge, USA.

Kanerva, P. 1993. Sparse distributed memory and related models. pp. 50-76. *In:* M.H. Hassoun [ed.]. Associative Neural Memories: Theory and Implementation. Oxford University Press, New York, USA.

Kanerva, P. 1994. The spatter code for encoding concepts at many levels. pp. 226-229. *In:* M. Marinaro and P.G. Morasso [eds.]. Proceedings of

International Conference on Artificial Neural Networks 1994 (ICANN.94). Sorrento, Italy. Springer.

Kanerva, P. 1996. Binary spatter-coding of ordered k-tuples. pp. 869-873. *In:* C. von der Malsburg, W. von Seelen, J. Vorbruggen and B. Sendhoff [eds.]. Proceedings of the International Conference on Artificial Neural Networks (ICANN96), Bochum, Germany. Springer.

Kanerva, P. 1997. Fully distributed representation, 358-365. *In* Proceedings of the 1997 Real World Computing Symposium (RWC'97), Tokyo, Japan. Real World Computing Partnership.

Kanerva, P. 2009. Hyperdimensional computing: an introduction to computing in distributed representation with high-dimensional random vectors. Cognitive Computation 1: 139-159.

Kanitscheider, B. 2006. Chaos and self-organization in science and humanities. pp. 66-90. *In:* M.-T. Huett and A.M. Freund [eds.]. Selbstorganisation. Ein Denksystem für Natur und Gesellschaft. Böhlau, Köln, DE. [German]

Kaplan, D. and C.F. Craver. 2011. The explanatory force of dynamical and mathematical models in neuroscience: a mechanistic perspective. Philosophy of Science 78: 601-627.

Kaplansky, I. 1977. Set Theory and Metric Spaces. AMS Chelsea Publishing, New York, USA.

Kasabov, N. 1998. Foundations of Neural Networks, Fuzzy Systems and Knowledge Engineering. 2nd Ed. A Bradford Book, The MIT Press, Cambridge, USA, London, UK.

Katok, A. and B. Hasselblatt. 1995. Introduction to the Modern Theory of Dynamical Systems. Cambridge University Press. Cambridge, UK.

Katz, J.J. and J.A. Fodor 1963. The structure of a semantic theory. Language 39: 170-210.

Katzner, S., I. Nauhaus, A. Benucci, V. Bonin, D.L. Ringach and M. Carandini. 2009. Local origin of field potentials in visual cortex. Neuron 61: 35-41.

Kauffman, S.A. 1993. The Origins of Order: Self-Organizing and Selection in Evolution. Oxford University Press. New York, USA.

Kauffman, S. 2000. Investigations. Oxford University Press, Oxford, UK.

Kaufmann, H. and H. Pape. 1996. Cluster analysis. pp. 437-536. *In:* L. Fahrmeir, A. Hamerle and G. Tutz [eds.]. Multivariate statistische Verfahren. 2nd Ed. Walter de Gruyter, Berlin, DE, New York, USA. [German]

Kavouras, M. and M. Kokla. 2007. Theories of Geographic Concepts: Ontological Approaches to Semantic Integration. CRC Press, Boca Raton, USA.

Kayser, C., R.F. Salazar and König. 2003. Responses to natural scenes in cat V1. Journal of Neurophysiology 90: 1910-1920.

Keller, J. 1990. Connectionism – a new paradigm for knowledge representation? Linguistische Berichte 128: 298-331. [German]

Kemke, C. 1988. The newer connectionism. Informatik Spektrum 11: 143-162. [German]

Kemmerling, A. 1991. Mental representations. Kognitionswissenschaft 1: 47-57. [German]

Khalil, H.K. 2002. Nonlinear Systems. Prentice Hall, Upper Saddle River, USA.

Kiefer, A.B. 2019. A Defense of Pure Connectionism. Ph.D. Thesis. The City University of New York. New York, USA.

Kilpatrick, Z.P. 2015. Stochastic synchronization of neural activity waves. Physical Review E 91: 040701(R).

Kirchhoff, M., T. Parr, E. Palacios, K. Friston and J. Kiverstein. 2018. The Markov blankets of life: autonomy, active inference and the free energy principle. Journal of the Royal Society Interface 15: 20170792.

Kirschfeld, K. 2001. Photoreception (peripheral visual organs). pp. 385-405. In: J. Dudel, R. Menzel and R.F. Schmidt [eds.]. Neurowissenschaft. Vom Molekül zur Kognition. 2nd. Ed. Springer-Verlag, Berlin, DE. [German]

Kirsh, D. 1991. When is information explicitly represented? pp. 340-365. In: P. Hanson [ed.]. Information, Language and Cognition. UBC Press, Vancouver, CA.

Kleene, S.C. 1967. Mathematical Logic. John Wiley and Sons, New York, USA.

Klir, G.J. 1969. An Approach to General Systems Theory. Van Nostrand Reinhold Company, New York, USA.

Klir, G.J. 1991. Facets of Systems Science. Plenum Press, New York, USA, London, UK.

Knieling, S. 2007. Introduction to the Modeling of Artificial Neural Networks. WiKu-Verlag für Wissenschaft und Kultur, Duisburg, DE. [German]

Knill, D.C. and A. Pouget. 2004. The Bayesian brain: the role of uncertainty in neural coding and computation. Trends in Neurosciences 27: 712-719.

Koch, C. 1999. Biophysics of Computation. Information Processing in Single Neurons. Oxford University Press, New York, USA.

Koch, C. 2004. The Quest for Consciousness. A Neurobiological Approach. Roberts, Denver, USA.

Koch, C., R.J. Douglas and U. Wehmeier. 1990. Visibility of a synaptically induced conductance changes: theory and simulations of anatomically characterized cortical pyramidal cells. The Journal of Neuroscience 10: 1728-1744.

Koch, C. and H. Schuster. 1992. A simple network showing burst synchronization without frequency locking. Neural Computation 4: 211-223.

Köhle, M. 1990. Neural Nets. Springer-Verlag. Wien, AT, New York, USA. [German]

König, P. 1994. A method for the quantification of synchrony and oscillatory properties of neuronal activity. Journal of Neuroscience Methods 54: 31-37.

König, P. and T.B. Schillen. 1990. Segregation of oscillatory responses by conflicting timuli – desynchronizing connections in neural oscillator layers. pp. 117-120. *In:* R. Eckmiller, G. Hartmann and G. Hauske [eds.]. Parallel Processing in Neural Systems and Computers. Elsevier Science Inc., Amsterdam, NL.

König, P. and T.B. Schillen. 1991. Stimulus-dependent assembly formation of oscillatory responses. I. Synchronization. Neural Computation 3: 155-166.

König, P., B. Janosch and T.B. Schillen. 1993. Assembly formation and segregation by a self-organizing neuronal oscillator model. pp. 509-513. *In:* F.H. Eeckman and J.M. Bower [eds.]. Computation and Neural Systems. Kluwer Academic Publishers, Boston, USA, Dordrecht, NL, London, UK.

König, P., A.K. Engel and W. Singer. 1995a. The relation between oscillatory acitivity and long-range synchronization in cat visual cortex. Proceedings of the National Academy of Sciences of the United States of America 92: 290-294.

König, P., A.K. Engel, P.R. Roelfsema and W. Singer. 1995b. How precise is neuronal synchronization? Neural Computation 7: 469-485.

Königsberger, K. 2002. Analysis 2. 4th Ed. Springer-Verlag, Berlin, DE. [German]

Kohonen, T. 1982a. Analysis of a simple self-organizing process. Biological Cybernetics 44: 135-140.

Kohonen, T. 1982b. Clustering, taxonomy, and topological maps of patterns, 114-128. *In* Proceedings of the 6th International Conference of Pattern Recognition, Munich, Germany. IEEE Computer Society Press.

Kohonen, T. 1982c. Self-organized formation of topologically correct feature maps. Biological Cybernetics 43: 59-69. (reprinted in Kohonen 1988b.)

Kohonen, T. 1984. Self-Organization and Associative Memory. Springer-Verlag, New York, USA.

Kohonen, T. 1988a. Self-Organizing and Associative Memory. 2nd Ed. Springer-Verlag, Berlin, DE.

Kohonen, T. 1988b. Self-organized formation of topologically correct feature maps. pp. 511-522. *In:* J.A. Anderson and E. Rosenfeld [eds.]. Neurocomputing: Foundations of Research. Chapter 30. MIT Press, Cambridge, USA.

Kohonen, T. 1993. Physiological interpretation of the self-organizing map algorithm. Neural Networks 6: 895-905.

Kohonen, T. 1995. Self-Organizing Maps. Springer-Verlag, Berlin, DE.

Kohonen, T. 1998. The self-organizing map. Neurocomputing 21: 1-6 (Special Volume on Self-Organizing Maps, E. Oja [ed.]).

Kohonen, T. 2001. Self-Organizing Maps. 3rd Ed. Springer-Verlag, Berlin, DE.

Kohonen, T. 2002. Overture. pp. 1-12. *In:* U. Seiffert and L.C. Jain [eds.]. Self-Organizing Neural Networks. Recent Advances and Applications. Physica-Verlag, Heidelberg, DE, New York, USA.

Kolb, B. and I.Q. Whishaw. 2015. Fundamentals of Human Neuropsychology. 7th Ed. Worth Publisher, New York, USA.

Kolchinsky, A., M.P. van den Heuvel, A. Griffa, P. Hagmann, L.M. Rocha, O. Sporns and J. Goñi. 2014. Multi-scale integration and predictability in resting state brain activity. Frontier in Neuroinformatics 8: 66.

Kolen, J.F. 2001. Dynamical systems and iterated function Systems. pp. 83-102. *In:* J.F. Kolen and S.C. Kremer [eds.]. A Field Guide to Dynamical Recurrent Networks. IEEE Press, New York, USA.

Kolmogorov, A.N. 1968a. Three approaches to the quantitative definition of information. International Journal of Computer Mathematics 2: 157-168.

Kolmogorov, A.N. 1968b. Logical basis for information theory and probability theory. IEEE Transactions on Information Theory 14: 662-664.

Kolo, C., T. Christaller and E. Pöppel. 1999. Bioinformation. Problemlösungen für die Wissensgesellschaft. Physica-Verlag, Heidelberg, DE. [German]

Kondepudi, D. 2008. Introduction to Modern Thermodynamics. Wiley, Chichester, UK.

Kopell, N. 2000. We got rhythm: dynamical systems of the nervous system. Notices of the American Mathematical Society 47: 6-16.

Kopell, N. and B. Ermentrout. 1986. Symmetry and phaselocking in chains of weakly coupled oscillators. Communications on Pure and Applied Mathematics 39: 623-660.

Korb, K.B. 1996. Symbolism and connectionism. AI back at a join point. pp. 247-257. *In:* D.L. Dowe, K.B. Korb and J.J. Oliver [eds.]. Proceedings of the Conference on Information, Statistics and Induction in Science (ISIS'96), Melbourne, Australia. World Scientific Publishing.

Korndörfer, C., E. Ullner, J. García and G. Pipa. 2017. Cortical spike synchrony as measure of input familiarity. Neural Computation 29: 1-20.

Kornwachs, K. 2008. Non-classical systems and the problem of emergence. pp. 181-231. *In:* R. Breuninger [ed.]. Selbstorganisation. Humboldt-Studienzentrum. Universität Ulm. KIZ Medienzentrum. Ulm, DE. [German]

Kornwachs, K. and K. Jacoby [eds.] 1996. Information: New Questions to a Multidisciplinary Concept. Akademie Verlag, Berlin, DE.

Kosko, B. 1992. Neural Networks and Fuzzy Systems – A Dynamical Systems Approach to Machine Intelligence. Prentice-Hall, London, UK.

Kostal, L., P. Lansky and J.-P. Rospars. 2007. Neuronal coding and spiking randomness. European Journal of Neuroscience 26: 2693-2701.

Kotropoulos, C., I. Pitas, S. Fischer and B. Duc. 1997. Face authentication using morphological dynamic link architecture. pp. 169-176. *In:* J. Bigün, B. Chollet and G. Borgefors [eds.]. Proceedings of the First International Conference (AVBPA'97), Audio- and Video-based Biometric Person Authentication, Crans-Montana, Switzerland. Springer.

Kowalsky, H.-J. and G.O. Michler. 1995. Linear Algebra. 10th Ed. Walter de Gruyter. Berlin u.a., DE. [German]

Kozma, R. and W.J. Freeman. 2009. The KIV model of intentional dynamics and decision making. Neural Networks 22: 277-285.

Kralemann, B.C. 2006. Environment, Culture, Semantics – Reality. A Theory of Environmental- and Culture-Dependent Semantic Structures of Reality Based on the Modeling of Cognitive Processes by Neural Networks. Ph.D. Thesis, Leipziger Universit"atsverlag, Kiel, Schleswig-Holstein. [German]

Krasnosel'skiĭ, M.A. and A.V. Pokrovskiĭ. 1989. Systems with Hysteresis. Springer, Berlin, DE.

Kratky, K.W. 1990. The paradigm shift from external to self-organization. pp. 3-17. *In:* K.W. Kratky and F.Wallner [eds.]. Grundprinzipien der Selbstorganisation. Wissenschaftliche Buchgesellschaft, Darmstadt, DE. [German]

Krause, C.D. 2013. Psycholinguistics and Neurolinguistics. pp. 66-71. *In:* A. Stephan and S. Walter. [eds.]. Handbuch Kognitionswissenschaft. Metzler, Stuttgart, Weimar, DE. [German]

Kreiter, A.K. and W. Singer. 1992. Oscillatory neuronal responses in the visual cortex of the awake macaque monkey. European Journal of Neuroscience 4: 369-375.

Kreiter, A.K. and W. Singer. 1996. Stimulus-dependent synchronization of neuronal responses in the visual cortex of the awake macaque monkey. The Journal of Neuroscience 16: 2381-2396.

Kremkow, J., A. Kumar, S. Rotter and A. Aertsen. 2007. Emergence of population synchrony in a layered network of the cat visual cortex. Neurocomputing 70: 2069-2073.

Kreyssig, P. and P. Dittrich. 2011. Emergent control. pp. 67-78. *In:* C. Müller-Schloer, H. Schmeck and T. Ungerer [eds.]. Organic Computing – A Paradigm Shift for Complex Systems. Birkhäuser, Basel, CH.

Krieger, D.J. 1996. Introduction to General Systems Theory. Fink, München, DE. [German]

Krohn, W., G. Küppers and R. Paslack. 1987. Self-organization – the genesis and development of a scientific revolution. pp. 441-465. *In:* S.J. Schmidt [ed.]. Der Diskurs des Radikalen Konstruktivismus. Suhrkamp Verlag, Frankfurt, DE. [German]

Krohn, W. and G. Küppers [eds.] 1990. Self-Organization. Aspects of a Scientific Revolution. Vieweg, Braunschweig und Wiesbaden, DE. [German]

Krohn, W. and G. Küppers. 1992. Self-organization: A new paradigm for the sciences. Information Philosophy 20: 23-30. [German]

Krumke, S.O. 2009. Graph Theoretical Concepts and Algorithms. 2nd Ed. Vieweg + Teubner, Wiesbaden, DE. [German]

Kugler, P.N. and M.T. Turvey. 1987. Information, Natural Law, and the Self-Assembly of Rhythmic Movement: Theoretical and Experimental Investigations. Erlbaum, Hillsdale, USA.

Kuhn, T.S. 1962/2012. The Structure of Scientific Revolutions. University of Chicago Press, Chicago, USA.

Kumar, A., S. Rotter and A. Aertsen. 2008. Conditions for propagating synchronous spiking and asynchronous firing rates in a cortical network model. Journal of Neuroscience 28: 5268-5280.

Kuo, D. and C. Eliasmith. 2005. Integrating behavioral and neural data in a model of zebrafish network interaction. Biological Cybernetics 93: 178-187.

Kuratowski, K. 1967. Set Theory. North Holland, Amsterdam, NL.

Kurthen, M. 1992. Neurosemantics. Basics of a Praxiological Cognitive Neuroscience. F. Enke Verlag, Stuttgart, DE. [German]

Kurthen, M. 1999. Conscious behaviour explained. Consciousness and Cognition 8: 155-158.

Kvasnička, V. and J. Pospíchal. 2004. Holographic reduced representation in artificial intelligence and cognitive science. Faculty of Computer Science and Information Technologies. Slovak Technical University. [unpublished manuscript]

Kyselo, M. 2013. Enactivism. pp. 197-201. *In:* A. Stephan and S. Walter. [eds.]. Handbuch Kognitionswissenschaft. Metzler, Stuttgart, Weimar, DE. [German]

Laan, A., T. Gutnick, M.L. Kuba and G. Laurent. 2014. Behavioral analysis of cuttlefish traveling waves and its implications for neural control. Current Biology 24: 1737-1742.

Lades, M., J.C. Vorbrüggen, J. Buhmann, J. Lange, C. von der Malsburg, R.P. Würtz and W. Konen. 1993. Distortion invariant object recognition in the dynamic link architecture. IEEE Transactions on Computers 42: 300-310.

Ladyman, J., J. Lambert and K. Wiesner. 2013. What is a complex system? European Journal for Philosophy of Science 3: 33-67.

Lai, Y.-C. and C. Grebogi. 1996. Complexity in Hamiltonian-driven dissipative chaotic dynamical systems. Physical Review E 54: 4667-4675.

Lalisse, M. and P. Smolensky. 2018. Augmenting compositional models for knowledge base completion using gradient representations. arXiv preprint arXiv:1811.01062.

Lambert, A.J. and A.L. Chasteen. 1998. Social cognition. pp. 306-313. *In:* W. Bechtel and G. Graham [eds.]. A Companion to Cognitive Science. Blackwell Publisher, Malden, USA, Oxford, UK.

Lamme, V.A.F. and H. Spekreijse. 1998. Neuronal synchrony does not represent texture segregation. Nature 396: 362-366.

Landry, E. 2007. Shared structure need not be shared set-structure. Synthese 158: 1-17.

Lane, P.C.R. and J.B. Henderson. 1998. Simple synchrony networks: learning to parse natural language with temporal synchrony variable binding. pp. 615-620. *In:* L.F. Niklasson, M. Boden and T. Ziemke [eds.]. Proceedings of the 8th International Conference on Artificial Neural Networks (ICANN'98), Vol. 2, Skövde, Sweden. Springer.

Lang, C.B. and N. Pucker. 1998. Mathematical Methods in Physics. Spektrum Akademischer Verlag, Heidelberg, DE, Berlin, DE. [German]

Langacker, R.W. 1987. Foundations of Cognitive Grammar. Vol. 1. Stanford University Press, Stanford, USA.

Langacker, R.W. 1991. Foundations of Cognitive Grammar. Vol. 2. Stanford University Press, Stanford, USA.

Lange, T.E. 1992. Hybrid connectionist models. Temporary bridges over the gap between the symbolic and the subsymbolic. pp. 237-290. *In:* J. Dinsmore [ed.]. The Symbolic and Connectionist Paradigms: Closing the Gap. Lawrence Erlbaum, Hillsdale, USA.

Lappi, O. and A.-M. Rusanen. 2011. Turing machines and causal mechanisms in cognitive science. pp. 224-239. *In:* P. McKay Illari, F. Russo and J. Williamson [eds.]. Causality in the Sciences. Oxford University Press, Oxford, UK.

Laughlin, R.B. 2005. A Different Universe. Reinventing Physics from the Bottom Down. Basic Books, Cambridge, USA.

Laurent, G. 1996 Dynamical representation of odors by oscillating and evolving neural assemblies. Trends in Neurosciences 19; 489-496.

Laurent, G. 2002. Olfactory network dynamics and the coding of multidimensional signals. Nature Reviews Neuroscience 3: 884-895.

Laurent, G. and H. Davidowitz. 1994. Encoding of olfactory information with oscillating neural assemblies. Science 265: 1872-1875.

Lazar, A., G. Pipa and J. Triesch. 2007. Fading memory and time series prediction in recurrent networks with different forms of plasticity. Neural Networks 20: 312-322.

Lazar, A., G. Pipa and J. Triesch. 2009. SORN: a self-organizing recurrent neural network. Frontiers in Computational Neuroscience 3: 23.

Leahey, T.H. 1991. A History of Modern Psychology. Prentice-Hall, Englewood Cliffs, USA.

Lazar, A., G. Pipa and J. Triesch. 2011. Emerging Bayesian priors in a selforganizing recurrent network. pp. 127-134. *In:* T. Honkela [ed.]. Proceedings of the 21th International Conference on Artificial Neural Networks and Machine Learning (ICANN'2011), Part II, Espoo, Finland. Springer.

Lebiere, C. and J.R. Anderson. 1993. A connectionist implementation of the ACT-R production system, 635-640. *In* Proceedings of the 15th Annual Conference of the Cognitive Science Society. Boulder, USA. Lawrence Erlbaum.

Lecoutre, C. 2009. Constraint Networks. Techiques and Algorithms. ISTE, London, UK.

LeCun, Y., B. Boser, J.S. Denker, D. Henderson, R.E. Howard,W. Hubbard and L.D. Jackel. 1989. Backpropagation applied to handwritten zip code recognition. Neural Computation 1: 541-551.

LeCun, Y., Y. Bengio and G. Hinton. 2015. Deep learning. Nature 521: 436.

Lee, M., X. He, W.-T. Yih, J. Gao, L. Deng and P. Smolensky. 2015. Reasoning in vector space: an explanatory study of question answering. arXiv preprint arXiv:1511.06426.

Legenstein, R., C.H. Papadimitriou, S. Vempala and W. Maass. 2016. Assembly pointers for variable binding in networks of spiking neurons. arXiv preprintarXiv: 1611.03698.

Leitgeb, H. 2005. Interpreted dynamical systems and qualitative laws: from neural network to evolutionary systems. Synthese 146: 189-202.

Lenk, H. 1975. Philosophical and scientific comments on systems theory. pp. 247-267. *In:* H. Lenk [ed.]. Pragmatische Philosophie. Plädoyers und Beispiele für eine praxisnahe Philosophie und Wissenschaftstheorie. Hoffmann und Campe Verlag, Hamburg, DE. [German]

Lenk, H. 1978. Philosophy of science and systems theory. pp. 239-269. *In:* H. Lenk and G. Ropohl [eds.]. Systemtheorie als Wissenschaftsprogramm. Athenäum Verlag, Königstein/Ts, DE. [German]

Lenzen, M. 2002. Natural and Artificial Intelligence. Introduction to Cognitive Science. Campus Verlag, Frankfurt, DE, New York, USA. [German]

Lepore, E. and Z.W. Pylyshyn. [Eds.] 1999. What is Cognitive Science? Blackwell Publishers, Malden, USA, Oxford, UK.

Lestienne, R. 1996. Determination of the precision of spike timing in the visual cortex of anaesthetised cats. Biological Cybernetics 74: 55-61.

Levelt, W.J.M. 1991. The connectionist style. Sprache & Kognition 10: 61-72. [German]

Leven, R.W., B.-P. Koch and B. Pompe. 1994. Chaos in Dissipative Systems. 2nd Ed. Akademie-Verlag, Berlin, DE. [German]

Levine, J. 1983. Materialism and qualia: the explanatory gap. Pacific Philosophical Quarterly 64: 354-361.

Levy, S.D. 2007a. Changing semantic role representations with holographic memory. In: C.T. Morrison and T. Oates [eds.]. Computational Approaches to Representation Change during Learning and Development: Papers from the 2007 AAAI Symposium. AAAI Press, MenloPark, USA.

Levy, S.D. 2007b. Analogical integration of semantic roles with vector symbolic architectures. In: A. Schwering, U. Krumnack, K.-U. Kühnberger and H. Gust [eds.]. Proceedings of the Workshop on Analogies: Integrating Multiple Cognitive Abilities (AnICA07), Nashville, United States of America, Publication Series of the Institute of Cognitive Science, University of Osnabrück.

Levy, S.D. 2010. Becoming recursive: toward a computational neuroscience account of recursion in language and thought. pp. 371-392. In: H. van der Hulst [ed.]. Recursion and Human Language. De Gruyter Mouton, Göttingen, DE.

Levy, S.D. and S. Kirby. 2006. Evolving distributed representations for language with self-organizing maps. pp. 57-71. In: P. Vogt, Y. Sugita, E. Tuci and C. Nehaniv [eds.] Proceedings of the Third International Symposium on the Emergence and Evolution of Linguistic Communication (EELC), Symbol grounding and beyond, Rome, Italy. Springer.

Levy, S.D. and R. Gayler. 2008. Vector symbolic architectures: a new building material for artificial general intelligence. pp. 414-418. In: P. Wang, B. Goertzel and S. Franklin [eds.]. Proceedings of the First Conference on Artificial General Intelligence (AGI-08). Memphis, United States of America. IOS Press.

Lewin, K. 1936. Principles of Topological Psychology. MacGraw-Hill, New York, USA.

Lewis, R.L. 1999. Cognitive modeling, symbolic. pp. 141-143. In: R.A. Wilson and F.C. Keil [eds.]. The MIT Encyclopedia of the Cognitive Sciences. The MIT Press, Cambridge, USA, London, UK.

Liaw, J.-S. and T.W. Berger. 1996. Dynamic synapse: a new concept of neural representation and computation. Hippocampus 6: 591-600.

Lindsay, P.H. and D.A. Norman. 1972/1977. Human Information Processing. An Introduction to Psychology. Academic Press, New York, USA.

Linke, A., M. Nussbaumer and P.R. Portmann. 2001. Textbook Linguistics. 4th Ed. Max Niemeyer Verlag, T¨ubingen, DE. [German]

Lipinsky, J., S. Schneegans, Y. Sandamirskaya, J.P. Spencer and G. Schöner. 2012. A neurobehavioral model of flexible spatial language behaviors. Journal for Experimental Psychology: Learning, Memory and Cognition 38: 1490-1511.

Litz, H.P. 2000. Multivariate Statistical Methods and their Application in Economics and Social Sciences. R. Oldenbourg Verlag, München, DE, Wien, AT. [German]

Lloyd, D. 2003. Representation, philosophical issues about. pp. 934-940. *In:* L. Nadel. [ed.]. Encyclopedia of Cognitive Science. Vol. 3. Natur Publishing Group. London, UK, New York, USA and Tokyo, JP.

Löwel, S. and W. Singer. 1992. Selection of intrinsic horizontal connections in the visual cortex by correlated neuronal activity. Science 255: 209-212.

Logothetis, N.K., J. Pauls and T. Poggio. 1995. Shape representation in the inferior temporal cortex of monkeys. Current Biology 5: 552-563.

Lomp, O., M. Richter, S.K.U. Zibner and G. Schöner. 2016. Developing dynamic field theory architectures for embodied cognitive systems with cedar. Frontiers in Neurorobotics 10: 14.

Lück, H.E. 2013. History of Psychology. Trends, Schools, Developments. 6th Ed. Kohlhammer, Stuttgart, DE. [German]

Lukoševičius, M. and H. Jaeger. 2009. Reservoir computing approaches to recurrent neural network training. Computer Science Review 3: 127-149.

Lukoševičius, M., H. Jaeger and B. Schrauwen. 2012. Reservoir computing trends. KI – Künstliche Intelligenz 26: 365-371.

Lumer, E.D., G.M. Edelman and G. Tononi. 1997a. Neural dynamics in a model of the thalamocortical system, 1: layers, loops, and the emergence of fast synchronous rhythms. Cerebral Cortex 7: 207-227.

Lumer, E.D., G.M. Edelman and G. Tononi. 1997b. Neural dynamics in a model of the thalamocortical system, 2: the role of neural synchrony tested through perturbations of spike timing. Cerebral Cortex 7: 228-236.

Lungarella, M., G. Metta, R. Pfeifer and G. Sandini. 2003. Developmental robotics: a survey. Connection Science 15: 151-190.

Lycan, W.G. 1991. Homuncular functionalism meets PDP. pp. 259-286. *In:* W. Ramsey, S.P. Stich and D.E. Rumelhart [eds.]. Philosophy and Connectionist Theory. Lawrence Erlbaum, Hillsdale, USA.

Lyre, H. 2002. Information Theory. A Philosophical-Scientific Introduction. Wilhelm Fink Verlag, München, DE. [German]

Lyre, H. 2006. Structural realism. Information Philosophie 4: 32-37. [German]

Lyre, H. 2013. Embodied and embedded cognition. pp. 186-192. *In:* A. Stephan and S. Walter. [eds.]. Handbuch Kognitionswissenschaft. Metzler, Stuttgart, Weimar, DE. [German]

Lyre, H. and S. Walter. 2013. Situated Cognition. pp. 184-185. *In:* A. Stephan and S. Walter. [eds.]. Handbuch Kognitionswissenschaft. Metzler, Stuttgart, Weimar, DE. [German]

Maass, W. 1995. On the computational complexity of networks of spiking neurons. pp. 183-190. *In:* G. Tesauro [ed.]. Eight Annual Conference on Neural Information Processing Systems (NIPS), Denver, United Staes of America. MIT Press.

Maass, W. 1996. Lower bounds for the computational power of networks of spiking neurons. Neural Computation 8: 1-40.

Maass, W. 1997. Networks of spiking neurons: the third generation of neural network models. Neural Networks 10: 1659-1671.

Maass, W. 1999. Computation with spiking neurons. pp. 55-85. *In:* W. Maass and C.M. Bishop [eds.]. Pulsed Neural Networks. MIT Press, Cambridge, USA.

Maass, W. 2002. Computing with spikes. Special Issue on Foundations of Information Processing of TELEMATIK 8: 32-36.

Maass, W. 2003. Computation with spiking neurons. pp. 1080-1083. *In:* M.A. Arbib [ed.]. The Handbook of Brain Theory and Neural Networks. 2nd Ed. The MIT Press. Cambridge, USA, London, UK.

Maass, W. 2015. To spike or not to spike: That is the question. Proceedings of the IEEE 103: 2219-2224.

Maass, W. 2016. Searching for principles of brain computation. Current Opinion in Behavioral Sciences 11: 81-92.

Maass, W. and A.M. Zador. 1998. Computing and learning with dynamic synapses. pp. 321-336. *In:* W. Maass and C.M. Bishop [eds.]. Pulsed Neural Networks. MIT Press, Cambridge, USA.

Maass, W. and A.M. Zador. 1999. Dynamic stochastic synapses as computational units. Neural Computation 11: 903-917.

Maass, W., T. Natschläger and H. Markram. 2002. Real-time computing without stable states: a new framework for neural computation based on perturbations. Neural Computation 14: 2531-2560.

MacDonald, C. and G. MacDonald. [eds.] 1995. Connectionism: Debates on Psychological Explanation. Vol. 2. Blackwell Publishers. Oxford/UK, Cambridge, USA.

Machamer, P., L. Darden and C. Craver. 2000. Thinking about mechanisms. Philosophy of Science 67: 1-25.

MacKay, W.A. 1997. Synchronized neuronal oscillations and their role in motor processes. Trends in Cognitive Sciences 1: 176-183.

Mac Lane, S. 1996. Structure in mathematics. Philosophia Mathematica 4: 174-183.

MacLeod, K. and G. Laurent. 1996. Distinct mechanisms for synchronization and temporal patterning of odor-encoding neural assemblies. Science 274: 976-979.

Mainzer, K. 1992. What is life. Denkanstöße 93: p. 43. [German]

Mainzer, K. 1993. Artificial intelligence, neuroinformatics and the task of philosophy. pp. 118-131. *In:* G. Kaiser [ed.]. Kultur und Technik im 21. Jahrhundert. Campus Verlag, Frankfurt, DE, New York, USA. [German]

Mainzer, K. 1994. Tasks, Aims and Limits of Neurophilosophy. pp. 131-151. *In:* G. Kaiser, D. Matejoski and J. Fedrowitz [eds.]. Neuroworlds: Gehirn – Geist – Kultur. Campus Verlag, Frankfurt, DE, New York, USA. [German]

Mainzer, K. 1999. Complex Systems and Nonlinear Dynamics in Nature and Society. pp. 3-29. *In:* K. Mainzer [ed.]. Komplexe Systeme und nichtlineare Dynamik in Natur und Gesellschaft. Komplexit"atsforschung in Deutschland auf dem Weg ins n"achste Jahrhundert. Springer-Verlag, Berlin, DE. [German]

Mainzer, K. 2003. AI – Artificial Intelligence. Fundamentals of Intelligent Systems. Wissenschaftliche Buchgesellschaft, Darmstadt, DE [German]

Mainzer, K. 2004. System: an introduction to systems science. pp. 28-39. *In:* L. Floridi [ed.]. The Blackwell Guide to the Philosophy of Computing and Information. Blackwell, Malden, USA.

Mainzer, K. 2005. What are complex systems? Complexity research as an integrative science. pp. 37-77. *In:* Gottfried Wilhelm Leibniz Gemeinschaft [ed.]. 1. Symposium zur Gründung der Deutsch-Japanischen Gesellschaft für Integrative Wissenschaft. J.H. Röll-Verlag, Bonn, DE. [German]

Mainzer, K. 2007a. Thinking in Complexity. The Complex Dynamics of Matter, Mind and Mankind. 5th Ed. Springer-Verlag, Berlin, DE.

Mainzer, K. 2007b. The emergence of self-conscious systems. From symbolic AI to embodied robotics. pp. 1-6. *In:* L. Lewis and T. Metzler [eds.]. Human Implications of Human-Robot Interaction. Templeton Foundation Press. Philadelphia, USA.

Mainzer, K. 2008. Organic computing and complex dynamical systems. Conceptual foundations and interdisciplinary perspectives. pp. 105-122. *In:* R.P. Würtz [ed.]. Organic Computing. Springer-Verlag, Berlin, DE.

Mainzer, K. 2010. Life as a Machine? From Systems Biology to Robotics and Artificial Intelligence. Mentis Verlag, Paderborn, DE. [German]

Mainzer, K. and L. Chua. 2013. Local Activity Principle. Imperial College Press, London, UK, Singapore, SG.

Makuuchi, M., J. Bahlmann, A. Anwander and A.D. Friederici. 2009. Segregating the core computational faculty of human language from working memory. Proceedings of the National Academy of Sciences of the United States of America 106: 8362-8367.

Mallot, H.A. 2013. Computational Neuroscience. A First Course. Springer, Heidelberg, DE.

Mallot, H.A., J. Kopecz and W. von Seelen. 1992. Neuroinformatics as an empirical science. Kognitionswissenschaft 3: 12-23. [German]

Mallot, H.A., W. Hübner and W. Stürzl. 2000. Neuronal nets. pp. 84-124. *In:* G. Görz, C.-R. Rollinger and J. Schneeberger [eds.]. Handbuch der Künstlichen Intelligenz. 3rd Ed. Oldenbourg Verlag, M"unchen, DE, Wien, AT. [German]

Malmgren, H. 2006. Presentations, re-presentations and learning. Philosophical Communications. Web Series. No. 35, Department of Philosophy, Göteborg University, Göteborg, SE: 163-182pp.

Mangold, R. 1996. The simulation of learning processes in connectionistic networks. pp. 389-444. *In:* N. Birbaumer, D. Frey, J. Kuhl, W. Schneider and R. Schwarzer [eds.]. Enzyklopädie der Psychologie. Themenbereich C: Theorie und Forschung. Serie 2: Kognition. Band 7: Lernen. Hogrefe, Göttingen, DE. [German]

Mani, D.R. and L. Shastri. 1993. Reflexive reasoning with multiple instantiation in a connectionist reasoning system with a type hierarchy. Connection Science 5: 205-242.

Manjunath, B.S., G.M. Haley, W.-Y. Ma and S.D. Newsam. 2005. Multiband techniques for texture classification and segmentation. pp. 455-470. *In:* A. Bovik [ed.]. Handbook of Image and Video Processing. 2nd Ed. Elsevier Academic Press. Burlington, USA, San Diego, USA, London, UK.

Marcus, G. 1998. Rethinking eliminative connectionism. Cognitive Psychology 37: 243-282.

Marcus, G.F. 2001. The Algebraic Mind. Integrating Connectionism and Cognitive Science. Bradford Book. The MIT Press, Cambridge, USA.

Marcus, G.F., A. Marblestone and T. Dean. 2014a. The atoms of neural computation: does the brain depend on a set of elementary, reusable computations? Science 346: 551–552.

Marcus, G.F., A. Marblestone and T. Dean. 2014b. Frequently asked questions for: the atoms of neural computation. arXiv 1410.8826.

Mareschal, D., M.H. Johnson, S. Sirois, M. Spratling, M. Thomas and G. Westermann. 2007. Neuroconstructivism. Vol. 1: How the Brain Constructs Cognition. Oxford University Press, Oxford, UK.

Marinell, G. 1995. Multivariate Procedures. 4th Ed. R. Oldenbourg Verlag, München, DE, Wien, AT. [German]

Markman, A.B. 2003. Representation formats in psychology. pp. 930-933. *In:* L. Nadel. [ed.]. Encyclopedia of Cognitive Science. Vol. 3. Natur Publishing Group, London, UK, New York, USA and Tokyo, JP.

Markram, H., Y. Wang and M. Tsodyks. 1998. Differential signaling via the same axon of neocortical pyramidal neurons. Proceedings of the National Academy of Sciences of the United States of America 95: 5323-5328.

Marr, D. 1982. Vision. A Computational Investigation into Human Representation and Processing of Visual Information. W.H. Freeman and Company, San Francisco, USA.

Martinás, K. 1999. Entropy and information. pp. 265-275. *In:* W. Hofkirchner and P. Fleissner [eds.]. The Quest of a Unified Theory of Information. Proceedings of the Second Conference on Foundations of Information Science, Vienna, Austria, Gordon and Breach Publishers.

Marx, M.H. 1994. Connectionism. pp. 301-302. *In:* R.J. Corsini [ed.]. Encyclopedia of Psychology. 2nd Ed. Vol. 1. John Wiley & Sons, New York, USA.

Massimini, M. and G. Tononi. 2018. Sizing up Consciousness: Towards an Objective Measure of the Capacity for Experience. Oxford University Press, Oxford, UK.

Mathar, R. 1996. Information Theory, Discrete Models and Procedures. Teubner-Verlag, Stuttgart, DE. [German]

Matthews, R.J. 1994. Three-concept monte: explanation, implementation and systematicity. Synthese 101: 347-363.

Matthews, R.J. 2001. Can connectionists explain systematicity? Mind and Language 12: 154-177.

Matthews, R.J. 2003. Connectionism and systematicity. pp. 687-690. *In:* L. Nadel [ed.]. Encyclopedia of Cognitive Science. Vol. 1. Natur Publishing Group. London, UK, New York, USA and Tokyo, JP.

Maurer, H. 2004/2009. The Architecture Types of the "Self-Organizing (Feature) Map (SO(F)M)" according to Teuvo Kohonen. B.Sc. Thesis (Studienarbeit). Wilhelm-Schickard-Institut für Informatik. Universität Tübingen. BoD-Verlag, Norderstedt, DE. [German]

Maurer, H. 2006/2009. Paul Smolensky's Subsymbolic Paradigm against the Background of the Symbolism vs. Connectionism Debate. M.A. Thesis (Magisterarbeit). Philosophisches Seminar. Universität Tübingen. BoD-Verlag, Norderstedt. DE. [German]

Maurer, H., M. Bogdan and W. Rosenstiel. 2007. Architecture Types of T. Kohonens Self-Organizing (Feature) Map (SO(F)M). Universität Tübingen, Tübingen, DE. [unpublished manuscript]

Maurer, H. 2009. Book review: P. Smolensky and G. Legendre: The harmonic mind. From neural computation to optimality-theoretic grammar. Vol. 1: Cognitive architecture. Vol. 2. Linguistic and philosophical implications. Cambridge, MAand London. A Bradford Book. The MIT Press. 2006. Journal for General Philosophy of Science 40: 141-147.

Maurer, H. 2014a. Integrative (Synchronization) Mechanisms of (Neuro-)Cognition against the Background of (Neo-)Connectionism, the Theory of Nonlinear Dynamic Systems, Information Theory and the Self-Organization Paradigm. Ph.D. Thesis. Universität Tübingen. BoD-Verlag, Norderstedt, DE. [German]

Maurer, H. 2014b. The (computer simulation) model of connectionism as fiction according to Hans Vaihinger. pp. 223-246. *In:* M. Neuber [ed.]. Fiktion und Fiktionalismus. Beiträge zu Hans Vaihingers Philosophie des Als Ob. Königshausen & Neumann, Würzburg, DE. [German]

Maurer, H. 2016. Integrative synchronization mechanisms in connectionist cognitive neuroarchitectures. Computational Cognitive Science 2: 3.

Maurer, H. 2017. Metaanalysis of the Paradigm of Self-Organization including the Nonlinear Dynamic Complex Systems. A Short Introduction to Philosophy of Science and the Natural Sciences. BoD-Verlag. Norderstedt, DE. [German]

Maurer, H. 2018. Connectionist Neuroarchitectures in Cognition and Consciousness Theory. Modeling Integrative (Phase) Synchronization Mechanisms: A Brief Introduction without Formulas. Universität Tübingen, Tübingen, DE. [unpublished manuscript]

Maurer, H. 2019. The neurocognitive soliton (NCS) hypothesis (poster presentation). pp. 117. *In:* A. Newen [ed.]. The European Conference for Cognitive Science 2019 (EuroCogSci 2019). Situated Minds and Flexible Cognition, Bochum, Germany. [unpublished manuscript]

Maye, A. 2002. Neuronal synchrony, temporal binding and perception. Ph.D. Thesis. Fakultät für Elektrotechnik und Informatik. Technische Universität Berlin, Berlin, DE. [German]

Maye, A. 2003. Correlated neuronal activity can represent multiple binding solutions. Neurocomputing 52-54: 73-77.

Maye, A. and M. Werning. 2004. Temporal binding of non-uniform objects. Neurocomputing 58-60: 941-948.

Maye, A. and M. Werning. 2007. Neuronal synchronization: from dynamics feature binding to compositional representations. Chaos and Complexity Letters 2: 315-325.

Maye, A. and A.K. Engel. 2012. Neuronal assembly models of compositionality. pp. 616-632. *In:* W. Hinzen, E. Machery and M. Werning [eds.]. The Oxford Handbook of Compositionality. Oxford University Press, Oxford, UK.

Maye, A., P. Wang, J. Daume, X. Hu and A.K. Engel. 2019. An oscillator ensemble model of sequence learning. Frontiers in Integrative Neuroscience 13: 43.

Mayner, W.G.P., W. Marshall, L. Albantakis, G. Findlay, R. Marchman and G. Tononi. 2018. PyPhi: a toolbox for integrated information theory. Plos Computational Biology 14: e1006343.

McCauley, R.N. 1998. Levels of explanation and cognitice architecture. pp. 611-624. *In:* W. Bechtel and G. Graham [eds.]. A Companion to Cognitive Science. Blackwell Publisher, Malden, USA, Oxford, UK.

McClelland, J.L. 1999. Cognitive modeling, connectionist. pp. 137-141. *In:* R.A. Wilson and F.C. Keil [eds.]. The MIT Encyclopedia of the Cognitive Sciences. The MIT Press, Cambridge, USA, London, UK.

McClelland, J.L. 2009. The place of modeling in cognitive science. Topics in Cognitive Science 1: 11-38.

McClelland, J.L. and J.L. Elman. 1986. The TRACE model of speech perception. Cognitive Psychology 18: 1-86.

McClelland, J.L., D.E. Rumelhart and G.E. Hinton. 1986. The appeal of parallel distributed processing. pp. 3-44. *In:* D.E. Rumelhart and J.L. McClelland [eds.]. Parallel Distributed Processing: Explorations in the Microstructure of Cognition. Vol. 1: Foundations. MIT Press. A Bradford Book, Cambridge, USA.

McClelland, J.L. and G. Vallabha. 2009. Connectionist models of development: mechanistic dynamical models with emergent dynamical properties. pp. 3-24. *In:* J.P. Spencer, M.S.C. Thomas, and J.L. McClelland. [eds.]. Toward a Unified Theory of Development: Connectionism and Dynamic Systems Theory ReConsidered. Oxford University Press, Oxford, UK.

McClelland, J.L., M.M. Botvinick, D.C. Noelle, D.C. Plaut, T.T. Rogers, M.S. Seidenberg and L.B. Smith. 2010. Letting structure emerge: connectionist and dynamical systems approaches to cognition. Trends in Cognitive Sciences 14: 348-356.

McClosky, M. 1991. Networks and theories: the place of connectionism in cognitive science. Psychological Science 2: 387-395.

McCulloch, W.S. and W. Pitts. 1943. A logical calculus of the ideas immanent in nervous activity. The Bulletin of Mathematical Biophysics 5: 115-133.

McCulloch, W.S. and W. Pitts. 1948. The statistical organization of nervous activity. Biometrics 4: 91-99.

McGovern, K. and B.J. Baars. 2007. Cognitive theories of consciousness. pp. 177-205. *In:* P.D. Telazo, M. Moscovitch and E. Thompson [eds.]. The Cambridge Handbook of Consciousness. Chap. 26. Cambridge University Press, Cambridge, UK.

McIlwain, J.T. 2001. Population coding: a historical scetch. pp. 3-7. *In:* M.A.L. Nicolelis [ed.]. Advances in Neural Population Coding. Elsevier, Amsterdam, NL.

McLaughlin, B.P. 1993a. The connectionism/classicism battle to win souls. Philosophical Studies 71: 163-190.

McLaughlin, B.P. 1993b. Systematicity, conceptual truth, and evolution. pp. 217-234. *In:* C. Hookway and D. Peterson [eds.]. Philosophy and Cognitive Science. Cambridge University Press, Cambridge, UK.

McLaughlin, B.P. 1997. Classical constituents in Smolensky's ICS architecture. pp. 331-343. *In:* M.L. Dalla Chiara, K. Doets, D. Mundici and J. van Benthem [eds.]. Volume Two of the Tenth International Congress of Logic, Methodology and Philosophy of Science, Structures and Norms in Science, Florence, Italy. Kluwer Academic Publishers.

McLaughlin, B.P. 1998. Connectionism. pp. 166-167. *In:* E. Craig [ed.]. Concise Routledge Encyclopedia of Philosophy. Routledge, London, UK, New York, USA.

McLaughlin, B.P. 2014. Can an ICS architecture meet the systematicity and productivity challenges? pp. 31-76. *In:* P. Calvo and J. Symons [eds.]. The Architecture of Cognition. Rethinking Fodor and Pylyshyn's Systematicity Challenge. MIT Press, Cambridge, USA, London, UK.

Mehring, C., U. Hehl, M. Kubo, M. Diesmann and A. Aertsen. 2003. Activity dynamics and propagation of synchronous spiking in locally connected random networks. Biological Cybernetics 88: 395-408.

Meibauer, J. 2002. Introduction to German Linguistics. J.B. Metzlersche Verlagsbuchhandlung und Carl Ernst Poeschel Verlag, Stuttgart, DE. [German]

Menge, H. [ed.] 1913/2001. Langenscheidt's Dictionary of Ancient Greek. Ancient Greek – German. 30*th* Ed. Langenscheidt. Berlin, DE. [German]

Menge, H. [ed.] 1986/1993. Langenscheidt. Pocket Dictionary Ancient Greek. Part 1. Ancient Greek – German. Langenscheidt. Berlin, DE. [German]

Mesarovic, M.D. and Y. Takahara. 1975. General Systems Theory: Mathematical Foundations. Academic Press, New York, USA.

Metcalfe Eich, J. 1982. A composite holographic associative recall model. Psychological Review 89: 627-661.

Metzinger, T. 1995. Faster than thought. Holism, homogeneity and temporal coding. pp. 425-457. *In:* T. Metzinger [ed.]. Conscious Experience. Schöningh, Paderborn, DE.

Metzinger, T. 1998. Anthropology and Cognitive Science. pp. 326-372. *In:* A. Engel and P. Gold [eds.]. Der Mensch in der Perspektive der Kognitionswissenschaft. Suhrkamp Verlag, Frankfurt am Main, DE. [German]

Metzler,W. 1998. Nonlinear Dynamics and Chaos. An Introduction. B.G. Teubner, Stuttgart, Leipzig, DE. [German]

Mielke, R. 2001. Psychology of Learning. An Introduction. Kohlhammer, Stuttgart, DE, Berlin, DE, Köln, DE. [German]

Miłkowski, M. 2018. From computer metapher to computational modeling. The evolution of computationalism. Minds and Machines 28: 515-541.

Miller, G. 2003. The cognitive revolution. Trends in Cognitive Sciences 7: 141-144.

Miller, G.A., E. Galanter and K.H. Pribram. 1960/1970. Plans and the Structure of Behavior. Holt, Rinehart and Winston, London, UK, New York, USA, Sydney, AU, Toronto, CA.

Miller, P.H. 2016. Theories of Developmental Psychology. 6th Ed. San Francisco State University, San Francisco, USA.

Milner, P.M. 1974. A model for visual shape recognition. Psychological Review 81: 521-535.

Minsky, M. 1975. A framework for representing knowledge. pp. 211-277. In: P.H. Winston [ed.]. The Psychology of Computer Vision. McGraw-Hill, New York, USA.

Minsky, M. and Papert, S. 1969/1988. Perceptrons. An Introduction to Computational Geometry. 3rd Expanded Ed. MIT Press, Cambridge, USA.

Mitchell, J.C. 2003. Concepts in Programming Languages. Cambridge University Press, Cambridge, UK.

Mittelstrass, J. 2003. Transdisciplinarity: Scientific Future and Institutional Reality. Universitätsverlag Konstanz, Konstanz, DE. [German]

Montemurro, M.A., M.J. Rasch, Y. Murayama, N.K. Logothetis and S. Panzeri. 2008. Phase-of-firing coding of natural visual stimuli in primary visual cortex. Current Biology 18: 375-380.

Moore, B. 1989. ART 1 and pattern clustering. pp. 174-185. In: D. Touretzky, G.E. Hinton and T.J. Sejnowski [eds.] Proceedings of the 1988 Connectionist Models Summer School. Pittsburgh, United States of America. Morgan Kaufmann.

Moore, W.J. 1998. Physical Chemistry. 5th Ed. Longman Publishing Group, London, UK.

Morfill, G. and H. Scheingraber. 1991. Chaos is everywhere ... and it Works. A New World View. Ullstein, Frankfurt am Main, Berlin, DE. [German]

Morin, E. 2008. On Complexity. Hampton Press, Cresskill, USA.

Morrison, A., C. Mehring, T. Geisel, A. Aertsen and M. Diesmann. 2005. Advancing the boundaries of high connectivity network simulation with distributed computing. Neural Computation 17: 1776-1801.

Müller, B., J. Reinhardt and M.T. Strickland. 1995. Neural Networks. An Introduction. Springer-Verlag, Berlin, Heidelberg, DE.

Müller, M.G., C.H. Papadimitriou, W. Maass and R. Legenstein. 2020. A model for structured information representation in neural networks of the brain. eNeuro 7: 3.

Munro, P.W. and J.A. Anderson. 1988. Tools for connectionist modeling: the dynamical systems methodology. Behavior Research Methods, Instruments, and Computers 20: 276-281.

Murdock, B.B. 1982. A theory for the storage and retrieval of item and associative information. Psychological Review 89: 316-338.

Murthy, V.N. and E.E. Fetz. 1992. Coherent 25- to 35-Hz oscillations in the sensorimotor cortex of awake behaving monkeys. Proceedings of the National Academy of Sciences of the United States of America 89: 5670-5674.

Nadeau, S.E. 2014. Attractor basins: a neural basis for the conformation of knowledge. pp. 305-333. *In:* A. Chatterjee [ed.]. The Roots of Cognitive Neuroscience. Behavioral Neurology and Neuropsychology. Oxford University Press, Oxford, UK.

Nadel, L. [ed.] 2003. Encyclopedia of Cognitive Science. Vol. 1-4. Natur Publishing Group. London, UK, New York, USA, and Tokyo, JP.

Nakamura, E.R. and T. Mori. 1999. What is complexity? pp. 89-100. *In:* K. Mainzer [ed.]. Komplexe Systeme und Nichtlineare Dynamik in Natur und Gesellschaft. Komplexitätsforschung in Deutschland auf dem Weg ins nächste Jahrhundert. Springer-Verlag. Berlin, DE. [German]

Nase, G., W. Singer, H. Monyer and A.K. Engel. 2003. Features of neuronal synchrony in mouse visual cortex. Journal of Neurophysiology 90: 1115-1123.

Neelakanta, P.S. and D.F. De Groff. 1994. Neural Network Modeling. Statistical Mechanics and Cybernetic Perspective, CRC Press, Boca Raton, USA.

Negrello, M., M. Hülse and F. Pasemann. 2008. Adaptive neurodynamics. pp. 85-111. *In:* Y. Shan and A. Yang [eds.]. Applications of Complex Adaptive Systems. IGI Publishing, Hershey, USA.

Neisser, U. 1967. Cognitive Psychology. Appleton-Century-Crofts Educational Division Meredith, New York, USA.

Neisser, U. 1974. Cognitive Psychology. Ernst Klett Verlag, Stuttgart, DE. [German]

Nelken, I. 1988. Analysis of the activity of single neurons in stochastic settings. Biological Cybernetics 59: 201-215.

Nelson, J.I. 1995. Binding in the visual system. pp. 157-159. *In:* M.A. Arbib [ed.]. The Handbook of Brain Theory and Neural Networks. The MIT Press, Cambridge, USA, London, UK.

Nelson, J.I., P.A. Salin, M.H.J. Munk, M. Arzi and J. Bullier. 1992. Spatial and temporal coherence in cortico-cortical connections: a cross-correlation study in areas 17 and 18 in the cat. Visual Neuroscience 9: 21-37.

Neuenschwander, S. and W. Singer. 1996. Long-range synchronization of oscillatory light responses in the cat retina and lateral geniculate nucleus. Nature 379: 728-733.

Neuenschwander, S., A.K. Engel, P. König, W. Singer and F.J. Varela. 1996. Synchronization of neuronal responses in the optic tectum of awake pigeons. Visual Neuroscience 13: 575-584.

Neumann, O. 1985. Information processing, artificial intelligence and the perspectives of cognitive psychology. pp. 3-37. *In:* O. Neumann [ed.]. Perspektiven der Kognitionspsychologie. Springer, Berlin, DE. [German]

Neuser, W. 1998. On the logic of self-organization. pp. 15-34. *In:* K. Gloy, W. Neuser and P. Reisinger [eds.]. Systemtheorie. Philosophische Betrachtungen und ihre Anwendungen. Bouvier Verlag, Bonn, DE. [German]

Neven, H. and A. Aertsen. 1992. Rate coherence and event coherence in the visual cortex: a neuronal model of object recognition. Biological Cybernetics 67: 309-322.

Newell, A. 1973. Artificial intelligence and the concept of mind. pp. 1-60. *In:* R.C. Schank and K.M. Colby [eds.]. Computer Models of Thought and Language. Freeman. San Francisco, USA.

Newell, A. 1980. Physical symbol systems. Cognitive Science 4: 135-183.

Newell, A. 1990. Unified Theories of Cognition. Harvard University Press, Cambridge, USA.

Newell, A.C. 1977. Synchronized solitons. Journal of Mathematical Physics 18: 922-926.

Newell, A. and H.A. Simon. 1976. Computer science as empirical inquiry: symbols and search. Communications of the Association for Computing Machinery 19: 113-126.

Newell, A., P.S. Rosenbloom and J.E. Laird. 1989. Symbolic architectures for cognition. pp. 93-131. *In:* M.I. Posner [ed.]. Foundations of Cognitive Science. MIT Press, Cambridge, USA.

Newhouse, S.E. 1984. Understanding chaotic dynamics. pp. 1-11. *In:* J. Chandra. [ed.]. Chaos in Nonlinear Dynamical Systems. SIAM, Philadelphia, USA.

Newman, J. and B.J. Baars. 1993. A neural attentional model for access to consciousness: a global workspace perspective. Concepts in Neuroscience 4: 255-290.

Nicolis, G. and I. Prigogine. 1977. Self-Organization in Non-Equilibrium Systems. From Dissipative Structures to Order through Fluctuations. Wiley. New York, USA.

Nicolis, G. and I. Prigogine. 1989. Exploring Complexity: An Introduction. W.H. Freeman, San Francisco, USA.

Nieder, A. 2013. Coding of abstract quantity by number neurons of the primate brain. Journal of Comparative Physiology A 199: 1-16.

Nieder, A. 2016. The neuronal code for number. Nature Reviews Neuroscience 17: 366-382.

Nieder, A., D.J. Freedman and E.K. Miller. 2002. Representation of the quantity of visual items in the primate prefrontal cortex. Science 297: 1708-1711.

Niegel, W. 1992. Self-organization – approaching a concept.. pp. 1-18. In: W. Niegel and P. Molzberger [eds.]. Aspekte der Selbstorganisation. Springer-Verlag. Berlin, DE. [German]

Niegel, W. and P. Molzberger [eds.] 1992. Aspects of Self-Organization. Springer-Verlag. Berlin, DE. [German]

Nielson, M. 2015. Neural Networks and Deep Learning. Online book. http://neuralnetworksanddeeplearning.com/.

Nikolić, D., P. Fries and W. Singer. 2013. Gamma oscillations: precise temporal coordination without a metronome. Trends in Cognitive Sciences 17: 54-55.

Nolfi, S. and D. Floreano. 2001. Evolutionary Robotics. The Biology, Intelligence, and Technology of Self-Organizing Machines. MIT Press, Bradford Books, Cambridge, USA.

Nolting, W. 2016a. Theoretical Physics 1. Classical Mechanics. Springer International Publishing, Basel, CH.

Nolting, W. 2016b. Theoretical Physics 2. Analytical Mechanics. Springer International Publishing, Basel, CH.

Nolting, W. 2017a. Theoretical Physics 4. Special Theory of Relativity. Springer International Publishing, Basel, CH.

Nolting, W. 2017b. Theoretical Physics 5. Thermodynamics. Springer International Publishing, Basel, CH.

Norman, D.A. 1968. Toward a theory of memory and attention. Psychological Review 75: 522-536.

Norman, K.A., E.L. Newman and A.J. Perotte. 2005. Methods for reducing interference in the complementary learning systems model: oscillating inhibition and autonomous memory rehearsal. Neural Networks 18: 1212-1228.

Norris, J.R. 1998. Markov Chains. Cambridge University Press, Cambridge, UK.

Northoff, G. 2014. Minding the Brain. A Guide to Philosophy and Neuroscience. Palgrave, Basingstoke, UK.

Norton, A. 1995. Dynamics: an introduction. pp. 45-68. *In:* R.F. Port and T.J. van Gelder [eds.]. Mind as Motion. Explorations in the Dynamics of Cognition. A Bradford Book. MIT Press, Cambridge, USA, London, UK.

Nyquist, H. 1924. Certain factors affecting telegraph speed. Bell System Technical Journal 3: 324-346.

O'Grady, W. 1997. Syntax: the analysis of sentence structure. pp. 181-244. *In:* W. O'Grady, M. Dobrovolsky and F. Katamba [eds.]. Contemporary Linguistics. An Introduction. 3rd Ed. Addison Wesley Longman, Harlow, UK.

O'Hare, G.M.P. [ed.] 1996. Foundations of Distributed Artificial Intelligence. Wiley, New York, USA.

Oizumi, M., L. Albantakis and G. Tononi. 2014. From the phenomenology to the mechanisms of consciuosness: integrated information theory 3.0. PLoS Computational Biology 10: e1003588.

Opwis, K. and G. Lüer. 1996. Models of representation of knowledge. pp. 337-431. *In:* N. Birbaumer, D. Frey, J. Kuhl, W. Schneider and R. Schwarzer [eds.]. Enzyklopädie der Psychologie. Themenbereich C: Theorie und Forschung. Serie 2: Kognition. Band 4: Gedächtnis. Hogrefe, Göttingen, DE. [German]

Oram, M.W., M.C. Wiener, R. Lestienne and B.J. Richmond. 1999. Stochastic nature of precisely timed spike patterns in visual system neuronal responses. Journal of Neurophysiology 81: 3021-3033.

O'Reilly, R.C., R.S. Busby and R. Soto. 2003. Three forms of binding and their neural substrates: alternatives to temporal synchrony. pp. 168-190. *In:* A. Cleeremans [ed.]. The Unity of Consciousness: Binding, Integration, and Dissociation. Oxford University Press, Oxford, UK.

O'Searcoid, M. 2007. Metric Spaces. Springer, London, UK.

Osgood, C.E. 1957. A behavioristic analysis of perception and language as cognitive phenomena. pp. 75-118. *In:* S. Bruner et al. [eds.]. Contemporary Approaches to Cognition. A Symposium held at the University of Colorado. Harvard University Press. Cambridge, USA.

Osherson, D.N. [ed.] 1995-1998. An Invitation to Cognitive Science. 2nd Ed. Part I–IV. MIT Press, Cambridge, USA.

Ott, E. 2002. Chaos in Dynamical Systems. Cambridge University Press, Cambridge, UK.

Pacherie, É. 2004. Cognitivism. p. 57. *In:* O. Houdé. [ed.]. Dictionary of Cognitive Science. Neuroscience, Psychology, Artificial Intelligence, Linguistic, and Philosophy. Psychology Press, New York, USA, Hove, UK.

Padulo, L. and M.A. Arbib. 1974. System Theory: A Unified State-Space Approach to Continuous and Discrete Systems. W.B. Saunders Co., Philadelphia, USA.

Pagin, P. and D. Westerståhl. 2008. Compositionality. pp. 96-123. *In:* K. von Heusinger, C. Maienborn and P. Portner [eds.]. Semantics. An International Handbook of Natural Language Meaning. Vol. 1. Mouton de Gruyter, Berlin, DE.

Pagin, P. and D. Westerståhl. 2010. Compositionality I. Definitions and variants. Philosophy Compass 5: 265-282.

Palanca, B.J.A. and G.C. DeAngelis. 2005. Does neuronal synchrony underlie visual feature grouping. Neuron 46: 333-346.

Palm, G. 1982. Neural Assemblies. An Alternative Approach to Artificial Intelligence. Springer-Verlag, Berlin, DE.

Palm, G. 1990. Cell assemblies as a guideline for brain research. Concepts in Neuroscience 1: 133-137.

Palmer, S.E. 1999. Vision science: photons to phenomenology. MIT Press, Cambridge, USA.

Palmigiano, A., T. Geisel, F. Wolf and D. Battaglia. 2017. Flexible information routing by transient synchrony. Nature Neuroscience 20: 1014-1022.

Papoulis, A. 1991. Probability, Random, Variables, and Stochastic Processes. 4th Ed. McGraw-Hill, New York, USA.

Parasuraman, R. 1986. Vigilance, monitoring and search. pp. 41-49. *In:* J.R. Boff, L. Kaufmann and J.P. Thomas [eds.]. Handbook of Human Perception and Performance. Vol. 2. Cognitive Processes and Performance.Wiley, New York, USA.

Pareigis, B. 2000. Linear Algebra for Computer Scientists. Springer-Verlag. Berlin, DE [German]

Pareti, G. and A. De Palma. 2004. Does the brain oscillate? The dispute on neuronal synchronization. Neurological Sciences 25: 41-47.

Pascanu, R. and H. Jaeger. 2011. A neurodynamical model for working memory. Neural Networks 24: 199-207.

Pasemann, F. 1995. Neuromodules: a dynamical systems approach to brain modelling. pp. 331-348. *In:* H.J. Herrmann, D.E.Wolf and E. Pöppel [eds.].Workshop on Supercomputing in Brain Research. From Tomography to Neural Networks. Jülich, Germany, World Scientific Publishing.

Pasemann, F. 1996. Representation without representation. Consideration on the neurodynamics of modular cognitive systems. pp. 42-91. *In:* G. Rusch, S.J. Schmidt and O. Breidbach [eds.]. Interne Repräsentationen – Neue Konzepte der Hirnforschung. Suhrkamp Verlag, Frankfurt/Main, DE. [German]

Pasemann, F. 1998. Structures and dynamics of recurrent neuromodules. Theory in Biosciences 117: 1-17.

Pasemann, F. 1999. Driving neuromodules into synchronous chaos. pp. 377-384. *In:* J. Mira and J.V. Sanchez-Andres [eds.]. International Work-Conference on Artificial and Natural Neural Networks (IWANN'99), Vol. I, Alicante, Spain. Springer.

Pasemann, F. 2002. Complex dynamics and the structure of small neural networks. Network: Computation in Neural Systems 13: 195-216.

Pasemann, F. 2017. Neurodynamics in the sensorimotor loop: Representing behavior relevant external situations. Frontiers in Neurorobotics 11: 5.

Pasemann, F. 2018. Synchronization cores and dynamical complexity of modular neural networks. Preprint. [unpublished manscript]

Pasemann, F. and N. Stollenwerk. 1998. Attractor switching by neural control of chaotic neurodynamics. Network: Computation in Neural Systems 9: 549-561.

Pasemann, F. and T. Wennekers. 2000. Generalized and partial synchronization of coupled neural networks. Network: Computation in Neural Systems 11: 41-61.

Pasemann, F., M. Hild and K. Zahedi. 2003. SO(2)-Networks as Neural Oscillators. pp. 144-151. *In:* J. Mira and J.R. Alvarez [eds.]. Computational Methods in Neural Modeling. Springer, Berlin, DE.

Pasemann, F., C.W. Rempis and A. von Twickel. 2012. Evolving humanoid behaviors for language games. pp. 67-86. *In:* L. Steels and M. Hild [eds.]. Language Grounding in Robots. Springer, New York, USA.

Paslack, A. 1991. Prehistory of Self-Organization. On the Archaeology of a Scientific Paradigm. Vieweg Verlag, Braunschweig, Wiesbaden, DE. [German]

Pearl, J. 1988. Probabilistic Reasoning in Intelligent Systems: Networks of Plausible Inference. Morgan Kaufmann, San Fransisco, USA.

Peitgen, H.-O., H. Jürgens and D. Saupe. 1994. Chaos. Building Blocks of Order. Springer-Verlag, Berlin, DE. [German]

Pelz, H. 2002. Linguistics. An Introduction. 7th Ed. Hoffmann und Campe, Hamburg, DE. [German]

Perez-Orive, J., O. Mazor, G.C. Turner, S. Cassenaer, R.I. Wilson and G. Laurent. 2002. Oscillations and sparsening of odor representations in the mushroom body. Science 297: 359-365.

Perkel, D.H. and T.H. Bullock. 1968a. Neural coding: a report based on an NRP work session. Neurosciences Research Program Bulletin 6: 219-349.

Perkel, D.H. and T.H. Bullock. 1968b. Neural Coding. pp. 405-527. *In:* F.O. Schmitt, T. Melnechuk, G.C. Quarton and G. Adelman [eds.]. Neurosciences Research Program Symposium Summaries. Vol. III. MIT Press, Cambridge, USA.

Perko, L. 2009. Differential Equations and Dynamical Systems. 3rd Ed. Springer, New York, USA.

Perlovsky, L.I. 1998. Conundrum of combinatorial complexity. IEEE Transactions on Pattern Analysis and Machine Intelligence 20: 666-670.

Perlovsky, L.I. and R. Kozma. 2007. Neurodynamics of cognition and consciousness, pp. 1-8. *In:* L.I. Perlovsky and R. Kozma [eds.]. Neurodynamics of Cognition and Consciousness. Springer, Berlin, DE.

Peschl, M.F. 1996a. Representation in natural and artificial (connectionistic) neuronal systems. pp. 579-580. *In:* G. Strube, B. Becker, C. Freksa, U. Hahn, K. Opwis und G. Palm [eds.]. Wörterbuch der Kognitionswissenschaft. Klett-Cotta Verlag, Stuttgart, DE. [German]

Peschl, M.F. 1996b. Epistemological and methodological questions on the traditional concept of representation in classical cognitive science. pp. 119-138. *In:* A. Ziemke and O. Breidbach. [eds.]. Repr¨asentationismus – was sonst? Eine kritische Auseinandersetzung mit dem repräsentationalistischen Forschungsprogramm in den Neurowissenschaften. Vieweg, Braunschweig, DE. [German]

Peschl, M.F. 1997. The representational relation between environmental structures and neural systems. Autonomy and environmental dependency in neural knowledge representation. Nonlinear Dynamics, Psychology, and Life Sciences 2: 99-121.

Petermann, F., K. Niebank and H. Scheithauer. 2004. Development Science. Developmental Psychology – Genetics – Neuropsychology. Springer-Verlag, Berlin, DE. [German]

Peters, A. and B.R. Payne. [eds.] 2002. The Cat Primary Visual Cortex. Academic Press, San Diego, USA.

Petersen, W. and M. Werning. 2007. Conceptual fingerprints: lexical decomposition by means of frames – a neuro-cognitive model. pp. 415-428. *In:* U. Priss, S. Polovina and R. Hill [eds.]. Conceptual Structures: Knowledge Architectures for Smart Applications. Springer-Verlag, Heidelberg, DE.

Petitot, J. 1991. Why connectionism is such a good thing: a criticism of Fodor and Pylyshyn's criticism of Smolensky. Philosophica (Belgium) 47: 49-79

Petitot, J. 1993. Natural dynamical models for cognitive grammars. pp. 81-104. *In:* F.D. Manjali [ed.]. Language and Cognition. Bahri Publications, New Delhi, IN.

Petitot, J. 1994. Dynamical constituency. An epistemological analysis. Sémiotiques 6: 187-225.

Petitot, J. 1995. Morphodynamics and attractor syntax: constituency in visual perception and cognitive grammar. pp. 227-281. *In:* R.F. Port and T. van Gelder [eds.]. Mind as Motion. Explorations in the Dynamics of Cognition. A Bradford Book. MIT Press, Cambridge/MA, USA and London, UK.

Petitot, J. 2011. Cognitive Morphodynamics. Dynamical Morphological Models of Constituency in Perception and Syntax. Peter Lang, Bern, CH, Berlin, DE.

Pfeifer, R. and C. Scheier. 1999. Understanding Intelligence. MIT Press, Cambridge, USA.

Pfeifer, R., M. Lungarella and O. Sporns. 2008. The synthetic approach to embodied cognition. A primer. pp. 121-137. *In:* O. Calvo and A. Gomila [eds.]. Handbook of Cognitive Science. Elsevier, Amsterdam, NE.

Phillips, S. and W.H. Wilson. 2016. Systematicity and a categorical theory of cognitive architecture: universal construction in context. Frontiers in Psychology 7: 1139.

Phillips, W.A. and W. Singer. 1997. In search of common foundations for cortical computation. The Behavioral and Brain Sciences 20: 657-722.

Piaget, J. 1970. Genetic Epistemology. Columbia University Press, New York. USA.

Piaget, J. and B. Inhelder. 1969. The Psychology of the Child. Basic Books, New York, USA.

Piccinini, G. 2007. Computational explanation and mechanistic explanation of mind. pp. 23-36. *In:* F. Ferretti, M. Marraffa and M. De Caro [eds.]. Cartographies of the Mind: The Interface Between Philosophy and Cognitive Science. Springer, Dordrecht, NE.

Piccinini, G. 2009. Computationalism in the philosophy of mind. Philosophy Compass 4: 515-532.

Piccinini, G. 2012. Computationalism. pp. 222-249. *In:* E. Margolis, R. Samuels and S. Stich [eds.]. The Oxford Handbook of Philosophy of Cognitive Science. Oxford University Press, Oxford, UK.

Piccinini, G. and C. Craver. 2011. Integrating psychology and neuroscience: functional analyses as mechanism sketches. Synthese 183: 283-311.

Pikovsky, A., M. Rosenblum and J. Kurths. 2001. Synchronization. A universal concept in nonlinear sciences. Cambridge University Press, Cambridge, UK.

Pina, J.E., M. Bodner and B. Ermentrout. 2018. Oscillations in working memory and neural binding: a mechanism for multiple memories and their interation. Plos Computational Biology: 14:e1006517.

Pinel, J.P.J., S.J. Barnes and P. Pauli. 2018. Biopsychology. 10th Ed. Pearson. Harlow, UK.

Pipa, G. 2006. The neuronal code: development of tools and hypotheses for understanding the role of synchronization of neuronal activity. Ph.D. Thesis. University of Technology. Berlin, DE.

Pipa, G. 2010a. Self-organized information processing in the brain. Habilitation Thesis, University of Technology Darmstadt, Darmstadt, DE.

Pipa, G. 2010b. Our brain plays jazz. Information processing in a self-organized and multi-scale system. Video. Redwood Center for Theoretical Neuroscience, University of California, Berkeley, USA.

Pipa, G. 2013. Theoretical Neuroscience. pp. 85-88. *In:* A. Stephan and S. Walter. [eds.]. Handbuch Kognitionswissenschaft. Metzler, Stuttgart, Weimar, DE. [German]

Plate, T. 1991. Holographic reduced representations. Technical Report CRGTR-91-1. Department of Computer Science, University of Toronto, Toronto, CA.

Plate, T. 1993. Holographic recurrent networks. Advances in Neural Information Processing Systems 5: 34-41.

Plate, T. 1994. Distributed representations and nested compositional structure. Ph.D. Thesis, Department of Computer Science. University of Toronto. Toronto, CA.

Plate, T. 1995. Holographic reduced representations. IEEE Transactions on Neural Networks 6: 623-641.

Plate, T.A. 1997a. Structure matching and transformation with distributed representations. pp. 309-327. *In:* R. Sun and F. Alexandre [eds.]. Connectionist-Symbolic Integration: From Unified to Hybrid Approaches. Lawrence Erlbaum, Mahwah, USA.

Plate, T.A. 1997b. A common framework for distributed representation schemes for compositional structure. pp. 15-34. *In:* F. Maire, R. Hayward and J. Diederich [eds.]. Connectionist Systems for Knowledge Representation and Deduction. Queensland University of Technology Press, Brisbane, AU.

Plate, T. 2003a. Distributed representations. pp. 1002-1010. *In:* L. Nadel. [ed.]. Encyclopedia of Cognitive Science. Vol. 1. Natur Publishing Group. London, UK, New York, USA, and Tokyo, JP.

Plate, T. 2003b. Holographic Reduced Representations. Distributed Representation for Cognitive Structures. Center for the Study of Language and Information (CSLI) Publications, Leland Stanford Junior University, Stanford, USA.

Plate, T.A. 2006. Convolution-based memory models. pp. 824-828. *In:* L. Nadel. [ed.]. Encyclopedia of Cognitive Science. Vol. 1. Natur Publishing Group. London, UK, New York, USA, and Tokyo, JP.

Plaut, D.C. 2000. Connectionist modeling. pp. 265-268. *In:* A. Kasdin [ed.]. Encyclopedia of Psychology. Vol. 2. American Psychological Association and Oxford University Press, Washington/DC, New York, USA.

Plaut, D.C. and J.L. McClelland. 2010. Locating object knowledge in the brain: a critique of Bower's (2009) attempt to revive the grandmother cell hypothesis. Psychological Review 117: 284-290.

Pockett, S., G.E.J. Bold and W.J. Freeman. 2009. EEG synchrony during a perceptual-cognitive task: widespread phase synchrony at all frequencies. Clinical Neurophysiology 120: 695-708.

Poggio, T. and S. Edelman. 1990. A network that learns to recognize 3D objects. Nature 343: 263-266.

Polk, T.A. and C.M. Seifert. [eds.] 2002. Cognitive Modeling. MIT Press, Cambridge, USA.

Pollak, J.B. 1990. Recursive distributed representations. Artificial Intelligence 46: 77-105.

Pompe, B. 2005. Introduction to Information Theory. Universität Greifswald. Hansestadt Greifswald, DE. [unpublished manuscript] [German]

Port, R.F. 2003. Dynamical system hypothesis in cognitive science. pp. 1027-1032. In: L. Nadel [ed.]. Encyclopedia of Cognitive Science. Vol. 1. Natur Publishing Group. London, UK, New York, USA, and Tokyo, JP.

Posner, M.J. [ed.] 1989. Foundations of Cognitive Science. MIT Press. Cambridge, USA.

Posner, M.I., C.R.R. Snyder and B.J. Davidson. 1980. Attention and the detection of signals. Journal of Experimental Psychology: General 109: 160-174.

Pospeschill, M. 2004. Connectionism and Cognition. An Introduction. Kohlhammer Verlag, Stuttgart, DE. [German]

Pouget, A. and P.E. Latham. 2003. Population codes. pp. 893-897. In: M.A. Arbib [ed.]. The Handbook of Brain Theory and Neural Networks. 2nd Ed. The MIT Press. Cambridge, USA, London, UK.

Prechtl, J.C. 1994. Visual motion induces synchronous oscillations in turtle visual cortex. Proceedings of the National Academy of Sciences of the United States of America 91: 12467-12471.

Price, C.J. and K.J. Friston. 2005. Functional ontologies for cognition: the systematic definition of structure and function. Cognitive Neuropsychology 22: 262-275.

Prigogine, I. 1980. From Being to Becoming. Freeman, San Francisco, USA.

Prigogine, I. 1985. New perspectives on complexity. In: S. Aida et al. [eds.]. The Science and Praxis of Complexity: Contributions to the Symposium held at Montpellier, France, 9-11 May, 1984. United Nations University, Tokyo, JP. (reprinted in Prigogine 1991.)

Prigogine, I. 1991. New perspectives on complexity. pp. 483-492. In: G.J. Klir [ed.]. Facets of Systems Science. Plenum Press, New York, USA, London, UK.

Prigogine, I. and I. Stengers. 1981/1993. Dialogue with Nature. New Ways of Scientific Thinking. 7th Ed. Piper, München, DE, Z¨urich, CH. [German]

Prigogine, I. and I. Stengers. 1984. Order out of Chaos. Man's New Dialogue with Nature. Bantam Books, Toronto, CA.

Prigogine, I. and I. Stengers. 1993. The Paradox of Time. Time, Chaos and Quanta. Piper. München u.a., DE. [German]

Prince, A. and P. Smolensky. 1991. Connectionism and harmony theory in linguistics. Technical Report CU-CS-533-91. Department of Computer Science, University of Colorado, Boulder, USA: 62pp.

Prinz, W. 1976. Cognition, cognitive. pp. 866-878. *In:* J. Ritter und K. Gründer [eds.]. Historisches Wörterbuch der Philosophie. Band 4. Wissenschaftliche Buchgesellschaft, Darmstadt, DE. [German]

Probst, D., H. Maass, H. Markman and M.O. Gewaltig. 2012. Liquid computing in a simplified model of cortical layer IV: learning to balance a ball. pp. 209-216. *In:* A.E. Villa, W. Duch, P. Erdi, F. Masulli and G. Palm [eds.]. Proceedings of the 22nd International Conference on Artificial Neural Networks and Machine Learning (ICANN'2012), Lausanne, Switzerland, Springer.

Prut, Y., E. Vaadia, H. Bergmann, I. Haalman, H. Slovin and M. Abeles. 1998. Spatiotemporal structure of cortical activity. Properties and behavioral relevance. Journal of Neurophysiology 79: 2857-2874.

Pulvermüller, F. 1999. Word's in the brain's language. Behavioral and Brain Sciences 22: 253-270.

Puntel, L.B. 2006. Structure and Being. Mohr Siebeck, Tübingen, DE. [German]

Purves, D., E.M. Brannon, R. Cabeza, S.H. Huettel, K.S. Labar, M.L. Platt and M. Woldorff [eds.]. 2013. Principles of Cognitive Neuroscience. 2nd Ed. Sinauer Associates, Sunderland, USA.

Pylyshyn, Z.W. 1980. Computation and cognition: issues in the foundations of cognitive science. Behavioral and Brain Sciences 3: 111-169.

Pylyshyn, Z.W. 1984. Computation and Cognition: Toward a Foundation for Cognitive Science. MIT Press, A Bradford Book, Cambridge, USA.

Pylyshyn, Z.W. 1985. Computation and Cognition: Toward a Foundation for Cognitive Science. 2nd Ed. MIT Press. A Bradford Book, Cambridge, USA.

Pylyshyn, Z.W. 1989. Computing in cognitive science. *In:* M.I. Posner [ed.]. Foundations of Cognitive Science. MIT Press, Cambridge, USA.

Qiu, F.T., T. Sugihara and R. von der Heydt. 2007. Figure-ground mechanisms provide structure for selective attention. Nature Neuroscience 10; 1492-1499.

Quian Quiroga, R., G. Kreiman, C. Koch and I. Fried. 2008. Sparse but not "Grandmother-Cell" coding in the medial temporal lobe. Trends in Cognitive Sciences 12: 87-91.

Quian Quiroga, R. and S. Panzeri. 2009. Extracting information from neural populations: information theory and decoding approaches. Nature Reviews Neuroscience 10: 173-185.

Quian Quiroga, R. and G. Kreiman. 2010. Measuring sparseness in the brain: comment on Bowers (2009). Psychological Review 117: 291-299.

Quine, W.V.O. 1940/1981. Mathematical Logic. Rev. Ed. Harvard University Press. Cambridge, USA.

Quine, W.V.O. 1970. Philosophy of Logic. Prentice-Hall, Englewood Cliffs, USA.

Quinlan, P.T. 1991. Connectionism and Psychology: A Psychological Perspective on New Connectionist Research. Harvester Wheatsheaf, New York, USA.

Rachkovskij, D.A. and E.M. Kussul. 2001. Binding and normalization of binary sparse distributed representations by context-dependent thinning. Neural Computation 13: 411-452.

Ramsey, W. 1999. Connectionism, philosophical issues. pp. 186-188. *In:* R.A. Wilson and F.C. Keil [eds.]. The MIT Encyclopedia of the Cognitive Sciences. The MIT Press, Cambridge, USA, London, UK.

Ramsey, W., S. Stich and J. Garon. 1990. Connectionism, eliminativism and the future of folk psychology. Philosophical Perspectives 4: 499-533.

Ranhel, J., E. Del Moral Hernandez and M.L. Netto. 2017. How complex behavior emerges from spikes. pp. 197-218. *In:* F. Adams, O. Pessoa Jr. and J.E. Kogler Jr. [eds.]. Cognitive Science. Recent Advances and Recurring Problems. Vernon Press, Wilmington, USA, Malaga, ES.

Rapaport, A. 1986. General System Theory. Essential Concepts & Applications. Abacus Press. Tunbridge Wells, UK.

Rapaport, W.J. 2000. Cognitive science. pp. 227-233. *In:* A. Ralston, E.D. Reilly, and D. Hemmindinger [eds.]. Encyclopedia of Computer Science. 4th Ed. Nature Publishing Group, New York, USA.

Rasmussen, D. 2019. NengoDL: combining deep learning and neuromorphic modelling methods. Neuroinformatics 17: 611-628.

Rasmussen, D. and C. Eliasmith. 2013. Modeling brain function: current developments and future prospects. JAMA Neurology 70: 1325-1329.

Rathgeber, B. 2011. Modelling in the Cognitive Sciences. 2nd Ed. LIT Verlag. Berlin, DE. [German]

Rauterberg, M. 1989. About the phenomenon: "Information." pp. 219-241. *In:* B. Becker [ed.]. Zur Terminologie in der Kognitionsforschung. Arbeitspapiere der Gesellschaft für Mathematik und Datenverarbeitung (GMD) Nr. 385. Sankt Augustin, Germany. [German]

Ray, S. and J.H.R. Maunsell. 2010. Differences in gamma frequencies across visual cortex restrict their possible use in computation. Neuron 67: 885-896.

Ray, S. and J.H.R. Maunsell. 2015. Do gamma oscillations play a role in cerebral cortex? Trends in Cognitive Science 19: 78-85.

Read, S.J., E.J. Vanman and L.C. Miller. 1997. Connectionism, parallel constraint satisfaction processes, and Gestalt principles: (re)introducing cognitive dynamics to social psychology. Personality and Social Psychology Review 1: 26-53.

Rechenberg, P. 2003. On the concept of information in information theory. Informatik Spektrum 26: 317-326. [German]

Regier, T. 2003. Computational models of cognition: constraining. pp. 611-615. *In:* L. Nadel. [ed.]. Encyclopedia of Cognitive Science. Vol. 1. Natur Publishing Group. London, UK, New York, USA, and Tokyo, JP.

Reichert, D.P. and T. Serre. 2014. Neuronal synchrony in complex-valued deep networks. *In:* Y. Bengio and Y. LeCun [eds.]. Proceedings of the 2nd International Conference on Learning Representations (ICLR'2014), Banff, Canada.

Reichl, L.E. 2009. A Modern Course in Statistical Physics. 3rd Ed. Wiley-VCH Verlag, Weinheim, DE.

Reid, R.C. and J.M. Alonso. 1995. Specificity of monosynaptic connections from thalamus to visual cortex. Nature 387: 281-284.

Reid, R.C. and W.M. Usrey. 2008. Vision. pp. 637-659. *In:* L. Squire, D. Berg, F.E. Bloom, S. Du Lac, A. Ghosh and N.C. Spitzer [eds.]. Fundamental Neuroscience. 3rd Ed. Elsevier Academic Press, Amsterdam, NL, Heidelberg, DE.

Reinhart, R.M.G. and J.A. Nguyen. 2019. Working memory revived in older adults by synchronizing rhythmic brain circuits. Nature Neurosience 22: 820-827.

Rempis, C., H. Toutounji and F. Pasemann. 2013a. Controlling the learning of behaviors in the sensorimotor loop with neuromodulators in self-monitoring neural networks. *In* Proceedings of the IEEE International Conference on Robotics and Automation (ICRA), Autonomous Learning Workshop, Karlsruhe, Germany.

Rempis, C., H. Toutounji and F. Pasemann. 2013b. Enhancing the Neuro-Controller Design Process for the Myon Humanoid Robot. Technical Report. University of Osnabrück, Osnabrück, Germany: 35pp.

Rey, G. 2003. Language of Thought. pp. 753-760. *In:* L. Nadel. [ed.]. Encyclopedia of Cognitive Science. Vol. 2. Natur Publishing Group London, UK, New York, USA and Tokyo, JP.

Rey, G.D. and K.F. Wender. 2011. Neural Networks. An Introduction to the Basics, Applications and Data Analysis. 2nd Ed. Huber, Bern, CH. [German]

Reyes, A.D. 2003. Synchrony-dependent propagation of firing rate in iteratively constructed networks *in vitro*. Nature Neuroscience 6: 593-599.

Reyes, A.D. and E.E. Fetz. 1993. Effects of transient depolarizing potentials on the firing rate of neocortical neurons. Journal of Neurophysiology 69: 1673-1683.

Richardson, K.A., S.J. Schiff and B.J. Gluckman. 2005. Control of traveling waves in the mammalian cortex. Physical Review Letters 94: 028103.

Riedl, R. 1975/1990. The Order of the Living. System Conditions of Evolution. Piper, München, DE, Z¨urich, CH. [German]

Riedl, R. 1992. Schrödinger's negentropy concept and biology. pp. 59-69. *In:* J. Götschl [ed.]. Erwin Schr¨odinger's World View. The Dynamics of Knowledge and Reality. Kluwer, Dordrecht, NL.

Riehle, A., S. Grün, M. Diesmann and A. Aertsen. 1997. Spike synchronization and rate modulation differentially involved in motor cortical function. Science 278: 1950-1953.

Rieke, F., D. Warland, R. de Ruyter van Steveninck and W. Bialek. 1997. Spikes: Exploring the Neural Code. A Bradford Book, The MIT Press, Cambridge, USA, London, UK.

Riesenhuber, M. and T. Poggio. 1999a. Hierarchical models of object recognition in cortex. Nature Neuroscience 2: 1019-1025.

Riesenhuber, M. and T. Poggio. 1999b. Are cortical models really bound by the "Binding Problem"? Neuron 24: 87-93.

Riley, M.A., K. Shockley and G. Van Orden. 2012. Learning from the body about the mind. Topics in Cognitive Science 4: 21-34.

Riley, M.S. and P. Smolensky. 1984. A parallel model of (sequential) problem solving. pp. 286-292. *In:* W. Kintsch [ed.] Proceedings of the Sixth Annual Conference of the Cognitive Science Society, Boulder, United States of America. Erlbaum. Hillsdale/NJ.

Rioul, O. 2018. This is IT: a primer on Shannon's entropy and information. Séminaire Poincaré 23: 43-77.

Rissanen, J. 1996. Information theory and neural nets. pp. 567-602. *In:* P. Smolensky, M. Mozer and D.E. Rumelhart [eds.]. Mathematical Perspectives on Neural Networks. Lawrence Erlbaum, Mahwah, USA.

Ritter, H. and T. Kohonen. 1989. Self-organizing semantic maps. Biological Cybernetics 61: 241-254.

Ritter, H., T. Martinetz and K. Schulten. 1992. Neural Computation and Self-Organizing Maps: An Introduction. Addison-Wesley, Reading, USA.

Robinson, C. 2009. Dynamical Systems. Stability, Symbolic Dynamics, and Chaos. 2nd Ed. CRC Press, Boca Raton, USA.

Robinson, D.J.S. 2003. An Introduction to Abstract Algebra. Walter de Gruyter, Berlin, DE.

Robinson, R.C. 2004. An Introduction to Nonlinear Dynamical Systems. Continuous and Discrete. Pearson Prentice Hall, Upper Saddle River, USA.

Robinson, R.C. 2012. An Introduction to Dynamical Systems. Continuous and Discrete. 2nd Ed. American Mathematical Society, Providence, USA.

Rockwell, W.T. 2005. Attractor spaces as modules: a semi-eliminative reduction of symbolic AI to dynamic systems theory. Minds and Machines 15: 23-55.

Rodriguez, E., N. George, J.-P. Lachaux, J. Martinerie, B. Renault and F.J. Varela. 1999. Perception's shadow: long-distance synchronization of human brain activity. Nature 397: 430-433.

Rodriguez-Molina, V.M., A. Aertsen and D. Heck. 2007. Spike timing and reliability in cortical pyramidal neurons: effects of EPSC kinetics, input synchronization and background noise on spike timing. PLoS ONE 2(3): e319.

Roelfsema, P.R., P. König, A.K. Engel, R. Sireteanu and W. Singer. 1994. Reduced synchronization in the visual cortex of cats with strabismic amblyopia. European Journal of Neuroscience 6: 1645-1655.

Roelfsema, P.R., A.K. Engel, P. König and W. Singer. 1995. Interareal synchronization between the visual, parietal and motor cortex of the awake cat. European Journal of Neuroscience, Supplement 8: 112.

Roelfsema, P.R., V.A. Lamme and H. Spekkreijse. 2004. Synchrony and covariation of firing rates in the primary visual cortex during contour grouping. Nature Neuroscience 7: 982-991.

Rösler, F. 2011. Psychophysiology of Cognition. An Introduction to Cognitive Neuroscience. Spektrum Akademischer Verlag, Heidelberg, DE. [German]

Rohde, M. 2013. Evolutionary robotics, organic computing and artificial life. pp. 180-183. In: A. Stephan and S. Walter. [eds.]. Handbuch Kognitionswissenschaft. Metzler, Stuttgart, Weimar, DE. [German]

Rojas, R. 1993. Theory of Neuronal Networks. A Systematic Introduction. Springer-Verlag, Berlin, DE. [German]

Rojas, R. and U. Hashagen [eds.] 2000. The First Computers. History and Architectures. MIT Press, Cambridge, USA.

Romba, M. 2001. Cognitive Structuring and Symbol-oriented Connectionism. Comparative Representation of Selected Cognitive Processes with Symbol Processing and Connectionist Models. A Model-Theoretical Investigation. Rainer Hampp Verlag, München/Mering, DE. [German]

Ropohl, G. 1978. Introduction to General Systems Theory. pp. 9-49. *In:* H. Lenk and G. Ropohl [eds.]. Systemtheorie als Wissenschaftsprogramm. Athenäum Verlag, Königstein/Ts, DE. [German]

Ropohl, G. 1979. A Systems Theory of Technology. The Foundation of the General Technology. Carl Hanser Verlag,München, DE,Wien, AT. [German]

Rosenblatt, F. 1958. The Perceptron. A probabilistic model for information storage and organization in the brain. Psychological Reviews 65: 386-408. (reprinted in Rosenblatt 1988.)

Rosenblatt, F. 1962. Principles of Neurodynamics: Perceptrons and the Theory of Brain Mechanism. Spartan Books, Washington D.C., USA.

Rosenblatt, F. 1988. The Perceptron. A probabilistic model for information storage and organization in the brain. pp. 92-114. *In:* J.A. Anderson and E. Rosenfeld [eds.]. Neurocomputing: Foundations of Research. Chapter 8. MIT Press, Cambridge, USA.

Roskies, A.L. 1999. Introduction: the binding problem. Neuron 24: 7-9.

Roth, G. 1992. Cognition: the formation of meaning in the brain. pp. 104-133. *In:* W. Krohn and G. K¨uppers [eds.]. Emergenz: Die Entstehung von Ordnung, Organisation und Bedeutung. Suhrkamp Verlag, Frankfurt/Main, DE. [German]

Roth, G. 1994. The Brain and its Reality. Suhrkamp Verlag, Frankfurt/Main, DE [German]

Rothkopf, C.A. 2013. Cognitive Neuroscience. pp. 78-84. *In:* A. Stephan and S. Walter [eds.]. Handbuch Kognitionswissenschaft. Metzler, Stuttgart, Weimar, DE. [German]

Rotter, S. and A. Aertsen. 1998. Accurate spike synchronisation in cortex. Zeitschrift für Naturforschung 53C: 686-689.

Rougier, N.P. and G.I. Detorakis. 2013. Self-organizing dynamic neural fields. pp. 281-288. *In:* Y. Yamaguchi [ed.]. Advances in Cognitive Neurodynamics (III). Proceedings of the Third International Conference on Cognitive Neurodynamics – 2011, Springer.

Ruiz, Y., S. Pockett, W.J. Freeman, E. Gonzales and L. Guang. 2010. A method to study global spatial patterns related to sensory perception in scalp EEG. Journal of Neuroscience Methods 191: 110-118.

Ruiz-Mirazo, K. and A. Moreno. 2004. Basic autonomy as a fundamental step in the synthesis of life. Artificial Life 10: 235-259.

Ruiz-Mirazo, K., J. Peretó and A. Moreno. 2004. A universal definition of life: autonomy and open-ended evolution. Origins of Life and Evolution of the Biosphere 34: 323-346.

Rumelhart, D.E. 1980. Schemata: the building blocks of cognition. pp. 33-58. *In:* R.J. Spiro, B.C. Bruce and W.F. Brewer [eds.]. Theoretical Issues in Reading Comprehension. Erlbaum, Hillsdale, USA.

Rumelhart, D.E. 1989. The architecture of mind: a connectionist approach. pp. 133-159. *In:* M.I. Posner [ed.]. Foundations of Cognitive Science. MIT Press, Cambridge, USA. (reprinted in Rumelhart 1997.)

Rumelhart, D.E. 1997. The architecture of mind: a connectionist approach. pp. 205-232. *In:* J. Haugeland [ed.]. Mind Design II. MIT Press, Cambridge, USA.

Rumelhart, D.E. and J.L. McClelland [eds.] 1986a. Parallel Distributed Processing: Explorations in the Microstructure of Cognition. Vol. 1: Foundations. MIT Press. A Bradford Book, Cambridge, USA.

Rumelhart, D.E. and J.L. McClelland [eds.] 1986b. Parallel Distributed Processing: Explorations in the Microstructure of Cognition. Vol. 2: Psychological and Biological Models. MIT Press, A Bradford Book, Cambridge, USA.

Rumelhart, D.E., G.E. Hinton and R.J. Williams. 1986a. Learning internal representations by error propagation. pp. 318-362. *In:* D.E. Rumelhart and J.L. McClelland [eds.]. Parallel Distributed Processing: Explorations in the Microstructure of Cognition. Vol. 1: Foundations. MIT Press. A Bradford Book, Cambridge, USA.

Rumelhart, D.E., G.E. Hinton and J.L. McClelland. 1986b. A general framework for parallel distributed processing. pp. 45-76. *In:* D.E. Rumelhart and J.L. McClelland [eds.]. Parallel Distributed Processing: Explorations in the Microstructure of Cognition. Vol. 1: Foundations. MIT Press. A Bradford Book, Cambridge, USA.

Rumelhart, D.E., P. Smolensky, G.E. Hinton and J.L. McClelland. 1986c. Schemata and sequential thought processes in PDP models. pp. 7-57. *In:* D.E. Rumelhart and J.L. McClelland [eds.]. Parallel Distributed Processing: Explorations in the Microstructure of Cognition. Vol. 2: Psychological and Biological Models. MIT Press, A Bradford Book, Cambridge, USA.

Russell, B. 1918-1919. The Philosophy of Logical Atomism. Open Court. LaSalle (reprinted in Russell, B. 1986.)

Russell, B. 1986. The philosophy of logical atomism. pp. 157-244. *In:* J.G. Slater [ed.]. Bertrand Russell. The Philosophy of Logical Atomism and other Essays 1914-19. The Collected Papers. Vol. 8. George Allen & Unwin, London, UK.

Salakhutdinov, R. and G. Hinton. 2009. Deep Boltzmann machines, 448-455. *In* Proceedings of the 12th International Conference on Artificial Intelligence and Statistics (AISTATS), Vol. 5, Clearwater, United States of America.

Sakurai, Y. 1999. How do cell assemblies encode information in the brain? Neuroscience Biobehavioral Reviews 23: 785-796.

Sandstede, B. 2007. Evans functions and nonlinear stability of travelling waves in neuronal network models. International Journal of Bifurcation and Chaos 17: 26932704.

Salari, N. and A. Maye. 2008. Brain Waves: How Synchronized Neuronal Oscillations can Explain the Perception of Illusory Objects. VDM Verlag Dr. Müller, Saarbrücken, DE.

Salin, P.A. and J. Bullier. 1995. Corticocortical connections in the visual system: structure and function. Physiological Reviews 75: 107-154.

Samuels, R., E. Margolis and S.P. Stich. 2012. Introduction: philosophy and cognitive science. pp. 3-18. In: E. Margolis, R. Samuels and S. Stich. [eds.]. The Oxford Handbook of Philosophy of Cognitive Science. Oxford University Press, Oxford, UK.

Samuelson, L.K., L.B. Smith, L.K. Perry and J.P. Spencer. 2011. Grounding word learning in space. PLoS ONE 6: e28095.

Samuelson, L.K. and C. Faubel. 2016. Grounding word learning in space and time. pp. 297-336. In: G. Schöner, J.P. Spencer and the DFT Research Group [eds.]. Dynamic Thinking: A Primer on Dynamic Field Theory. Oxford University Press, Oxford, UK, New York, USA.

Santos, B.A., X.E. Barandiaran and P. Husbands. 2012. Synchrony and phase relation dynamics underlying sensorimotor coordination. Adaptive Behavior 20: 321-336.

Sapojnikova, E. 2004. ART-Based Fuzzy Classifiers. ART Fuzzy Networks for Automatic Classification. Cuvillier Verlag, Göttingen, DE.

Sato, T. 1989. Interactions of visual stimuli in the receptive fields of inferior temporal neurons in awake monkeys. Experimental Brain Research 77: 23-30.

Schank, R.C. and R. Abelson. 1977. Scripts, Plans, Goals and Understanding. Erlbaum, Hillsdale, USA.

Schechter, B. 1996. How the brain gets rhythm. Science 274: 339-340.

Scheerer, E. 1988. Towards a history of cognitive science. International Social Science Journal 115: 7-18.

Scheerer, E. 1992. Mental representation in an interdisciplinary perspective. Report No. 72/1992 der Forschungsgruppe "Mind and Brain" des Zentrums für interdisziplinäre Forschung (ZiF), Universität Bielefeld, Bielefeld, DE: 45pp. [German]

Scheinerman, E.R. 2000. Invitation to Dynamical Systems. Department of Mathematical Sciences. The Johns Hopkins University. Internet Version.

Scherer, A. 1997. Neuronal Networks. Fundamentals and Applications. Vieweg, Braunschweig, Wiesbaden, DE. [German]

Scherz, U. 1999. Quantum Mechanics. An Introduction with Applications to Atoms, Molecules and Solids. B.G. Teubner, Stuttgart, DE, Leipzig, DE. [German]

Schiepek, G. and G. Strunk. 1994. Dynamic Systems. Fundamentals and Analysis Methods for Psychologists and Psychiatrists. Roland Asanger Verlag, Heidelberg, DE. [German]

Schiepek, G. and W. Tschacher [eds.] 1997. Self-Organization in Psychology and Psychiatry. Vieweg Verlag, Braunschweig, DE. [German]

Schierwagen, A. 1993. Models of neuroinformatics as mediators between neuroscientific facts and cognition theories. pp. 131-152. In: J.F. Maas [ed.]. Das sichtbare Denken. Modelle und Modellhaftigkeit in der Philosophie und denWissenschaften. Editions Rodopi B.V., Amsterdam, NL, Atlanta, USA. [German]

Schillen, T.B. and P. König. 1990a. Coherency detection by coupled oscillatory responses – synchronizing connections in neural oscillator layers. pp. 139-142. In: R. Eckmiller, G. Hartmann and G. Hauske [eds.]. Parallel Processing in Neural Systems and Computers. Elsevier Science Inc., Amsterdam, NL.

Schillen, T.B. and P. König. 1990b. Coherency detection and response segregation by synchronizing and desynchronizing delay connections in a neuronal oscillator model, 387-395. In IEEE Neural Networks Council [ed.] International Joint Conference on Neural Networks (IJCNN'90). Vol. II, San Diego, United States of America.

Schillen, T.B. and P. König. 1991a. Temporal coding by coherent oscillations as a potential solution to the binding problem: neural network simulations. pp. 153-171. In: H.G. Schuster [ed.]. Nonlinear Dynamics and Neuronal Networks. VCH Weinheim, New York, USA, Basel, CH, Cambridge, UK.

Schillen, T.B. and P. König. 1991b. Stimulus-dependent assembly formation of oscillatory responses. II. Desynchronization. Neural Computation 3: 167-177.

Schillen, T.B. and P. König. 1993. Temporal structure can solve the binding problem for multiple feature domains. pp. 503-507. In: F.H. Eeckman and J.M. Bower [eds.]. Computation and Neural Systems. Kluwer Academic Publishers, Boston, USA, Dordrecht, NL, London, UK.

Schillen, T.B. and P. König. 1994. Binding by temporal structure in multiple feature domains of an oscillatory neuronal network. Biological Cybernetics 70: 397-405.

Schlesinger, M. 2003. A lesson from robotics: modeling infants as autonomous agents. Adaptive Behavior 11: 97-107.

Schlesinger, M. 2004. Evolving agents as a metaphor for the developing child. Developmental Science 7: 154-168.

Schlesinger, M. 2009. The robot as a new frontier for connectionism and dynamic systems theory. pp. 182-199. In: J.P. Spencer, M.S.C. Thomas, and J.L.

Mc-Clelland. [eds.]. Toward a Unified Theory of Development: Connectionism and Dynamic Systems Theory ReConsidered. Oxford University Press, Oxford, UK.

Schlesinger, M. and D. Parisi. 2001. The agent-based approach: a new direction for computational models of development. Developmental Review 21: 121-146.

Schlesinger, M. and D. Parisi. 2007. Connectionism in an artificial life perspective: simulating motor, cognitive, and language development. pp. 129-158. *In:* D. Mareschal, S. Sirois, G. Westermann and M. Johnson [eds.]. Neuroconstructivism. 2. Perspectives and Prospects. Oxford University Press, Oxford, UK.

Schmeck, H., C. Müller-Schloer, E. Çakar, M. Mnif and U. Richter. 2011. Adaptivity and self-organisation in organic computing systems. pp. 5-37. *In:* C. Müller-Schloer, H. Schmeck and T. Ungerer [eds.]. Organic Computing – A Paradigm Shift for Complex Systems. Birkhäuser, Basel, CH.

Schmid, U. and Kindsmüller, M.C. 1996. Cognitive Modeling. An Introduction to the Logical and Algorithmic Foundations. Spektrum Akademischer Verlag, Heidelberg, DE. [German]

Schmidhuber, J. 2015. Deep learning in neural networks: an overview. Neural Networks 61: 85-117.

Schmidt, J.C. 2008. Instability in Nature and Science. A Philosophy of Science of Postmodern Physics. Walter de Gruyter, Berlin, DE, New York, USA. [German]

Schneegans, S. and G. Schöner. 2008. Dynamic field theory as a framework for understanding embodied cognition. pp. 241-270. *In:* P. Calvo and A. Gomilla [eds.]. Handbook of Cognitive Science. An Embodied Approach. 1st Ed. Elsevier, Amsterdam, NL.

Schöner, G. 2001. Neural systems and behavior: dynamical systems approaches. pp. 10573-10577. *In:* N.J. Smelser and P.B. Baltes. [eds.]. International Encyclopedia of the Social and Behavioral Sciences. Vol. 15. Elsevier Science, Oxford, UK.

Schöner, G. 2008. Dynamical systems approaches to cognition. pp. 101-126. *In:* R. Sun [ed.]. The Cambridge Handbook of Computational Psychology. Cambridge University Press, Cambridge, UK.

Schöner, G. 2009. Development as change of systems dynamics: stability, instability, and emergence. pp. 25-31. *In:* J.P. Spencer, M.S.C. Thomas and J.L. McClelland [eds.]. Toward a Unified Theory of Development: Connectionism and Dynamic Systems Theory ReConsidered. Oxford University Press, Oxford, UK.

Schöner, G. 2013. Theory of Dynamic Systems. pp. 175-179. *In:* A. Stephan and S. Walter [eds.]. Handbuch Kognitionswissenschaft. Metzler, Stuttgart, Weimar, DE. [German]

Schöner, G. 2019. The dynamics of neural populations capture the laws of the mind. Topics in Cognitive Science: DOI: 10.1111/tops.12453.

Schöner, G., J.P. Spencer and the DFT Research Group. 2016. Dynamic Thinking: A Primer on Dynamic Field Theory. Oxford University Press, Oxford, UK, New York, USA.

Schöning, U. 2008. Theoretical Computer Science – In Brief. 5th Ed. Spektrum Akademischer Verlag, Heidelberg, Berlin, DE. [German]

Scholz, O.R. 2013. Social and distributed cognition. pp. 202-206. *In:* A. Stephan and S. Walter [eds.]. Handbuch Kognitionswissenschaft. Metzler, Stuttgart, Weimar, DE. [German]

Schrauwen, B., D. Verstraeten and J. Van Campenhout. 2007. An overview of reservoir computing: theory, applications and implementations. pp. 471-482. *In:* M. Verleysen [ed.] Proceedings of the 15th European Symposium on Artificial Neural Networks (ESANN'2007), Bruges, Belgium.

Schröder, B. 2013. Computational Linguistics. pp. 71-75. *In:* A. Stephan and S. Walter [eds.]. Handbuch Kognitionswissenschaft. Metzler, Stuttgart, Weimar, DE. [German]

Schrödinger, E. 1944/2012. What is Life? The Physical Aspect of the Living Cell. Cambridge University Press, Cambridge, UK.

Schumacher, J., H. Toutounji and G. Pipa. 2013. An analytical approach to single node delay-coupled reservoir computing. pp. 26-33. *In:* V. Mladenov, P. Koprinkova-Hristova, G. Palm, A. Villa, B. Apolloni and N.K. Kasabov [eds.]. Proceedings of the 23rd International Conference on Artificial Neural Networks (ICANN'2013), Sofia, Bulgaria. Springer.

Schumacher, J., H. Toutounji and G. Pipa. 2015. An introduction to delay-coupled reservoir computing. pp. 63-90. *In:* P. Koprinkova-Hristova, V. Mladenov and N.K. Kasabov [eds.]. Artificial Neural Networks. Methods and Applications in Bio-/Neuroinformatics. Springer International Publishing Switzerland, Cham, CH, Heidelberg, DE, New York, USA, Dordrecht, NL, London, UK.

Schunn, C.D. and D. Klahr. 1998. Production system. pp. 542-551. *In:* W. Bechtel and G. Graham [eds.]. A Companion to Cognitive Science. Blackwell Publisher, Malden, USA, Oxford, UK.

Schuster, H. and P. Wagner. 1990. A model for neuronal oscillations in the visual cortex. Biological Cybernetics 64: 77-82.

Schuster, H.G. 2007. Conscious or Unconscious? Wiley-VCH Verlag, Weinheim, DE. [German]

Schuster, H.G. and W. Just. 2005. Deterministic Chaos: An Introduction. 4th Ed. Wiley-VCH Verlag, Weinheim, DE.

Schwabl, F. 2006. Statistical Mechanics. 3rd Ed. Springer-Verlag, Berlin, DE, Heidelberg, DE. [German]

Schweitzer, F. 1997. Self-organization and information. pp. 99-129. *In:* H. Krapp and T. Wagenbaur [eds.]. Komplexität und Selbstorganisation – Chaos in Natur und Kulturwissenschaften. Wilhelm Fink Verlag, München, DE. [German]

Schwender, D., C. Madler, S. Klasing, K. Peter and E. Pöppel. 1994. Anesthetic control of 40-Hz brain activity and implizit memory. Consciousness and Cognition 3: 129-147.

Scott, A.C. 1999. Nonlinear Science: Emergence and Dynamics of Coherent Structures. Oxford University Press, Oxford, UK.

Scott, A.C. [ed.] 2005. Encyclopedia of Nonlinear Science. Routledge, Taylor & Francis Group. New York, USA, Oxford, UK.

Scott, A.C. 2007. The Nonlinear Universe. Chaos, Emergence, Life. Springer-Verlag, Berlin, Heidelberg, DE.

Scott Jordan, J., N. Srinivasan and C. Van Leeuwen 2015. The role of complex systems theory in cognitive science. Cognitive Processing 16: 315-317.

Seiffert, H. 1985. Introduction to the Philosophy of Science. Vol. 3: Theory of Action – Modal Logic – Ethics – Systems Theory. Beck Verlag, München, DE [German]

Seiler, T. 1996. Recursive autoassociative memory and holographically reduced representation. M.Sc. Thesis (Diplomarbeit). Fakultät für Informatik. Technische Universität Dresden, Dresden, DE. [German]

Sejnowski, T.J. 1986. Open questions about computation in cerebral cortex. pp. 372-389. *In:* D.E. Rumelhart and J.L. McClelland [eds.]. Parallel Distributed Processing: Explorations in the Microstructure of Cognition. Vol. 2: Psychological and Biological Models. MIT Press. A Bradford Book, Cambridge, USA.

Sejnowski, T.J. 1999. Computational neuroscience. pp. 166-168. *In:* R.A. Wilson and F.C. Keil [eds.]. The MIT Encyclopedia of the Cognitive Sciences. The MIT Press, Cambridge, USA, London, UK.

Sejnowski, T.J. 2018. The Deep Learning Revolution. The MIT Press, Cambridge, USA.

Sejnowski, T.J. 2020. The unreasonable effectiveness of deep learning in artificial intelligence. Proceedings of the National Academy of Sciences of the United States of America. https://doi.org/10.1073/pnas.1907373117 .

Sejnowski, T.J. and C. Rosenberg. 1986. NETtalk: a parallel network that learns to read aloud. Technical Report 86-01. Department of Electrical Engineering and Computer Science, Johns Hopkins University, Baltimore, USA: 32pp. [unpublished manuscript]

Sengupta, B., M.B. Stemmler and K.J. Friston. 2013. Information and efficiency in the nervous system – a synthesis. PLoS Computational Biology 9: E1003157.

Senkowski, D., T.R. Schneider, J.J. Foxe and A.K. Engel. 2008. Crossmodal binding through neural coherence: implications for multisensory processing. Trends in Neurosciences 31: 401-409.

Shadlen, M.N. 2003. Rate versus temporal coding models. pp. 819-825. *In:* L. Nadel. [ed.]. Encyclopedia of Cognitive Science. Vol. 3. Natur Publishing Group. London, UK, New York, USA and Tokyo, JP.

Shadlen, M.N. and W.T. Newsome. 1994. Noise, neural codes and cortical organization. Current Opinion in Neurobiology 4: 569-579.

Shadlen, M.N. and W.T. Newsome. 1998. The variable discharge of cortical neurons: implications for connectivity, computation, and information coding. The Journal of Neuroscience 18: 3870-3896.

Shadlen, M.N. and J.A. Movshon. 1999. Synchrony unbound: a critical evaluation of the temporal binding hypothesis. Neuron 24: 67-77.

Shalizi, C.R. and K.L. Shalizi. 2005. Quantifying self-organization in cyclic cellular automata. pp. 108-117. *In:* L. Schimansky-Geier, D. Abbott, A. Neiman, C. van den Broeck [eds.]. Noise in Complex Systems and Stochastic Dynamics. SPIE Press, Bellingham, USA.

Shanahan, M. 2003. The frame problem. pp. 144-150. *In:* L. Nadel [ed.]. Encyclopedia of Cognitive Science. Vol. 2. Natur Publishing Group. London, UK, New York, USA and Tokyo, JP.

Shannon, C.E. 1948. A mathematical theory of communication. The Bell System Technical Journal 27: 379-423, 623-655.

Shannon, C.E. and W. Weaver. 1949/1963. The Mathematical Theory of Communication. University of Illinois Press, Urbana, USA.

Shapiro, L. 2011. Embodied Cognition. Routledge, London, UK, New York, USA.

Sharkey, N.E. 1991. Connectionist representation techniques. Artificial Intelligence Review 5: 143-167.

Sharma, S., S. Aubin and C. Eliasmith. 2016. Large-scale cognitive model design using the Nengo neural simulator. Biologically Inspired Cognitive Architectures 2016: 86-100.

Shastri, L. 1996. Temporal synchrony, dynamic bindings, and SHRUTI: a representational but non-classical model of reflexive reasoning. Behavioral and Brain Sciences 19: 331-337.

Shastri, L. 1999. Advances in SHRUTI – a neurally motivated model of relational knowledge representation and rapid inference using temporal synchrony. Applied Intelligence 11: 79-108

Shastri, L. 2007. SHRUTI: a neurally motivated architecture for rapid, scalable inference. pp. 183-203. *In:* B. Hammer and P. Hitzler [eds.]. Perspectives of Neural-Symbolic Integration. Springer-Verlag. Berlin, DE, Heidelberg, DE.

Shastri, L. and V. Ajjanagadde. 1993. From simple associations to systematic reasoning: a connectionist representation of rules, variables and dynamic bindings using temporal synchrony. Behavioral and Brain Sciences 16: 417-494.

Shea, N. 2007. Content and its vehicles in connectionist systems. Mind and Language 22: 246-269.

Shiffrin, R.M. 2010. Perspectives on modeling in cognitive science. Topics in Cognitive Science 2: 736-750.

Shmiel, T., R. Drori, O. Shmiel, Y. Ben-Shaul, Z. Nadasdy, M. Shemesh, M. Teicher and M. Abeles. 2005. Neurons of the cerebral cortex exhibit precise inter-spike timing in correspondence to behavior. Proceedings of the National Academy of Sciences of the United States of America 102: 18655-18657.

Shmiel, T., R. Drori, O. Shmiel, Y. Ben-Shaul, Z. Nadasdy, M. Shemesh, M. Teicher and M. Abeles. 2006. Temporally precise cortical firing patterns are associated with distinct action segments. Journal of Neurophysiology 96: 2645-2652.

Siebert, C. 1998. Qualia. The phenomenal as a problem of philosophical and of empirical theories of consciousness. Ph.D. Thesis. Philosophische Fakultät. Humboldt-Universität zu Berlin, Berlin, DE. [German]

Silberstein, M. and A. Chemero 2012. Complexity and extended phenomenological-cognitive systems. Topics in Cognitive Science 4: 35-50.

Simon, D. and K.J. Holyoak. 2002. Structural dynamics of cognition: from consistency theories to constraint satisfaction. Personality and Social Psychology Review 6: 283-294.

Simon, H.A. 1962. The architecture of complexity. Proceedings of the American Philosophical Society 106: 467-482.

Simon, H.A. 1999. Production systems. pp. 676-678. In: R.A. Wilson and F.C. Keil [eds.]. The MIT Encyclopedia of the Cognitive Sciences. The MIT Press, Cambridge, USA, London, UK.

Simon, H.A. 2003. Computational models: why build them? pp. 621-623. In: L. Nadel [ed.]. Encyclopedia of Cognitive Science. Vol. 1. Natur Publishing Group. London, UK, New York, USA, and Tokyo, JP.

Simon, H.A. and A. Newell. 1964. Information processing in computer and man. The American Scientist 52: 281-300.

Simon, H.A. and C.A. Kaplan. 1989. Foundations of cognitive science. pp. 1-47. In: M.I. Posner. [ed.]. Foundations of Cognitive Science. MIT Press, Cambridge, USA.

Singer, W. 1990. Search for coherence: a basic principle of cortical self-organization. Concepts in Neuroscience 1: 1-26.

Singer, W. 1993. Synchronization of cortical activity and its putative role in information processing and learning. Annual Review of Physiology 55: 349-374.

Singer, W. 1994a. The role of synchrony in neocortical processing and synaptic plasticity. pp. 141-173. *In:* E. Domany, J.L. van Hemmen and K. Schulten [eds.]. Models of Neural Networks II. Temporal Aspects of Coding and Information Processing in Biological Systems. Chap. 4. Springer-Verlag, New York, USA.

Singer, W. 1994b. Coherence as an organizing principle of cortical functions. pp. 153-183. *In:* O. Sporns and G. Tononi [eds.]. Selectionism and the Brain. International Review of Neurobiology. Vol. 37. Academic Press, San Diego, USA.

Singer, W. 1995. Synchronization of neuronal responses as a putative binding mechanism. pp. 960-964. *In:* M.A. Arbib [ed.]. The Handbook of Brain Theory and Neural Networks. The MIT Press, Cambridge, USA, London, UK.

Singer, W. 1996. Neuronal synchronization: a solution to the binding problem. pp. 100-130. *In:* R.R. Llinás and P.S. Churchland [eds.]. The Mind-Brain Continuum. Sensory Processes. MIT Press, Cambridge, USA.

Singer, W. 1997. Consciousness, something "new, hitherto outrageous". Berichte und Abhandlungen. Berlin-Brandenburgische Akademie der Wissenschaften 4: 175-190. [German]

Singer, W. 1999a. Binding by neural synchrony. pp. 81-84. *In:* R.A. Wilson and F.C. Keil [eds.]. The MIT Encyclopedia of the Cognitive Sciences. The MIT Press, Cambridge, USA, London, UK.

Singer, W. 1999b. Neuronal synchrony: a versatile code for the definition of relations. Neuron 24: 49-65.

Singer, W. 1999c. The image in the mind – a paradigm shift. pp. 267-278. *In:* D. Ganten, E. Meyer-Galow, H.-H. Ropers, H. Scheich, H. Schwarz, E. Truscheit and K. Urban [eds.]. Gene, Neurone, Qubits & Co. Unsere Welten der Information. Gesellschaft Deutscher Naturforscher und Ärzte. Stuttgart, DE, Heidelberg, DE. [German]

Singer, W. 1999d. Time as coding space? Current Opinion in Neurobiology 9: 189-194.

Singer, W. 2000. Response synchronization, a neural code for relatedness. pp. 35-48. *In:* J.J. Bolhuis [ed.]. Brain, Perception, Memory. Advances in Cognitive Neuroscience. Oxford University Press, Oxford, UK.

Singer, W. 2001. Neuronal synchrony as a binding mechanism. pp. 10567-10570. *In:* N.J. Smelser and P.B. Baltes [eds.]. International Encyclopedia of the Social & Behavioral Sciences. Vol. 15. Elsevier Science, Oxford, UK.

Singer, W. 2002a. The observer in the brain. pp. 144-170. *In:* W. Singer [ed.]. Der Beobachter im Gehirn. Essays zur Hirnforschung. Suhrkamp Verlag, Frankfurt/M., DE. [German]

Singer, W. 2002b. Brain development or the search for coherence. Determinants of brain development. pp. 120-143. *In:* W. Singer [ed.]. Der Beobachter im Gehirn. Essays zur Hirnforschung. Suhrkamp Verlag, Frankfurt/M., DE. [German]

Singer, W. 2002c. Neurobiological remarks on the constructivism discourse. pp. 87-111. *In:* W. Singer [ed.]. Der Beobachter im Gehirn. Essays zur Hirnforschung. Suhrkamp Verlag, Frankfurt/M., DE. [German]

Singer, W. 2002d. From brain to consciousness. pp. 60-76. *In:* W. Singer [ed.]. Der Beobachter im Gehirn. Essays zur Hirnforschung. Suhrkamp Verlag, Frankfurt/M., DE. [German]

Singer, W. 2002e. Response synchronization, Gamma oscillations, and perceptual binding in cat primary visual cortex. pp. 521-559. *In:* A. Peters and B.R. Payne [eds.]. The Cat Primary Visual Cortex. Academic Press, San Diego, USA.

Singer, W. 2003a. Synchronization, binding and expectancy. pp. 1136-1143. *In:* M.A. Arbib [ed.]. The Handbook of Brain Theory and Neural Networks. 2nd Ed. The MIT Press. Cambridge, USA, London, UK.

Singer, W. 2003b. Unser Menschenbild im Spannungsfeld von Selbsterfahrung und neurobiologischer Fremdbeschreibung. KIZ Universität Ulm, Ulm, DE. [German]

Singer, W. 2004. Synchrony, oscillations and relational codes. pp. 1665-1681. *In:* L.M. Chalupa and J.S. Werner [eds.]. The Visual Neurosciences. 2nd Ed. The MIT Press. Cambridge, USA.

Singer, W. 2005. The brain – an orchestra without a conductor. Max Planck Forschung. Das Wissenschaftsmagazin der Max-Planck-Gesellschaft 2: 15-18. [German]

Singer, W. 2009. Neural synchrony and feature binding. pp. 253-259. *In:* L.R. Squire [ed.]. Encyclopedia of Neuroscience. Vol. 6. Academic Press, Oxford, UK.

Singer, W. 2013. Cortical dynamics revisited. Trends in Cognitive Sciences 17: 616-626.

Singer, W. 2018. Neuronal oscillations: unavoidable and useful? European Journal of Neuroscience 48: 2389-2399.

Singer, W., C.M. Gray, A.K. Engel, P. König, A. Artola and S. Bröcher. 1990. Formation of cortical cell assemblies. pp. 939-952. *In:* [none]. Cold Spring Harbor Symposia on Quantitative Biology. Vol. 55: The Brain. Cold Spring Harbor Laboratory Press, Cold Spring Harbor, USA.

Singer, W. and C.M. Gray. 1995. Visual feature integration and the temporal correlation hypothesis. Annual Review of Neuroscience 18: 555-586.

Singer, W., A.K. Engel, A.K. Kreiter, M.H.J. Munk, S. Neuenschwander and P.R. Roelfsema. 1997. Neuronal assemblies: necessity, signature and detectability. Trends in Cognitive Sciences 1: 252-261.

Singer, W. and A. Lazar. 2016. Does the cerebral cortex exploit high-dimensional, non-linear dynamics for information processing? Frontiers in Computational Neuroscience 10: 99.

Singh, R. and C. Eliasmith. 2006. Higher-dimensional neurons explain the tuning and dynamics of working memory cells. Journal of Neuroscience 26: 3667-3678.

Sipser, M. 2013. Introduction to the Theory of Computation. 3rd Ed. Thomson, Boston, USA.

Skarda, C.A. and W.J. Freeman. 1987. How brains make chaos in order to make sense of the world. Behavioral and Brain Sciences 10: 161-195.

Skinner, B.F. 1953. Science and Human Behavior. Macmillan, New York, USA.

Skirke, U. 1997. Technology and self-organization. On the problem of a sustainable concept of progress. Ph.D. Thesis, Universität Hamburg, Hamburg, DE. [German]

Skowronski, M.D. and J.G. Harris. 2007. Automatic speech recognition using a predictive echo state network classifier. Neural Networks 20: 414-423.

Slaby, J. 2013. Critical neuro- and cognitive science. pp. 523-528. *In:* A. Stephan and S. Walter [eds.]. Handbuch Kognitionswissenschaft. Metzler, Stuttgart, Weimar, DE. [German]

[SLOAN Foundation] Miller, G.A. and E. Walker [eds.] 1978. Cognitive Science 1978. Report of The State of the Art Committee to The Advisors of The Alfred P. Sloan Foundation. October 1, 1978. Alfred P. Sloan Foundation, University of California, Berkeley, USA: 249pp.

Sloman, S. 1999. Cognitive architecture. pp. 124-126. *In:* R.A. Wilson and F.C. Keil [eds.]. The MIT Encyclopedia of the Cognitive Sciences. The MIT Press, Cambridge, USA, London, UK.

Smith, L.B. and L.K. Samuelson. 2003. Different is good: connectionism and dynamic systems theory are complementary emergentist approaches to development. Developmental Science 6: 434-439.

Smith Churchland, P. 1986. Neurophilosophy: Toward a Unified Science of the Mind/Brain. The MIT Press, Cambridge, USA.

Smith Churchland, P. 2002. Brain-Wise: Studies in Neurophilosophy. MIT Press, Cambridge, USA.

Smith Churchland, P. and T.J. Sejnowski. 1989. Neural representation and neural computation. pp. 343-382. *In:* L. Nadel [ed.]. Philosophical Perspectives. MIT Press, Cambridge, USA.

Smith Churchland, P. and T.J. Sejnowski. 1992. The Computational Brain. MIT Press, Cambridge, USA.

Smolensky, P. 1983. Schema selection and stochastic inference in modular Environments. pp. 378-382. *In:* Proceedings of the Third National Conference on Artificial Intelligence (AAAI'83), Washington/DC, United States of America, American Association for Artificial Intelligence.

Smolensky, P. 1984a. Harmony theory: thermal parallel models in a computational context. *In:* P. Smolensky and M.S. Riley [eds.] Harmony Theory: Problem Solving, Parallel Cognitive Models, and Thermal Physics. Technical Report 8404. Institute for Cognitive Science, University of California, San Diego, USA: 12pp.

Smolensky, P. 1984b. The mathematical role of self-consistency in parallel computation. *In:* P. Smolensky and M.S. Riley [eds.] Harmony Theory: Problem Solving, Parallel Cognitive Models, and Thermal Physics. Technical Report 8404. Institute for Cognitive Science, University of California, San Diego, USA: 6pp.

Smolensky, P. 1986a. Information processing in dynamical systems: foundations of harmony theory. pp. 194-281. *In:* D.E. Rumelhart and J.L. McClelland [eds.]. Parallel Distributed Processing: Explorations in the Microstructure of Cognition. Vol. 1: Foundations. MIT Press. A Bradford Book, Cambridge, USA.

Smolensky, P. 1986b. Formal modeling of subsymbolic processes: an introduction to harmony theory. pp. 204-235. *In:* N.E. Sharkey [ed.]. Directions in the Science of Cognition. Ellis Horwood, New York, USA.

Smolensky, P. 1986c. Neural and conceptual interpretations of parallel distributed processing models. pp. 390-431. *In:* D.E. Rumelhart and J.L. McClelland [eds.]. Parallel Distributed Processing: Explorations in the Microstructure of Cognition. Vol. 2: Psychological and Biological Models. MIT Press. A Bradford Book, Cambridge, USA.

Smolensky, P. 1987a. On variable binding and the representation of symbolic structures in connectionist systems. Technical Report CU-CS-355-87. Department of Computer Science, University of Colorado, Boulder, USA: 68pp.

Smolensky, P. 1987b. A method for connectionist variable binding. Technical Report CU-CS-356-87. Department of Computer Science, University of Colorado, Boulder, USA: 10pp.

Smolensky, P. 1988a. On the proper treatment of connectionism. Behavioral and Brain Sciences 11: 1-74.

Smolensky, P. 1988b. The constituent structure of connectionist mental states: a reply to Fodor and Pylyshyn. *In:* T. Horgan and J. Tienson [eds.]. Spindel Conference 1987: Connectionism and the Philosophy of Mind. The Southern

Journal of Philosophy. Special Issue on Connectionism and the Foundations of Cognitive Science. Supplement 26: 137-161.

Smolensky, P. 1988c. Putting together connectionism – again. Behavioral and Brain Sciences 11: 59-74.

Smolensky, P. 1989a. Connectionist modeling: neural computation/mental connections. pp. 49-67. *In:* L. Nadel, L.A. Cooper, P. Culicover and R.M. Harnish [eds.]. Neural Connections. Mental Computation. The MIT Press, A Bradford Book, Cambridge, USA.

Smolensky, P. 1990. Tensor product variable binding and the representation of symbolic structures in connectionist systems. Artificial Intelligence 46: 159-216.

Smolensky, P. 1991. Connectionism, constituency, and the language of thought. pp. 201-227. *In:* B. Loewer and G. Rey [eds.]. Meaning in Mind. Fodor and his Critics. Blackwell, Cambridge, USA, Oxford, UK.

Smolensky, P. 1994. Computational models of mind. pp. 176-185. *In:* S. Guttenplan [ed.]. A Companion to the Philosophy of Mind. Blackwell Publishers, Oxford, UK, Cambridge, USA.

Smolensky, P. 1995. Reply: constituent structure and explanation in an integrated connectionist / symbolic cognitive architecture. pp. 223-290. *In:* C. MacDonald and G. MacDonald. [eds.]. Connectionism: Debates on Psychological Explanation. Vol. 2. Blackwell Publishers. Oxford/UK, Cambridge, USA.

Smolensky, P. 2012a. Symbolic functions from neural computation. Philosophical Transactions of the Royal Society of London A: Mathematical, Physical and Engineering Sciences 370: 3543-3569.

Smolensky, P. 2012b. Subsymbolic computation theory for the human intuitive processor. pp. 675-685. *In:* S.B. Cooper, A. Dawar and B. Löwe [eds.]. Proceedings of the Turing Centenary Conference and 8th Conference on Computability in Europe (CiE 2012), How the World Computes, Cambridge, United Kingdom. Springer.

Smolensky, P., G. Legendre and Y. Miyata. 1992. Principles for an integrated connectionist/symbolic theory of higher cognition. Technical Report CUCS-600-92. Department of Computer Science and Institute of Cognitive Science. University of Colorado, Boulder, USA: 75pp.

Smolensky, P., G. Legendre and Y. Miyata. 1994. Integrating connectionist and symbolic computation for the theory of language. pp. 509-530. *In:* V. Honavar and L. Uhr [eds.]. Artificial Intelligence and Neural Networks: Steps toward Principled Integration. Academic Press, San Diego, USA, London, UK.

Smolensky, P. and G. Legendre. 2006a. The Harmonic Mind: From Neural Computation to Optimality-Theoretic Grammar. Vol. 1: Cognitive Architecture. A Bradford Book, The MIT Press, Cambridge, USA, London, UK.

Smolensky, P. and G. Legendre. 2006b. The Harmonic Mind: From Neural Computation to Optimality-Theoretic Grammar. Vol. 2: Linguistic and Philosophical Implications. A Bradford Book, The MIT Press, Cambridge, USA, London, UK.

Smolensky, P., M. Lee, X. He,W.-T. Yih, J. Gao and L. Deng. 2016. Basic reasoning with tensor product representations. arXiv preprint arXiv:1601.02745.

Snooks, G.D. 2008. A general theory of complex living systems: exploring the demand side of dynamics. Complexity 13: 12-20.

Snyman, J.A. and D.N. Wilke. 2018. Practical Mathematical Optimization Basic Optimization Theory and Gradient-Based Algorithms. 2nd Ed. Springer International Publishing, Cham, CH.

Sobel, C.P. 2001. The Cognitive Sciences. An Interdisciplinary Approach. Mayfield, Mountain View, USA.

Sobel, C.P. and P. Li. 2013. The Cognitive Sciences. An Interdisciplinary Approach. 2nd Ed. SAGE, Los Angeles, USA.

Softky, W.R. 1995. Simple codes versus efficient codes. Current Opinion in Neurobiology 5: 239-247.

Solomonoff, R.J. 1964a. A formal theory of inductive inference. Part 1. Information and Control 7: 1-22.

Solomonoff, R.J. 1964b. A formal theory of inductive inference. Part 2. Information and Control 7: 224-254.

Solso, R.L. 2005. Cognitive Psychology. Springer-Verlag, Heidelberg, DE. [German]

Somers, D. and N. Kopell. 1993. Rapid synchronization through fast treshold modulation. Biological Cybernetics 68: 393-407.

Somers, D. and N. Kopell. 1995. Waves and synchrony in networks of oscillators of relaxation and non-relaxation type. Physica D: Nonlinear Phenomena 89: 169-183.

Sommers, F. 1989. Predication in the logic terms. Notre Dame Journal of Formal Logic 31: 106-126.

Sompolinsky, H. 1988. Statistical mechanics of neural networks. Physics Today 41: 70-80.

Sompolinsky, H., D. Golomb and D. Kleinfeld. 1990. Global processing of visual stimuli in a neural network of coupled oscillators. Proceedings of the National Academy of Sciences of the United States of America 87: 7200-7204.

Sontag, E.D. 1998. Mathematical Control Theory. 2nd Ed. Springer, New York, USA.

Sougné, J.P. 1999. INFERNET: a neurocomputational model of binding and inference. Ph.D. Université de Liège, Liège, BE.

Sougné, J.P. 2003. Binding problem. pp. 374-382. *In:* L. Nadel [ed.]. Encyclopedia of Cognitive Science. Vol. 1. Natur Publishing Group. London, UK, New York, USA and Tokyo, JP.

Spencer, J.P. and G. Schöner. 2003. Bridging the representational gap in the dynamic systems approach to development. Development Science 6: 392-412.

Spencer, J.P., E. Dineva and G. Schöner. 2009a. Moving toward a unified theory while valuing the importance of the initial conditions. pp. 354-372. *In:* J.P. Spencer, M.S.C. Thomas and J.L. McClelland [eds.]. Toward a Unified Theory of Development: Connectionism and Dynamic Systems Theory Re-Considered. Oxford University Press, Oxford, UK.

Spencer, J.P., S. Perone and J.S. Johnson. 2009b. The dynamic field theory and embodied cognitive dynamics. pp. 86-118. *In:* J.P. Spencer, M.S.C. Thomas and J.L. McClelland [eds.] 2009b. Toward a Unified Theory of Development: Connectionism and Dynamic Systems Theory Re-Considered. Oxford University Press, Oxford, UK.

Spencer, J.P., M.S.C. Thomas and J.L. McClelland [eds.] 2009c. Toward a Unified heory of Development: Connectionism and Dynamic Systems Theory Re-Considered. Oxford University Press, Oxford, UK.

Spitzer, M. 2000. Spirit in the Net. Models for Learning, Thinking and Acting. Spektrum Akademischer Verlag, Heidelberg, DE, Berlin, DE. [German]

Spivey, M. 2007. The Continuity of Mind. Oxford University Press, Oxford, UK.

Sporns, O. 1994. Selectionist and instructionist ideas in neuroscience. pp. 4-26. *In:* O. Sporns and G. Tononi [eds.]. Selectionism and the Brain. International Review of Neurobiology. Vol. 37. Academic Press, San Diego, USA.

Sporns, O. 2011. Networks of the Brain. The MIT Press, Cambridge, USA, London, UK.

Sporns, O. 2013. Network attributes for segregation and integration in the human brain. Current Opinion in Neurobiology 23: 162-171.

Sporns, O. and G. Tononi. [eds.] 1994. Selectionism and the Brain. International Review of Neurobiology. Vol. 37. Academic Press, San Diego, USA.

Squire, L.R., D. Berg, F.E. Bloom, S. Du Lac, A. Ghosh and N.C. Spitzer. [eds.] 2008. Fundamental Neuroscience. 3rd Ed. Elsevier Academic Press, Amsterdam, NL, Heidelberg, DE.

Stainton, R.J. 2006. Contemporary Debates in Cognitive Science. Blackwell, London, UK.

Stanley, G.B. 2013. Reading and writing the neural code. Nature Neuroscience 16: 259-263.

Stapf, H. 2009. Dorsch Psychological Dictionary. 15th Ed. Verlag Hans Huber, Hogrefe, Bern, CH. [German]

Stavropoulos, D.N. 2008. Oxford Greek-English Learner's Dictionary. Oxford University Press. Oxford, UK, New York, USA.

Steedman, M. 1996. Cognitive algorithms: questions of representations and computation in building a theory. pp. 173-210. *In:* D.N. Osherson [ed.]. An Invitation to Cognitive Science. 2nd Ed. Vol. 4. Methods, Models, and Conceptual Issues. MIT Press, Cambridge, USA.

Stegmüller, W. 1973. Personal and Statistical Probability. Problems and Results of Philosophy of Science and Analytical Philosophy. Part IV. First Half-Volume: Personal Probability and Rational Decision. Springer-Verlag, Berlin, DE. [German]

Stegmüller, W. 1987. Main Streams of Contemporary Philosophy. A Critical Introduction. Vol. III. 8th Ed. Alfred Kröner Verlag, Stuttgart, DE. [German]

Stegmüller, W. and M. Varga von Kibéd. 1984. Structure Types of Logic. Problems and Results of Philosophy of Science and Analytical Philosophy. Part III. Springer-Verlag, Berlin, DE. [German]

Stein, R.B., R.R. Gossen and K.E. Jones. 2005. Neuronal variability: noise or part of the signal? Nature Reviews Neuroscience 6: 389-397.

Steinbacher, K. 1990. System/system theory. p. 500. *In:* H.J. Sandkühler [ed.]. Europäische Enzyklopädie zu Philosophie und Wissenschaften. Band 4. Felix Meiner Verlag, Hamburg, DE. [German]

Stephan, A. 1999. Emergence. From Unpredictability to Self-Organization. Dresden Universitäts verlag, Dresden, DE. [German]

Stephan, A. 2003. Emergence. pp. 1108-1115. *In:* L. Nadel [ed.]. Encyclopedia of Cognitive Science. Vol. 1. Natur Publishing Group. London, UK, New York, USA, and Tokyo, JP.

Stephan, A. 2006. On the role of the concept of emergence in the philosophy of mind and in cognitive science. pp. 146-166. *In:* D. Sturma [ed.]. Philosophie und Neurowissenschaften. Suhrkamp Verlag, Frankfurt/Main, DE. [German]

Stephan, A. and S. Walter [eds.]. 2013. Handbook Cognitive Science. Metzler, Stuttgart, Weimar, DE. [German]

Sterelny, K. 1990. The Representational Theory of Mind. An Introduction. Basil Blackwell, Oxford, UK.

Stewart, T.C. and C. Eliasmith. 2008. Building production systems with realistic spiking neurons. pp. 1759-1764. *In:* B.C. Love, K. McRae and V.M. Sloutsky [eds.]. Proceedings of the 30th Annual Meeting of the Cognitive Science Society, Austin, United States of America.

Stewart, T.C., T. Bekolay and C. Eliasmith. 2011. Neural representations of compositional structures. Representing and manipulating vector spaces with spiking neurons. Connection Science 22: 145-153.

Stewart, T.C. and C. Eliasmith. 2012. Compositionality and biologically plausible models. pp. 596-615. *In:* M. Werning, W. Hinzen and E. Machery [eds.]. The Oxford Handbook of Compositionality. Oxford University Press, Oxford, UK.

Stewart, T.C. and C. Eliasmith. 2014. Large-scale synthesis of functional spiking neural circuits. Proceedings of the IEEE 102: 881-898.

Stillings, N.A., S.E. Weisler, C.H. Chase, M.H. Feinstein, J.L. Garfield, and E.L. Rissland. 1995. Cognitive Science: An Introduction. 2nd Ed. The MIT Press, Cambridge, USA.

Stollenwerk, N. and F. Pasemann. 1996. Control strategies for chaotic neuromodules. International Journal of Bifurcation and Chaos 6: 693-703.

Stone, G.O. 1986. An analysis of the delta rule and the learning of statistical associations. pp. 444-459. *In:* D.E. Rumelhart and J.L. McClelland [eds.]. Parallel Distributed Processing: Explorations in the Microstructure of Cognition. Vol. 1: Foundations. MIT Press. A Bradford Book, Cambridge, USA.

Stone, J.V. 2015. Information Theory. A Tutorial Introduction. Sebtel Press, Sheffield, UK.

Stonier, T. 1997. Information and Meaning: An Evolutionary Perspective. Springer-Verlag, London, UK.

Stopfer, M., S. Bhagavan, B. Smith and G. Laurent. 1997. Impaired odour discrimination on desynchronization of odour-encoding neural assemblies. Nature 390: 70-74.

Strasser, A. 2010. A functional view toward mental representations. pp. 15-25. *In:* D. Ifenthaler, P. Pirnay-Dummer and N.M. Seel [eds.]. Computer-Based Diagnostics and Systematic Analysis of Knowledge. Springer Science+Business Media. New York, USA, Heidelberg, DE.

Strogatz, S.H. 2018. Nonlinear Dynamics and Chaos. With Applications to Physics, Biology, Chemistry, and Engineering. 2nd Ed. CRC Press. Boca Raton, USA.

Strohner, H. 1995. Cognitive Systems. An Introduction to Cognitive Science. Westdeutscher Verlag, Opladen, DE. [German]

Strube, G. 1990. Neoconnectionism: A new basis for the theory and modeling of human cognition. Psychologische Rundschau 41: 129-143. [German]

Strube, G. 1996a. Cognition. p. 305. *In:* G. Strube, B. Becker, C. Freksa, U. Hahn, K. Opwis and G. Palm [eds.]. Wörterbuch der Kognitionswissenschaft. Klett-Cotta Verlag, Stuttgart, DE. [German]

Strube, G. 1996b. Cognitive Science. pp. 317-319. *In:* G. Strube, B. Becker, C. Freksa, U. Hahn, K. Opwis and G. Palm [eds.]. Wörterbuch der Kognitionswissenschaft. Klett-Cotta Verlag, Stuttgart, DE. [German]

Strube, G. 1996c. Symbol processing. p. 708. *In:* G. Strube, B. Becker, C. Freksa, U. Hahn, K. Opwis and G. Palm [eds.]. Wörterbuch der Kognitionswissenschaft. Klett-Cotta Verlag, Stuttgart, DE. [German]

Strube, G. 1996d. Algorithm. p. 7. *In:* G. Strube, B. Becker, C. Freksa, U. Hahn, K. Opwis and G. Palm [eds.]. Wörterbuch der Kognitionswissenschaft. Klett-Cotta Verlag, Stuttgart, DE. [German]

Strube, G., C. Habel, L. Konieczny and B. Hemforth. 2000. Cognition. pp. 19-71. *In:* G. Görz, C.-R. Rollinger and J. Schneeberger [eds.]. Handbuch der Künstlichen Intelligenz. 3rd Ed. Oldenbourg Verlag, München, DE, Wien, AT. [German]

Strunk, G. 2000. The theory of nonlinear dynamic systems - fundamentals – benefit – therapy. Systeme. Interdisziplinäre Zeitschrift für systemtheoretisch orientierte Forschung und Praxis in den Humanwissenschaften 14: 185-197. [German]

Strunk, G. and G. Schiepek. 2006. Systemic Psychology. An Introduction to the Complex Foundations of Human Behavior. Elsevier. Spektrum Akademischer Verlag, München, DE [German]

Stufflebeam, R.S. 1998. Representation and computation. pp. 636-648. *In:* W. Bechtel and G. Graham [eds.]. A Companion to Cognitive Science. Blackwell Publisher, Malden, USA, Oxford, UK.

Sturm, A.K. and P. König. 2001. Mechanisms to synchronize neuronal activity. Biological Cybernetics 84: 153-172.

Sturm, T. and H. Gundlach. 2013. On the history and historiography of the "cognitive revolution" – a reflection. pp. 7-21. *In:* A. Stephan and S. Walter [eds.]. Handbuch Kognitionswissenschaft. Metzler, Stuttgart, Weimar, DE. [German]

Sucharowski, W. 1996. Language and Cognition. New Perspectives in Linguistics. Westdeutscher Verlag. Opladen, DE. [German]

Sun, R. 1995. CONSYDERR: a two-level hybrid architecture for structuring knowledge for commonsense reasoning. pp. 247-281. *In:* R. Sun and L.A. Bookman [eds.]. Computational Architectures Integrating Symbolic and Connectionist Processing. A Perspective on the State of the Art. Kluwer Academic Publishers, Dordrecht, NL.

Sun, R. 1997. An introduction to hybrid connectionist-symbolic models. pp. 1-10. *In:* R. Sun and F. Alexandre [eds.]. Connectionist-Symbolic Integration: From Unified to Hybrid Approaches. Lawrence Erlbaum, Mahwah, USA.

Sun, R. 1998. Artificial intelligence. pp. 341-351. *In:* W. Bechtel and G. Graham [eds.]. A Companion to Cognitive Science. Blackwell Publisher, Malden, USA, Oxford, UK.

Sun, R. 2001. Artificial intelligence. Connectionist and symbolic approaches. pp. 783-789. *In:* N.J. Smelser and P.B. Baltes [eds.]. International Encyclopedia of the Social & Behavioral Sciences. Pergamon/Elsevier Science, Oxford, UK.

Sun, R. 2008. Introduction to computational cognitive modeling. pp. 3-19. *In:* R. Sun [ed.]. The Cambridge Handbook of Computational Psychology. Cambridge University Press. Cambridge, UK.

Suppes, P. 1957/1999. Introduction to Logic. Dover Publications, Mineola, USA.

Sutton, R.S. and A.G. Barto. 1998. Reinforcement Learning. An Introduction. A Bradford Book, The MIT Press, London, UK.

Tabor, W. 2009. Dynamical insight into structure in connectionist models. pp. 165-181. *In:* J.P. Spencer, M.S.C. Thomas and J.L. McClelland [eds.]. Toward a Unified Theory of Development: Connectionism and Dynamic Systems Theory ReConsidered. Oxford University Press, Oxford, UK.

Tacca, M.C. 2010. Seeing Objects: The Structure of Visual Representation. Mentis, Paderborn, DE.

Tallon, C., O. Bertrand, P. Bouchet and J. Pernier. 1995. Gamma-range activity evoked by coherent visual stimuli in humans. European Journal of Neuroscience 7: 1285-1291.

Tallon-Baudry, C. 2003. Oscillatory synchrony as a signature for the unity of visual experience in humans. pp. 153-167. *In:* A. Cleeremans [eds.]. The Unity of Consciousness: Binding, Integration, and Dissociation. Oxford University Press, Oxford, UK.

Tallon-Baudry, C. 2004. Attention and awareness in synchrony. Trends in Cognitive Science 8: 523-525.

Tallon-Baudry, C. 2009. The roles of gamma-band oscillatory synchrony in human visual cognition. Frontiers in Bioscience 14: 331-332.

Tallon-Baudry, C., O. Bertrand, C. Delpuech and J. Pernier. 1996. Stimulus specificy of phase-locked and non-phased-locked 40 Hz visual responses in human. Journal of Neuroscience 16: 4240-4249.

Tallon-Baudry, C., O. Bertrand, C. Delpuech and J. Pernier. 1997. Oscillatory gamma-band (30-70 Hz) activity induced by a visual search task in humans. Journal of Neuroscience 17: 722-734.

Tallon-Baudry, C., O. Bertrand, S. Peronnet and J. Pernier. 1998. Induced gamma-band activity during the delay of a visual short-term memory task in humans. Journal of Neuroscience 18: 4244-4254.

Tallon-Baudry, C., A. Kreiter and O. Bertrand. 1999. Sustained and transient oscillatory responses in the gamma and beta bands in a visual short-term memory task in humans. Visual Neuroscience 16: 449-459.

Tallon-Baudry, C. and O. Bertrand. 2003. Gamma oscillations in humans. pp. 255-260. *In:* L. Nadel [ed.]. Encyclopedia of Cognitive Science. Vol. 2. Natur Publishing Group. London, UK, New York, USA and Tokyo, JP.

Tanaka, K., H. Saito, Y. Fukada and M. Moriya. 1991. Coding visual images of objects in the inferotemporal cortex of the macaque monkey. The Journal of Neuroscience 66: 170-189.

Tanaka, T. and A. Weitzenfeld, A. 2002. Adaptive resonance theory. pp. 157-169. *In:* A. Weitzenfeld, M.A. Arbib and A. Alexander [eds.]. The Neural Simulation Language: A System for Brain Modeling. Bradford Books, MIT Press, Cambridge, USA.

Tani, J. 2014. Self-organization and compositionality in cognitive brains: a neurorobotics study. Proceedings of the IEEE. Special Issue on Cognitive Dynamic Systems 102: 586-605.

Tani, J. 2017. Exploring Robotic Minds: Actions, Symbols, and Consciousness as Self-Organizing Dynamic Phenomena. Oxford University Press, UK, New York, USA.

Tani, J., K. Friston and S. Haykin. 2014. Further thoughts on the paper by Tani: self-organization and compositionality in cognitive brains. Proceedings of the IEEE 102: 606-607.

Tesar, B.B. and P. Smolensky. 1994. Synchronous firing variable binding is a tensor product representation with temporal role vectors. pp. 870-875. *In:* A. Ram and K. Eiselt [eds.] Proceedings of the Sixteenth Annual Conference of the Cognitive Science Society, Atlanta, United States of America. Lawrence Erlbaum.

Teschl, G. 2011. Ordinary Differential Equations and Dynamical Systems. American Mathematical Society, Providence, USA. [unpublished manuscript]

Thagard, P. 1989. Explanatory coherence. Behavioral and Brain Sciences 12: 435-467.

Thagard, P. [ed.] 1998. Mind Readings. Introductory Selections on Cognitive Science. MIT Press, Cambridge, USA.

Thagard, P. 2000. Coherence in Thought and Action. MIT Press, Cambridge, USA, London, UK.

Thagard, P. 2005. Mind: An Introduction to Cognitive Science. 2nd Ed. MIT Press, Cambridge, USA, London, UK.

Thagard, P. 2012. Cognitive architectures. pp. 50-70. *In:* K. Frankish and W. Ramsey [eds.]. The Cambridge Handbook of Cognitive Science. Cambridge University Press, Cambridge, UK.

Thagard, P. 2014. Cognitive science. *In:* E.N. Zalta [ed.]. The Stanford Encyclopedia of Philosophy (July 11, 2014 Edition).

Thagard, P. and E. Millgram. 1995. Inference to the best plan: a coherence theory of decision. pp. 439-454. *In:* A. Ram and D.B. Leake [eds.]. Goal-Driven Learning. MIT Press, Cambridge, USA.

Thagard, P. and K. Verbeurgt. 1998. Coherence as constraint satisfaction. Cognitive Science 22: 1-24.

Thelen, E. 1995. Time-scale dynamics and the development of an embodied cognition. pp. 69-100. *In:* R.F. Port and T. van Gelder [eds.]. Mind as Motion. Explorations in the Dynamics of Cognition. A Bradford Book. MIT Press, Cambridge/MA, USA and London, UK.

Thelen, E. and L.B. Smith. 1993. A Dynamic Systems Approach to the Development of Cognition and Action. MIT Press, Cambridge, USA.

Thelen, E. and E. Bates. 2003. Connectionism and dynamic systems: are they really different? Development Science 6: 378-391.

Thelen, E. and L.B. Smith. 2006. Dynamic systems theories. pp. 258-312. *In:* W. Damon and R.M. Lerner. [eds.]. Handbook of Child Psychology. Vol. 1: Theoretical Models of Human Development. 6*th* Ed. John Wiley and Sons, New York, USA.

Theunissen, F. and J.P. Miller. 1995. Temporal encoding in nervous systems: a rigorous definition. Journal of Computational Neuroscience 2: 149-162.

Thiele, A. and G. Stoner. 2003. Neuronal synchrony does not correlate with motion coherence in cortical area MT. Nature 421: 366-370.

Thom, R. 1972/1980. Structural Stability and Morphogenesis. An Outline of a General Theory of Models. Benjamin/Cummings, Reading, USA.

Thom, R. 1975. Structural Stability and Morphogenesis. Benjamin, Reading, USA.

Thom, R. 1980. Mathematical Models of Morphogenesis. Christian Bourgois, Paris. [French]

Thom, R. 1983. Mathematical Models of Morphogenesis. Horwood, Chichester, UK.

Thom, 1989. Semiophysics. Addison-Wesley, Redwood City, USA.

Thomas, M.S.C. and J.L. McClelland. 2008. Connectionist models of cognition. pp. 23-58. *In:* R. Sun [ed.]. Cambridge Handbook of Computational Cognitive Modelling. Cambridge University. Cambridge, UK.

Thomas, M.S.C., J.L. McClelland, F.M. Richardson, A.C. Schapiro and F.D. Baughman. 2009. Dynamic and connectionist approaches to development: toward a future of mutually beneficial coevolution. pp. 337-353. *In:* J.P. Spencer, M.S.C. Thomas and J.L. McClelland [eds.]. Toward a Unified Theory of Development: Connectionism and Dynamic Systems Theory ReConsidered. Oxford University Press, Oxford, UK.

Thompson, E. and F.J. Varela. 2001. Radical embodiment: neural dynamics and consciousness. Trends in Cognitive Science 5: 418-425.

Thompson, J.M.T. and H.B. Stewart. 1986. Nonlinear Dynamics and Chaos: Geometrical Methods for Engineers and Scientists. Wiley, New York, USA.

Thorndike, E.L. 1911. Animal Intelligence: Experimental Studies. Macmillan, New York, USA.

Thorpe, S.J. 2003. Localized versus distributed representations. pp. 643-645. *In:* M.A. Arbib [ed.]. The Handbook of Brain Theory and Neural Networks. 2nd Ed. The MIT Press. Cambridge, USA, London, UK.

Tolman, E.C. 1932/1949. Purposive Behavior in Animals and Men. Cambridge University Press. London, UK.

Tolman, E.C. 1938. The determiners of behavior at a choice point. Psychological Review 45: 1-41.

Tolman, E.C. 1948. Cognitive Maps in Rats and Men. Psychological Review 55: 192-217.

Tononi, G. 2004a. An information integration theory of consciousness. BMC Neuroscience 5: 1-22.

Tononi, G. 2004b. Consciousness and the brain: theoretical aspects. *In:* G. Adelman and B. Smith [eds.]. Encyclopedia of Neuroscience. 3rd Ed. Elsevier, Amsterdam, NL, Oxford, UK.

Tononi, G. 2009. An integrated information theory of consciousness. pp. 403-416. *In:* W.P. Banks [ed.]. Encyclopedia of Consciousness. Academic Press, Oxford, UK, San Diego, USA.

Tononi, G. 2010. Information integration: its relevance to brain function and consciousness. Archives Italiennes De Biologie 148: 299-322.

Tononi, G. 2012. Integrated information theory of consciousness: an updated account. Archives Italiennes De Biologie 150: 56-90.

Tononi, G., O. Sporns and G.M. Edelman. 1992. Reentry and the program of integrating multiple cortical areas: simulation of dynamic integration in the visual system. Cerebral Cortex 2: 310-335.

Tononi, G., O. Sporns and G.M. Edelma. 1994. A measure for brain complexity: relating functional segregation and integration in the nervous system. Proceedings of the National Academy of Sciences of the United States of America 91: 5033-5037.

Tononi, G. and G.M. Edelman. 1998a. Consciousness and complexity. Science 282: 1846-1851.

Tononi, G. and G.M. Edelman. 1998b. Consciousness and the integration of information in the brain. pp. 245-279. *In:* H.H. Jasper, L. Descarries, V.F.

Castellucci and S. Rossignol [eds.]. Consciousness. At the Frontiers of Neuroscience. Plenum Press, New York, USA.

Tononi, G., A.R. McIntosh, D.P. Russell and G.M. Edelman. 1998a. Functional clustering: identifying strongly interactive brain regions in neuroimaging data. NeuroImage 7: 133-149.

Tononi, G., G.M. Edelman and O. Sporns. 1998b. Complexity and coherency: integrating information in the brain. Trends in Cognitive Sciences 2: 474-484.

Tononi, G. and O. Sporns. 2003. Measuring information integration. BMC Neuroscience 4: 1-20.

Tononi, G. and C. Koch. 2008. The neural correlates of consciousness: an update. Annals New York Academy of Science 1124: 239-261.

Tononi, G., M. Boly, M. Massimini and C. Koch. 2016. Integrated information theory: from consciousness to its physical substrate. Nature Reviews. Neuroscience 17: 450-461.

Touretzky, D.S. 1986. BoltzCONS: reconciling connectionism with the recursive nature of stacks and trees, 522-530. *In* Cognitive Science Society (U.S.) [ed.] Proceedings of the 8*th* Conference of the Cognitive Science Society. Amherst, Unites States of America. Lawrence Erlbaum.

Touretzky, D.S. 1991. Connectionism and compositional semantics. pp. 17-31. *In:* J.A. Barnden and J.B. Pollack [eds.]. High-Level Connectionist Models. Advances in Connectionist & Neural Computation Theory. Erlbaum, Hillsdale, USA.

Touretzky, D.S. 2003. Connectionist and symbolic representations. pp. 260-263. *In:* M.A. Arbib [ed.]. The Handbook of Brain Theory and Neural Networks. 2*nd* Ed. The MIT Press. Cambridge, USA, London, UK.

Touretzky, D.S. and S. Geva. 1987. A distributed connectionist representation for concept structures. Technical Report. Paper 1935. Computer Science Department. Carnegie Mellon University, Pittsburgh, Pennsylvania, USA: 10pp. [unpublished manuscript]

Touretzky, D.S and G.E. Hinton. 1988. A distributed connectionist production system. Cognitive Science 12: 423-466.

Toutounji, H. and F. Pasemann. 2014. Behavior control in the sensorimotor loop with short-term synaptic dynamics induced by self-regulating neurons. Frontiers in Neurorobotics 8: 19.

Toutounji, H. and G. Pipa. 2014. Spatiotemporal computations of an excitable and plastic brain: neuronal plasticity leads to noise-robust and noise-constructive computations. PLoS Computational Biology 10: e1003512.

Toutounji, H., J. Schumacher and G. Pipa. 2015. Homeostatic plasticity for node delay coupled reservoir computing. Neural Computation 27: 1159-1187.

Trappenberg, T.P. 2010. Fundamentals of Computational Neuroscience. 2nd Ed. Oxford University Press, Oxford, UK, New York, USA.

Traub, R.D., J.G. Jefferys and R. Miles. 1993. Analysis of the propagation of disinhibition induced after-discharges along the guineau-pig hippocampal slice *in vitro*. Journal of Physiology 472: 267-287.

Traub, R.D., M.A. Whittington, I.M. Stanford and J.G.R. Jefferys. 1996. A mechanism for generation of long-range synchronous fast oscillations in the cortex. Nature 382: 621-624.

Traub, R.D., G.R. Jefferys and A. Whittington. 1999. Fast Oscillations in Cortical Circuits. The MIT Press, Cambridge, USA.

Traub, R.D., N. Kopell, A. Bibbig, E.H. Buhl, F.E.N. Lebeau and M.A. Whittington. 2001. Gap junctions between interneuron dendrites can enhance synchrony of gamma oscillations in distributed networks. The Journal of Neuroscience 21(23): 9378-9386.

Trautner, H.M. 1991. Textbook of Developmental Psychology. Vol. 2: Theories and Findings. 2nd Ed. Hogrefe, Göttingen, DE. [German]

Treisman, A. 1977. Focused attention in the perception and retrieval of multidimensional stimuli. Perception and Psychophysics 22: 1-11.

Treisman, A. 1986. Features and objects in visual processing. Scientific American 254: 114-125.

Treisman, A. 1988. Features and objects. The fourteenth Bartlett memorial lecture. Quarterly Journal of Experimental Psychology 40A: 201-237.

Treisman, A. 1993. The perception of features and objects. pp. 5-35. *In:* A. Baddeley and L. Weiskrantz [eds.]. Attention: Selection, Awareness & Control. A Tribute to Donald Broadbent. Clarendon Press, Oxford, UK.

Treisman, A. 1996. The binding problem. Current Opinion in Neurobiology 6: 171-178.

Treisman, A. 1998. Feature binding, attention and object perception. Philosophical Transactions of the Royal Society. Biological Sciences 353: 1295-1306.

Treisman, A. 1999. Solutions to the binding problem: progress through controversy and convergence. Neuron 24: 105-110.

Treisman, A. 2006. Object tokens, binding, and visual memory. pp. 315-338. *In:* H.D. Zimmer, A. Mecklinger and U. Lindenberger [eds.]. Handbook of Binding and Memory. Perspectives from Cognitive Neuroscience. Oxford University Press, Oxford, UK.

Treisman, A. and G. Gelade. 1980. A feature-integration theory of attention. Cognitive Psychology 12: 97-136.

Treisman, A. and H. Schmidt. 1982. Illusory conjunctions in the perception of objects. Cognitive Psychology 14: 107-141.

Treisman, A. and S. Sato. 1990. Conjunction search revisited. Journal of Experimental Psychology. Human Perception and Performance 16: 459-476.

Triesch, J. and C. von der Malsburg. 2001. Democratic integration: self-organized integration of adaptive cues. Neural Computation 13: 2049-2074.

Troy, W.C. 2008a. Wave phenomena in neuronal networks. pp. 431452. *In:* N. Akhmediev and A. Ankiewicz [eds.]. Dissipative Solitons. From Optics to Biology and Medicine. Springer, Berlin, DE.

Troy, W.C. 2008b. Traveling waves and synchrony in an excitable large-scale neuronal network with asymmetric connections. SIAM Journal on Applied Dynamical Systems 7: 12471282.

Ts'o, D.Y. and C.D. Gilbert. 1988. The organization of chromatic and spatial interactions in the primate striate cortex. The Journal of Neuroscience 8: 1712-1727.

Tucker, D.M. 2001. Motivated anatomy: a core-and-shell model of corticolimbic architecture. pp. 125-160. *In:* G. Gainotti [ed.]. Handbook of Neuropsychology. 2nd Ed. Vol. 5: Emotional Behavior and its Disorders. Elsevier Science, Amsterdam, NL.

Turing, A.M. 1936. On computable numbers, with an application to the Entscheidungsproblem. Proceedings of the London Mathematical Society 2: 230-265.

Turing, A.M. 1938. On computable numbers, with an application to the Entscheidungsproblem: a correction. Proceedings of the London Mathematical Society 2: 544-546.

Tye, M. 1988. Representation in pictorialism and connectionism. *In:* T. Horgan and J. Tienson [eds.]. Spindel Conference 1987: Connectionism and the Philosophy of Mind. The Southern Journal of Philosophy. Special Issue on Connectionism and the Foundations of Cognitive Science. Supplement 26: 163-183.

Uhlhaas, P., G. Pipa, L. Lima, S. Melloni, S. Neuenschwander, D. Nikolic and W. Singer. 2009. Neural synchrony in cortical networks: history, concept and current status. Frontiers in Integrative Neuroscience 3: 1-19.

Uhlhaas, P., G. Pipa, S. Neuenschwander, M. Wibral and W. Singer. 2011. A new look at gamma? High- (>60 Hz) g-band activity in cortical networks: function, mechanisms and impairment. Progress in Biophysics and Molecular Biology 105: 14-28.

Ulich, D. 2000. Introduction to Psychology. 3rd Ed. Kohlhammer, Stuttgart, DE. [German]

Unbehauen, R. 2002. System Theory 1: General Principles, Signals and Linear Systems in Time and Frequency Range. 4th Ed. Oldenbourg, München, DE, Wien, AT. [German]

Unbehauen, R. 1969/1998. Systems Theory 2: Multidimensional, Adaptive and Nonlinear Systems. 4th Ed. Oldenbourg, München, DE, Wien, AT. [German]

Uran, C., A. Peter, A. Lazar, W. Barnes, J. Klon-Lipok, K. Shapcott, R. Roese, P. Fries, W. Singer and M. Vinck. 2020. Predictability in natural images determines V1 firing rates and synchronization: a deep neural network approach. bioRxiv. From: https://doi.org/10.1101/2020.08.10.242958. [unpublished manuscript]

Urchs, M. 2002. Machine – Body – Mind. An introduction to Cognitive Science. Vittorio Klostermann, Frankfurt am Main, DE. [German]

Vad´en, T. 1996. The Symbolic and Subsymbolic Theories in Cognitive Science. Tampereen Yliopisto, Tampere, FI.

van der Pol, B. 1926. On relaxation oscillation. Philosophical Magazine 2: 978-992.

van der Velde, F. and M. de Kamps. 2003. A neural blackboard architecture of sentence structure. Technical Report. Leiden University, Leiden, NL: 40pp. [unpublished manuscript]

van der Velde, F. and M. de Kamps. 2006a. Neural blackboard architectures of combinatorial structures in cognition. Behavioral and Brain Sciences 29: 37-70.

van der Velde, F. and M. de Kamps. 2006b. From neural dynamics to combinatorial structures. Behavioral and Brain Sciences 29: 88-108.

van de Wouw, N., E. Lefeber and I. Lopez Arteaga [eds.] 2017. Nonlinear Systems. Techniques for Dynamical Analysis and Control. Springer International Publishing, Basel, CH.

van Gelder, T. 1989. Distributed representation. Ph.D. Thesis, University of Pittsburgh, Pittsburgh, USA.

van Gelder, T. 1990a. Compositionality: a connectionist variation on a classical theme. Cognitive Science 14: 355-384.

van Gelder, T. 1990b. Why distributed representation is inherently non-symbolic. pp. 58-66. *In:* G. Dorffner. [ed.]. Konnektionismus in Artificial Intelligence und Kognitionsforschung. Springer-Verlag, Berlin u.a., DE.

van Gelder, T. 1991a. What is the "D" in "PDP"? A survey of the concept of distribution. pp. 33-59. *In:* W. Ramsey, S.P. Stich and D.E. Rumelhart [eds.]. Philosophy and Connectionist Theory. Lawrence Erlbaum, Hillsdale, USA.

van Gelder, T. 1991b. Classical questions, radical answers: connectionism and the structure of mental representations. pp. 355-381. *In:* T. Horgan and J. Tienson [eds.]. Connectionism and the Philosophy of Mind. Kluwer Academic Publisher, Dordrecht, NE.

van Gelder, T. 1992a. Defining "distributed representation". Connection Science. Special Issue on Philosophical Issues in Connectionist Modeling 4: 175-191.

van Gelder, T. 1992b. Making conceptual space. pp. 179-194. *In:* S. Davis [ed.]. Connectionism: Theory and Practice. Oxford University Press, New York, USA, Oxford, UK.

van Gelder, T. 1997. Dynamics and cognition. pp. 421-450. *In:* J. Haugeland [ed.]. Mind Design II. Philosophy – Psychology – Artificial Intelligence. Revised and Enlarged Edition. A Bradford Book. The MIT Press. Cambridge, USA, London, UK.

van Gelder, T. 1998a. Author's response: disentangling dynamics, computation and cognition. Behavioral and Brain Sciences 21: 654-661.

van Gelder, T. 1998b. The dynamical hypothesis in cognitive science. Behavioral and Brain Sciences 21: 615-628.

van Gelder, T. 1999a. Defending the dynamical hypothesis. pp. 13-28. *In:* W. Tschacher and J.-P. Dauwalder [eds.]. Dynamics, Synergetics, Autonomous Agents: Nonlinear Systems Approaches to Cognitive Psychology and Cognitive Science. World Scientific, Singapore, SG.

van Gelder, T. 1999b. Distributed vs. local representation. pp. 236-238. *In:* R.A. Wilson and F.C. Keil [eds.]. The MIT Encyclopedia of the Cognitive Sciences. The MIT Press, Cambridge, USA, London, UK.

van Gelder, T. 1999c. Revisiting the Dynamical Hypothesis. Preprint No. 2/99. pp. 1-21. University of Melbourne. Department of Philosophy. Australia. [unpublished manuscript]

van Gelder, T. 1999d. Dynamic approaches to cognition. pp. 243-245. *In:* R.A. Wilson and F.C. Keil [eds.]. The MIT Encyclopedia of the Cognitive Sciences. The MIT Press, Cambridge, USA, London, UK.

van Gelder, T. and R.F. Port [eds.]. 1995. It's about time: an overview of the dynamical approach to cognition. pp. 1-43. *In:* R.F. Port and T. van Gelder [eds.]. Mind as Motion. Explorations in the Dynamics of Cognition. A Bradford Book. MIT Press, Cambridge/MA, USA and London, UK.

Van Hulle, M.M. 2000. Faithful Representations and Topographic Maps – From Distortion- to Information-Based Self-Organization. John Wiley, New York, USA.

Vankov, I. and J. Bowers. 2019. Training neural networks to encode symbols enables combinatorial generalization. Philosophical Transactions of the Royal Society B 375: 20190309.

Van Leeuwen, M. 2005. Questions for the dynamicist: the use of dynamical Systems theory in the philosophy of cognition. Minds and Machines 15: 271-333.

Van Rullen, R. and S.J. Thorpe. 2001. Rate coding versus temporal order coding: what the retinal ganglion cells tell the visual cortex. Neural Computation 13: 1255-1283.

Van Rullen, R., R. Guyonneau and S.J. Thorpe. 2005. Spike times make sense. Trends in Neurosciences 28: 1-4.

Varela, F. 1975. A calculus for self-reference. International Journal of General Systems 2: 5-24.

Varela, F. 1979. Principles of Biological Autonomy. North Holland, New York, USA, Oxford, UK.

Varela, F.J. 1988/1993. Cognitive Science. A Cartography of Current Ideas. Editions du Seuil. Paris, FR.

Varela, F.J. 1993. Cognitive Science, Cognitive Techniques. A Sketch of Current Perspectives. 3rd Ed. Suhrkamp Verlag, Frankfurt am Main, DE. [German]

Varela, F.J. 1995. Resonant cell assemblies: a new approach to cognitive functions and neuronal synchrony. Biological Research 28: 81-95.

Varela, F., H.R. Maturana and R. Uribe. 1974. Autopoiesis: the organization of living systems, its characterization and a model. Biosystems 5: 187-196.

Varela, F.J. 2006. Neuronal synchrony and cognitive functions. pp. 95-108. In: B. Feltz, M. Crommelinck and P. Goujon [eds.]. Self-Organization and Emergence in Life Sciences. Springer-Verlag, Dordrecht, NL.

Varela, F.J., E. Thompson, and E. Rosch. 1993. The Embodied Mind – Cognitive Science and Human Experience. 3rd Pr. The MIT Press, Cambridge, USA.

Varela, F.J., J.P. Lachaux, E. Rodriguez and J. Martinerie. 2001. The brainweb: phase synchronization and large-scale integration. Nature Neuroscience 2: 229-237.

Varela, F.J. and E. Thompson. 2003. Neural synchrony and the unity of mind: a neurophenomenological perspective. pp. 266-287. In: A. Cleeremans [ed.]. The Unity of Consciousness: Binding, Integration, and Dissociation. Oxford University Press, Oxford, UK.

Vater, H. 2002. Introduction to Linguistics. 4th Ed. Wilhelm Fink Verlag, München, DE. [German]

Vec, M., M.-T. Huett and A.M. Freund [eds.] 2006. Self-Organization. A System of Thought for Nature and Society. Böhlau, Köln, DE. [German]

Vemulapalli, G.K. 2010. Invitation to Physical Chemistry. Imperial College Press, London, UK.

Verdejo, V.M. 2013. Computationalism, connectionism, dynamicism and beyond: looking for an integrated approach to cognitive science. pp. 405-416. In: V. Karakostas and D. Dieks [eds.]. EPSA11 Perspectives and Foundational Problems in Philosophy of Science. Springer, Cham, CH.

Vernon, D., G. Metta and G. Sandini. 2007. A survey of artificial cognitive systems: implications for the autonomous development of mental capabilities in computational agents. IEEE Transactions on Evolutionary Computation 11: 151-180.

Vicente, R., L.L. Gollo, C.R. Mirasso, I. Fischer and G. Pipa. 2009. Far in space and yet in synchrony: neuronal mechanisms for zero-lag long-range synchronization. pp. 143-167. *In:* K. Josic, J. Rubin, M. Matias and R. Romo [eds.]. Coherent Behaviour in Neuronal Networks. Springer-Verlag, New York, USA.

Vinck, M. and C.A. Bosman. 2016. More gamma more predictions: gammasynchronization as a key mechanism for efficient integration of classical receptive field inputs with surround predictions. Frontiers in Systems Neuroscience 10: 35.

Visser, S., R. Nicks, O. Faugeras and S. Coombes. 2017. Standing and travelling waves in a spherical brain model. Physica D 349: 27-45.

Voelker, A.R. 2019. Dynamical systems in spiking neuromorphic hardware. Ph.D. Thesis. University of Waterloo, Waterloo, CA.

von Bertalanffy, L. 1950a. The theory of open systems in physics and biology. Science 111: 23-29.

von Bertalanffy, L. 1950b/2010. An outline of general system theory. British Journal for the Philosophy of Science 1: 134-165.

von Bertalanffy, L. 1953. Biophysics of the Flow Equilibrium. Introduction to the Physics of Open Systems and its Application in Biology. Verlag Friedrich Vieweg & Sohn, Braunschweig, DE. [German]

von Bertalanffy, L. 1968. General System Theory. Foundations, Development, Applications. George Braziller, New York, USA.

von Bertalanffy, L. 1972a. The history and status of general systems theory. The Academy of Management Journal 15: 407-426.

von Bertalanffy, L. 1972b. On a general system theory. pp. 31-45. *In:* K. Bleicher [ed.]. Organisation als System. Gabler, Wiesbaden, DE. [German]

von Bertalanffy, L. 1975. Perspectives on General System Theory. Scientific-Philosophical Studies. George Braziller, New York, USA.

von Bertalanffy, L. and A. Rapaport. 1956. General system theory. pp. 1-10. *In:* L. von Bertalanffy and A. Rapaport. [eds.]. General Systems. Yearbook of the International Society for the Systems sciences. Vol. 1.Wiley, Chichester, UK.

von der Malsburg, C. 1973. Self-organization of orientation selective cells in the striate cortex. Kybernetik 14: 85-100.

von der Malsburg, C. 1981. The correlation theory of brain function. Internal Report 81-2, Department of Neurobiology, Max-Planck-Institute of Biophysikal Chemistry, Göttingen, DE: 26pp. (reprinted in von der Malsburg 1994.)

von der Malsburg, C. 1985. Nervous structures with dynamical links. Berichte der Bunsengesellschaft für Physikalische Chemie 89: 703-710.

von der Malsburg, C. 1986. Am I thinking assemblies? pp. 161-176. *In:* G. Palm and A. Aertsen [eds.]. Brain Theory. Springer-Verlag, Berlin, DE.

von der Malsburg, C. 1990. Network self-organization. pp. 421-432. *In:* S.F. Zornetzer, J. Davis and C. Lau [eds.]. An Introduction to Neural and Electronic Networks. Academic Press, San Diego, USA.

von der Malsburg, C. 1994. The correlation theory of brain function. pp. 95-119. *In:* E. Domany, J.L. van Hemmen and K. Schulten [eds.]. Models of Neural Networks II. Temporal Aspects of Coding and Information Processing in Biological Systems. Chap. 2. Springer-Verlag, New York, USA.

von der Malsburg, C. 1995a. Dynamic link architecture. pp. 329-331. *In:* M.A. Arbib [ed.]. The Handbook of Brain Theory and Neural Networks. The MIT Press, Cambridge, USA, London, UK.

von der Malsburg, C. 1995b. Binding in models of perception and brain function. Current Opinion in Neurobiology 5: 520-526.

von der Malsburg, C. 1995c. Network self-organization in the ontogenesis of the mammalian visual system. pp. 447-463. *In:* S.F. Zornetzer, J. Davis and C. Lau [eds.]. An Introduction to Neural and Electronic Networks. 2nd Ed. Academic Press, San Diego, USA.

von der Malsburg, C. 1996. The binding problem of neural networks. pp. 131-146. *In:* R.R. Llinás and P.S. Churchland [eds.]. The Mind-Brain Continuum. Sensory Processes. MIT Press, Cambridge, USA.

von der Malsburg, C. 1999. The what and why of binding: the modeler's perspective. Neuron 24: 95-104.

von der Malsburg, C. 2001. Binding problem, neural basis of. pp. 1178-1180. *In:* N.J. Smelser and P.B. Baltes [eds.]. International Encyclopedia of the Social & Behavioral Sciences. Vol. 15. Elsevier Science, Oxford, UK.

von der Malsburg, C. 2002a. Dynamic link architecture. pp. 365-368. *In:* A. Arbib [ed.]. The Handbook of Brain Theory and Neural Networks. 2nd Ed. The MIT Press, Cambridge, USA, London, UK.

von der Malsburg, C. 2002b. How are neural signals related to each other and to the world? Journal of Consciousness Studies 9: 47-60.

von der Malsburg, C. 2003a. Self-organization and the brain. pp. 1002-1005. *In:* M.A. Arbib [ed.]. The Handbook of Brain Theory and Neural Networks. 2nd Ed. The MIT Press. Cambridge, USA, London, UK.

von der Malsburg, C. 2003b. Neural model of object vision: Quick links for sharp images. NEUROrubin: 31-34. [German] von der Malsburg, C. 2018. Concerning the neural code. Journal of Cognitive Science 19: 511-550.

von der Malsburg, C. 2020. Example brain - boundary conditions for a cognitive architecture. pp. 3-30. *In:* E. Portmann and S. D'Onofrio [eds.]. Cognitive Computing. Theorie, Technik und Praxis. Springer Vieweg, Wiesbaden, DE. [German]

von der Malsburg, C. and D.J. Willshaw. 1976. How patterned neural connections can be set up by self-organization. Proceedings of the Royal Society of London B 194: 431-445.

von der Malsburg, C. and W. Schneider. 1986. A neural cocktail-party processor. Biological Cybernetics 54: 29-40.

von der Malsburg, C. and E. Bienenstock. 1987. A neural network for the retrieval of superimposed connection patterns. Europhysics Letters 3: 1243-1249.

von der Malsburg, C. and W. Singer. 1988. Principles of cortical network organization. pp. 69-99. *In:* P. Rakic and W. Singer [eds.]. Neurobiology of Neocortex. Life Sciences Research Report 42, DahlemWorkshop Reports. JohnWiley & Sons, Chichester, UK.

von Eckardt, B. 1993. What is Cognitive Science? MIT Press, Cambridge, USA.

von Eckardt, B. 1999. Mental representation. pp. 527-529. *In:* R.A. Wilson and F.C. Keil [eds.]. The MIT Encyclopedia of the Cognitive Sciences. The MIT Press, Cambridge, USA, London, UK.

von Eckardt, B. 2003. Cognitive science: philosophical issues. pp. 552-559. *In:* L. Nadel [ed.]. Encyclopedia of Cognitive Science. Vol. 1. Natur Publishing Group. London, UK, New York, USA, and Tokyo, JP.

von Eckardt, B. 2012. The representational theory of mind. pp. 29-49. *In:* K. Frankish and W. Ramsey [eds.]. The Cambridge Handbook of Cognitive Science. Cambridge University Press, Cambridge, UK.

von Foerster, H. 1960. On Self-Organization Systems and their Environments. pp. 31-50. *In:* M.C. Yovits and S. Cameron [eds.]. Self-Organizing Systems. Proceedings of an Interdisciplinary Conference, 5 and 6 May, 1959. Symposium Publications Division, Pergamon Press.

von Seelen, W. and K. Behrend. 2016. Principles of Neural Information Processing. Springer, Heidelberg, DE.

von Weizsäcker, C.F. 1974. The Unity of Nature. Studies. Deutscher Taschenbuch Verlag, München, DE. [German]

von Weizsäcker, C.F. 1988. Structure of Physics. Deutscher Taschenbuch Verlag. München, DE. [German]

Wachter, A. and H. Hoeber. 1998. Revision Book Theoretical Physics. Springer-Verlag, Berlin, DE. [German]

Walsh, V. and S. Laughlin. 2006. Representation. pp. 70-84. *In:* R. Morris [ed.]. Cognitive Systems: Information Processing Meets Brain Science. Elsevier Academic Press. Amsterdam, NL, Heidelberg, DE, San Diego, USA.

Walter, H. 2006. The neuronal foundations of consciousness. pp. 555-564. *In:* H.-O. Karnath and P. Thier [eds.]. Kognitive Neurowissenschaften. 2. Auflage. Springer-Verlag, Heidelberg, DE. [German]

Walter, H. and S. M̈uller. 2012. The neuronal foundations of consciousness. pp. 655-664. *In:* H.-O. Karnath and P. Thier [eds.]. Kognitive Neurowissenschaften. 3. Auflage. Springer-Verlag, Heidelberg, DE. [German]

Walter, H. 2013a. Neurophilosophy and philosophy of neuroscience. pp. 133-138. *In:* A. Stephan and S. Walter [eds.]. Handbuch Kognitionswissenschaft. Metzler, Stuttgart, Weimar, DE. [German]

Walter, S. 2013b. Extended cognition. pp. 193-197. *In:* A. Stephan and S. Walter [eds.]. Handbuch Kognitionswissenschaft. Metzler, Stuttgart, Weimar, DE. [German]

Walter, S. 2014. Cognition. Reclam, Stuttgart, DE. [German]

Walters, P. 1982. An Introduction to Ergodic Theory. Springer, New York, USA, Heidelberg, DE.

Wang, D.L. 2003. Visual scene segmentation. pp. 1215-1219. *In:* A. Arbib [ed.]. The Handbook of Brain Theory and Neural Networks. 2*nd* Ed. The MIT Press, Cambridge, USA, London, UK.

Wang, P., F. Göschl, U. Friese, P. König and A.K. Engel. 2019. Long-range functional coupling predicts performance: oscillatory EEG networks in multisensory processing. NeuroImage 196: 114-125.

Wang, S. and Y. Liu. 2005. Differences and commonalities between connectionism and symbolism. pp. 34-38. *In:* J. Wang, X. Liao and Z. Yi [eds.]. Proceedings of the Second International Symposium on Neural Networks. Advances in neural networks – ISNN 2005, Part I, Chongqing, China. Springer.

Wang, X.-J. 2003. Neural oscillations. pp. 272-280. *In:* L. Nadel [ed.]. Encyclopedia of Cognitive Science. Vol. 3. Natur Publishing Group. London, UK, New York, USA and Tokyo, JP.

Wang, X.-J. 2008. Attractor network models. pp. 667-679. *In:* L.R. Squire [ed.]. Encyclopedia of Neuroscience. Academic Elsevier, Amsterdam, NL.

Watson, J.B. 1919. Psychology as the behaviorist views it. Psychological Review 20: 158-177.

Weber, K. 1999. Simulation and Explanation. Cognitive Science and AI Research from a Philosophy of Science Perspective. Waxmann, Münster, DE. [German]

Weldle, H. 2011. Syntactic and referential language comprehension processes from a connectionist perspective. Ph.D. Thesis, Albert-Ludwigs-Universität Freiburg im Breisgau, Freiburg im Breisgau, DE. [German]

Wells, A.J. 1998. Turings analysis of computation and theories of cognitive architecture. Cognitive Science 22: 269-294.

Weng, J., J.L. McClelland, A. Pentland, O. Sporns, I. Stockmann and M. Sur. 2001. Artificial intelligence: autonomous mental development by robots and animals. Science 291: 599-600.

Wennekers, T. and F. Pasemann. 1996. Synchronous chaos in highdimensional modular neural networks. International Journal of Bifurcation and Chaos 6: 2055-2067.

Werbos, P.J. 1974. Beyond regression. New tools for prediction and analysis in the behavioral sciences. Ph.D. Thesis, Harvard University, Cambridge, USA.

Wermter, S. and R. Sun. 2000. An overview of hybrid neural systems. pp. 1-13. *In:* S. Wermter and R. Sun [eds.]. Hybrid Neural Systems. Springer-Verlag, Berlin, DE.

Werner, D. 2005. Functional Analysis. 5th Ed. Springer-Verlag. Berlin. DE. [German]

Werner, H. 1978. Introduction to General Algebra. Bibliographisches Institut, Mannheim, DE. [German]

Werning, M. 2001. How to solve the problem of compositionality by oscillatory networks. pp. 1094-1099. *In:* J.D. Moore and K.E. Stenning [eds.]. Proceedings of the Twenty-Third Annual Conference of the Cognitive Science Society. Edinburgh, Scotland. Lawrence Erlbaum Associates.

Werning, M. 2002. How to compose contents. A review of Jerry Fodor's In Critical Consition: Polemic Essays on Cognitive Science and the Philosophy of Mind. Psyche 8: 1-9.

Werning, M. 2003a. Synchrony and composition: toward a cognitive architecture between classicism and connectionism. pp. 261-278. *In:* B. Löwe, W. Malzkorn and T. Räsch [eds.]. Foundations of the Formal Sciences II. Applications of Mathematical Logic in Philosophy and Linguistics. Kluwer Academic Publishers. Dordrecht, NL, Boston, USA, London, UK.

Werning, M. 2003b. Ventral vs. dorsal pathway: the source of the semantic object/event and the syntactic noun/verb distinction. Commentary. *In:* J.R. Hurford. The neural basis of predicate-argument structure. The Behavioral and Brain Sciences 26: 299-300.

Werning, M. 2004. Compositionality, context, categories and the indeterminacy of translation. Erkenntnis 60: 145-178.

Werning, M. 2005a. The temporal dimension of thought: cortical foundations of predicative representation. Synthese 146: 203-224.

Werning, M. 2005b. Right and wrong reasons for compositionality. pp. 285-309. *In:* M. Werning, E. Machery and G. Schurz [eds.]. The Compositionality of Meaning and Content. Vol. I: Foundational Issues. Ontos Verlag, Frankfurt, DE.

Werning, M. 2005c. Neuronal synchronization, covariation, and compositional representation. pp. 283-312. *In:* M. Werning, E. Machery and G. Schurz [eds.]. The Compositionality of Meaning and Content. Vol. II: Applications to Linguistics, Psychology and Neuroscience. Ontos Verlag, Frankfurt, DE.

Werning, M. 2008. The "complex first paradox": why do semantically thick concepts so early lexicalize as nouns? Interaction Studies 9: 67-83.

Werning, M. 2012. Non-symbolic compositional representation and its neuronal foundation: towards an emulative semantics. pp. 633-654. *In:* M. Werning, W. Hinzen and E. Machery [eds.]. The Oxford Handbook of Compositionality. Oxford University Press, Oxford, UK.

Werning, M. and A. Maye. 2006. The neural basis of the object concept in ambiguous and illusionary perception. pp. 876-81. *In:* R. Sun and N. Miyake [eds.]. Proceedings of the Twenty-Eighth Annual Conference of the Cognitive Science Society, Vancouver, Canada. Lawrence Erlbaum Associates.

Westheimer, G. 2008. Was Helmholtz a Bayesian? Perception 39: 642-650.

Whitehead, A.N. and B. Russell. 1910-1913/1927. Principia Mathematica. Vol. 1-3. 2nd Ed. Cambridge University Press, Cambridge, UK.

Whittington, M.A., R.D. Traub and G.R. Jefferys. 1995. Synchronized oscillations in interneuron networks driven by metabotropic glutamate receptor activation. Nature 373: 612-615.

Whittington, M.A., H.C. Doheny, R.D. Traub, F.E.N. Lebeau and E.H. Buhl. 2001. Differential expression of synaptic and nonsynaptic mechanisms underlying stimulus-induced gamma oscillations in vitro. The Journal of Neuroscience 21: 1727-1738.

Wicki, W. 2010. Developmental Psychology. Ernst Reinhardt Verlag, München, DE, Basel, CH. [German]

Widrow, B. and M.E. Hoff, Jr. 1960. Adaptive switching circuits, 96-104. *In* [Institute of Radio Engineers] Proceedings of the IRE Western Electric Show and Convention (WESCON) Conference. Part 4, Los Angeles, Unites States of America.

Widrow, B. and S.D. Stearns. 1985. Adaptive Signal Processing. Prentice Hall. Englewood Cliffs, USA.

Wiener, N. 1948/1961. Cybernetics or Control and Communication in the Animal and the Machine. MIT Press, Cambridge, USA.

Wiener, N. 1965. Perspectives in cybernetics. pp. 399-408. *In:* N. Wiener and J.P. Schadé [eds.]. Cybernetics of the Nervous System. Elsevier Publishing Company, Amsterdam, NL.

Wildgen, W. 1985. Archetype Semantics. Fundamentals of a Dynamic Semantics based on Catastrophe Theory. Narr Verlag, Tübingen, DE. [German]

Wildgen, W. 1987. Part I: The Dynamic Paradigm in Linguistics. *In:* W.Wildgen and L. Mottron [eds.]. Dynamische Sprachtheorie. Sprachbeschreibung und Spracherklärung nach den Prinzipien der Selbstorganisation und der Morphogenese. Studienverlag Brockmeyer, Bochum, DE. [German]

Wildgen, W. 2010. The Linguistics of the 20th Century. An Attempt of a Résumé. Walter De Gruyter, Berlin, DE, New York, USA. [German]

Wildgen, W. and P.J. Plath. 2005. Catastrophe and chaos theory in linguistic modeling. pp. 688-705. *In:* R. Köhler, G. Altmann and R.G. Piotrowski [eds.]. Quantitative Linguistik. Quantitative Linguistics. Ein internationales Handbuch. An International Handbook. Walter de Gruyter, Berlin, DE, New York, USA. [German]

Wiles, J. and J. Hallinan. 2001. Guest editorial – evolutionary computation and cognitive science: modeling evolution and evolving models. IEEE Transactions on Evolutionary Computation 5: 89-92.

Willshaw, D. 1981. Holography, associative memory, and inductive generalization. pp. 83-104. *In:* G.E. Hinton and J.A. Anderson [eds.]. Parallel Models of Associative Memory. Lawrence Erlbaum Associates, Hillsdale, USA.

Willshaw, D. 2006. Self-organization in the nervous system. pp. 5-33. *In:* R. Morris [ed.]. Cognitive Systems: Information Processing Meets Brain Science. Elsevier Academic Press, Amsterdam, NL, Heidelberg, DE.

Willshaw, D.J., O.P. Buneman and H.C. Longuet-Higgins. 1969. Non-holographic associative memory. Nature 222: 960-962.

Wilson, H.R. 1999. Spikes, Decisions, and Actions: The Dynamical Foundations of Neuroscience. Oxford University Press. Oxford, UK, New York, USA.

Wilson, H.R. and J.D. Cowan. 1972. Excitatory and inhibitory interactions in localized populations of model neurons. Biophysical Journal 12: 1-24.

Wilson, H.R. and J.D. Cowan. 1973. A mathematical theory of the functional dynamics of cortical and thalamic nervous tissue. Kybernetik 13: 5580.

Wilson, M. 2002. Six views of embodied cognition. Psychonomic Bulletin & Review 9: 625-636.

Wilson, R.A. and F.C. Keil. [eds.] 1999. The MIT Encyclopedia of the Cognitive Sciences. The MIT Press, Cambridge, USA, London, UK.

Wilson, R.A. and L. Foglia. 2011. Embodied cognition. *In:* E.N. Zalta [ed.]. The Stanford Encyclopedia of Philosophy (July 25, 2011 Edition).

Wischmann, S., M. Hülse, J. Knabe and F. Pasemann. 2006. Synchronization of internal neural rhythms in multi-robotic systems. Adaptive Behavior 14: 117-127.

Wiskott, L. and C. von der Malsburg. 1996a. Face recognition by dynamic link matching. Internal Report 96 05. Institut für Neuroinformatik, Ruhr-Universit"at Bochum, Bochum: 15pp. (reprinted in Wiskott, L. and C. von der Malsburg 1996b)

Wiskott, L. and C. von der Malsburg. 1996b. Face recognition by dynamic link matching. *In:* J. Sirosh, R. Miikulainen and Y. Choe [eds.]. Lateral Interactions in the Cortex: Structure and Function. [eBook]

Wiskott, L. and C. von der Malsburg. 1999. Object recognition in a self-organizing neuronal system. pp. 169-188. *In:* K. Mainzer [ed.]. Komplexe Systeme und nichtlineare Dynamik in Natur und Gesellschaft. Springer-Verlag, Berlin, DE, Heidelberg, DE. [German]

Wittgenstein, L. 1921/1990. Tractatus logico philosophicus. pp. 7-86. *In:* J. Schulte [ed.]. Ludwig Wittgenstein. Werkausgabe. Vol. 1: Tractatus logicophilosophicus. Tageb"ucher 1914-16. Philosophische Untersuchungen. 7th Ed. Suhrkamp Verlag, Berlin, DE. [German]

Wittgenstein, L. 1929. Some remarks on logical form. Aristotelian Society Supplementary 9: 162-171. (reprinted in Wittgenstein, L. 1993.)

Wittgenstein, L. 1993. Some remarks on logical form. pp. 29-35. *In:* J.C. Klagge and A. Nordmann [eds.]. LudwigWittgenstein. Philosophical Occasions 1912-51. Hackett Publishing Company, Indianapolis, USA.

Wolfe, J.M. 1998. Visual search. pp. 14-73. *In:* H. Pashler [ed.]. Attention. Psychological Press, Hove, UK.

Wolfe, J.M. and K.R. Cave. 1999. The psychophysical evidence for a binding problem in human vision. Neuron 24: 11-17.

Wolff, M.P.H., P. Hauck, and W. Küchlin 2004. Mathematics for Informatics and Bioinformatics. Springer-Verlag. Berlin, Heidelberg u.a., DE [German]

Wolstenholme, E.F. 1990. System Enquiry. A System Dynamics Approach. John Wiley & Sons, Chichester, UK.

Womelsdorf, T., J.-M. Schoelen, R. Oostenveld, W. Singer, R. Desimone, A.K. Engel and P. Fries. 2007. Modulation of neuronal interactions through neuronal synchronization. Science 316: 1609-1612.

Wu, J.Y., L. Guan and Y. Tsau. 1999. Propagating activation during oscillations and evoked responses in neocortical slices. Journal of Neuroscience 19: 50055015.

Wussing, H. 2009. 6000 Years of Mathematics. A Cultural-Historical Time Travel. Springer-Verlag. Berlin, Heidelberg, DE. [German]

Yang, B.-S., T. Han and Y.-S. Kim. 2004. Integration of ART-Kohonen neural network and case-based reasoning for intelligent fault diagnosis. Expert System with Applications 26: 387-395.

Yao, Y. and W.J. Freeman. 1990. A model of biological pattern recognition with spatially chaotic dynamics. Neural Networks 3: 153-170.

Yegnanarayana, B. 1994. Artificial neural networks for pattern recognition. Sādhanā 19: 189-238.

Yue, X., I. Biederman, M.C. Mangini, C. von der Malsburg and O. Amir. 2012. Predicting the psychophysical similarity of faces and non-face complex shapes by image-based measures. Vision Research 55: 41-46.

Zabel, T. 2005. Classification with Neuronal Networks. CARTE. Cooperative Adaptive Resonance Theory Ensembles. Logos Verlag, Berlin, DE. [German]

Zadeh, L.A. 1962. From circuit theory to system theory. Proceedings of the Institute of Radio Engineers 50: 856-865. (reprinted in Zadeh 1991.)

Zadeh, L.A. 1965. Fuzzy sets. Information and Control 8: 338-353.

Zadeh, L.A. 1969. The concept of system, aggregate, and state in system theory. pp. 3-42. In: L.A. Zadeh and E. Polak. [eds.]. System Theory. McGraw-Hill, New York, USA.

Zadeh, L.A. 1991. From circuit theory to system theory. pp. 309-323. In: G.J. Klir [ed.]. Facets of Systems Science. Plenum Press, New York, USA, London, UK.

Zeeman, E.C. 1976. Catastrophe theory. Scientific American 234: 65-70, 75-83.

Zell, A. 2003. Simulation of Neuronal Networks. 2nd Ed. R. Oldenbourg Verlag, München, DE, Wien, AT. [German]

Zhang, T., D. Lengshi, W. You, W.J. Freeman and L. Guang. 2015. EEG spatiotemporal pattern classification of the stimuli on different fingers. pp. 147-153. In: H. Liljenström [ed.]. Proceedings of the Fourth International Conference on Cognitive Neurodynamics – 2013, Advances in Cognitive Neurodynamics (IV), Sigtuna, Sweden, Springer.

Zhou, H., H.S. Friedman and R. von der Heydt. 2000. Coding of border ownership in monkey visual cortex. Journal of Neuroscience 20: 6594-6611.

Zhu, J. and C. von der Malsburg. 2002. Synapto-synaptic interactions speed up dynamic link matching. Neurocomputing 44-46: 721-728.

Zhu, J. and C. von der Malsburg. 2003. Learning control units for invariant recognition. Neurocomputing 52-54: 447-453.

Zhu, J. and C. von der Malsburg. 2004. Maplets for correspondence-based object recognition. Neural Networks 17: 1311-1326.

Ziemke, A. and S. Cardoso de Oliveira. 1996. Neuronal representations. On the representationalist research program in cognition research. pp. 1-28. *In:* A. Ziemke and O. Breidbach [eds.]. Repräsentationismus – was sonst? Eine Auseinandersetzung mit dem repräsentationalistischen Forschungsprogramm in den Neurowissenschaften. Vieweg, Braunschweig, DE. [German]

Ziemke, T. 2003. What's that thing called embodiment? 1134-1139. *In:* R. Alterman and D. Kirsh [eds.] Proceedings of the 25th Annual Conference of the Cognitive Science Society. Boston, USA. Lawrence Erlbaum Associates.

Zimmermann, H.J. 1994. Fuzzy Set Theory and its Applications. 2nd Ed. Kluwer Academic, Boston, USA.

Zippelius, A. 1993. Statistical mechanics of neural networks. Physica A: Statistical Mechanics and its Applications 194: 471-481.

Zylberberg, A., S. Dehaene, P.R. Roelfsema and M. Sigman 2011. The human Turing machine: a neural framework for mental programs. Trends in Cognitive Sciences 15: 293-300.

Author Index

Subject Index

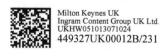

9 780367 638917